Teaching Clinical Reasoning

Books in the ACP Teaching Medicine Series

Theory and Practice of Teaching Medicine
Jack Ende, MD, MACP
Editor

Methods for Teaching Medicine
Kelley M. Skeff, MD, PhD, MACP
Georgette A. Stratos, PhD
Editors

Teaching in Your Office, A Guide to Instructing Medical Students and Residents, Second Edition
Patrick C. Alguire, MD, FACP
Dawn E. DeWitt, MD, MSc, FACP
Linda E. Pinsky, MD, FACP
Gary S. Ferenchick, MD, FACP
Editors

Teaching in the Hospital
Jeff Wiese, MD, FACP
Editor

Mentoring in Academic Medicine
Holly J. Humphrey, MD, MACP
Editor

Leadership Careers in Medical Education
Louis Pangaro, MD, MACP
Editor

Teaching Clinical Reasoning
Robert L. Trowbridge Jr, MD, FACP
Joseph J. Rencic, MD, FACP
Steven J. Durning, MD, PhD, FACP
Editors

Teaching Medicine Series

Jack Ende, MD, MACP
Series Editor

Teaching Clinical Reasoning

Robert L. Trowbridge Jr., MD, FACP
Joseph J. Rencic, MD, FACP
Steven J. Durning, MD, PhD, FACP
Editors

American College of Physicians • Philadelphia, Pennsylvania

Vice President, Publishing: Diane Scott-Lichter
Associate Publisher, Circulation, Licensing and Permissions: Aileen McHugh
Associate Publisher, New Product Development: Thomas McCabe
Digital Products Associate: Bernie Turner
Books Associate: Charles Graver
Copy Editing: Suzanne Meyers
Cover Design: Kate Nichols
Text Design: Michael Ripca
Composition: Cenveo Publisher Services

Printing/binding by Versa Press
Printed in the United States of America

ISBN: 978-1-938921-05-6

Library of Congress Cataloging-in-Publication Data

Teaching clinical reasoning / [edited by] Robert L. Trowbridge, Joseph J. Rencic,
Steven J. Durning.
    p. ; cm.
  Includes bibliographical references and index.
  ISBN 978-1-938921-05-6
I. Trowbridge, Robert L., Jr., editor. II. Rencic, Joseph J., editor. III. Durning, Steven J.,
editor. IV. American College of Physicians, issuing body.
  [DNLM: 1. Clinical Medicine–education. 2. Diagnosis, Differential. 3. Decision Making.
  4. Diagnostic Techniques and Procedures. 5. Teaching–methods. WB 18]
  RB38.25
  616.07'5076--dc23
                              2015009020

15 16 17 18 19 20 / 9 8 7 6 5 4 3 2 1

Contributors

Anthony R. Artino Jr., PhD
Associate Professor of Medicine,
    Department of Medicine
Uniformed Services University of the
    Health Sciences
Bethesda, Maryland

Gurpreet Dhaliwal, MD
Professor of Medicine
University of California, San Francisco
San Francisco
Veterans Affairs Medical Center
San Francisco, California

Steven J. Durning, MD, PhD, FACP
Professor of Medicine and Pathology
Uniformed Services University of the
    Health Sciences
Bethesda, Maryland

D. Michael Elnicki, MD, FACP
Professor of Medicine, Department of
    Medicine
University of Pittsburgh
Pittsburgh, Pennsylvania

Mark L. Graber, MD, FACP
Senior Fellow, RTI International
President, Society to Improve Diagnosis
    in Medicine

Eric Holmboe, MD, MACP
Accreditation Council for Graduate
    Medical Education
Chicago, Illinois

Jennifer R. Kogan, MD, FACP
Associate Professor of Medicine
Director of Undergraduate Education,
    Department of Medicine
Perelman School of Medicine at the
    University of Pennsylvania
Philadelphia, Pennsylvania

Jeffrey S. La Rochelle, MD, MPH, FACP
Associate Professor of Medicine,
    Department of Medicine
Uniformed Services University of the
    Health Sciences
Bethesda, Maryland

Valerie J. Lang, MD, FACP
Associate Professor of Medicine
University of Rochester Medical Center
Rochester, New York

Cynthia H. Ledford, MD, FACP
Associate Professor of Clinical Medicine
    and Clinical Pediatrics
Associate Vice Chair for Education,
    Department of Medicine
Assistant Dean of Evaluation and
    Assessment, College of Medicine
Ohio State University
Columbus, Ohio

L. James Nixon, MD, MHPE
Professor of Medicine and Pediatrics
Vice Chair for Education, Department
    of Medicine
Division of General Internal Medicine
University of Minnesota Medical School
Minneapolis, Minnesota

Temple A. Ratcliffe, MD, FACP
Assistant Professor of Medicine
Uniformed Services University of the
    Health Sciences
Bethesda, Maryland

James B. Reilly, MD, MS, FACP
Internal Medicine Residency Program
    Director
Allegheny Health Network
Pittsburgh, Pennsylvania
Assistant Professor of Medicine
Temple University School of Medicine
Philadelphia, Pennsylvania

Joseph J. Rencic, MD, FACP
Associate Professor of Medicine, Tufts
University School of Medicine
Internal Medicine Residency Associate
Program Director, Tufts Medical
Center
Boston, Massachusetts

Lambert Schuwirth, MD, PhD
Professor for Innovative Assessment,
Department of Educational
Development and Research,
Maastricht University,
The Netherlands, and
Distinguished Professor of Medical
Education, Chang Gung University,
Taoyuan, Taiwan

Dario M. Torre, MD, PhD, MPH, FACP
Associate Professor of Medicine,
Department of Medicine
Drexel University College of Medicine
Philadelphia, Pennsylvania

Robert L. Trowbridge Jr., MD, FACP
Assistant Professor of Medicine
Tufts University School of Medicine
Boston, Massachusetts
Department of Medicine
Maine Medical Center
Portland, Maine

Joan M. Von Feldt, MD, MSEd
Professor of Medicine
University of Pennsylvania
Philadelphia, Pennsylvania

To my wife, Nina, and children, Julia, Robbie, and Henry,
who keep me loved and laughing. To my parents for all of their support.
- R. Trowbridge

To my parents, Joseph and Mary Rencic, without whose sacrifices
I could never have had the life that I have today. To my wife, Varsha,
and my children, Satya and Mina, whose love and support sustain me.
- J. Rencic

To my wife, Kristen, and my two sons, Andrew and Daniel, for their
unwavering love and support. To my parents, and my in-laws for
their advice and encouragement.
- S. Durning

Acknowledgment

We wish to acknowledge the talent, dedication, and patience of the authors whose efforts and expertise resulted in this book. We also acknowledge the countless students, residents, colleagues, and patients who continue to challenge assumptions and tune our understanding of clinical reasoning, making the practice of medicine the privilege it is.

Contents

Visit www.acponline.org/teachingbooks
for additional information.

About the *Teaching Medicine* Series

This book series, *Teaching Medicine*, represents a major initiative from the American College of Physicians. It is intended for College members but also for the profession as a whole. Internists, family physicians, subspecialists, surgical colleagues, nurse practitioners, and physician assistants—indeed, anyone involved with medical education—should find this book series useful as they pursue one of the greatest privileges of the profession: the opportunity to teach and make a difference in the lives of learners and their patients. The series is composed of seven books:

- *Theory and Practice of Teaching Medicine*, edited by me, considers how medical learners learn (how to be doctors), how medical teachers teach, and how they (the teachers) might learn to teach better.

- *Methods for Teaching Medicine*, edited by Kelley M. Skeff and Georgette A. Stratos, builds on this foundation but focuses on the actual methods that medical teachers use. This book explores the full range of techniques that encourage learning within groups. The authors present a conceptual framework and guiding perspectives for understanding teaching; the factors that support choices for particular teaching methods (such as lecturing vs. small group discussion); and practical advice for preceptors, attendings, lecturers, discussion leaders, workshop leaders, and, finally, course directors charged with running programs for continuing medical education.

- *Teaching in Your Office, Second Edition*, edited by Patrick C. Alguire, Dawn E. DeWitt, Linda E. Pinsky, and Gary S. Ferenchick, will be familiar to many teaching internists. It has been reissued as part of this series. This book remains the office-based preceptor's single most useful resource for preparing to receive medical students and residents into an ambulatory practice setting or, among those already engaged in office-based teaching, for learning how to do it even better.

- *Teaching in the Hospital* is edited by Jeff Wiese and considers the challenges and rewards of teaching in that particular setting. Hospitalists as well as more traditional internists who attend on the inpatient service will be interested in the insightful advice that this book provides. This advice focuses not only on how to conduct rounds and encourage learning among students and house officers but also on how to frame and orient the content of rounds for some of the more frequently encountered inpatient conditions.

- *Mentoring in Academic Medicine,* edited by Holly J. Humphrey, considers professional development across the continuum of medical education, from issues pertaining to students to residents to faculty themselves, as well as issues pertaining to professional development of special populations. Here is where the important contributions of mentors and role models are explored in detail.

- *Leadership Careers in Medical Education,* edited by Louis Pangaro, this book is written for members of the medical faculty who are pursuing—or who are considering— careers as clerkship directors, residency program directors, or educational leaders of departments or medical schools, careers that require not only leadership skill but also a deep understanding of the organization and administration of internal medicine's educational enterprise. This book explores the theory and practice of educational leadership, including curricular design and evaluation; and offers insightful profiles of many of internal medicine's most prominent leaders.

- *Teaching Clinical Reasoning* concludes this series. Edited by Robert L. Trowbridge Jr., Joseph J. Rencic, and Steven J. Durning, this book explores one of clinical medicine's most fascinating questions, which happens also to be a question that is critical for medical education: "What, apart from medical knowledge, is essential for clinical expertise?" Related to that question, of course, and most germane for medical teachers are the questions, "How can teachers 'diagnose' the learner who appears to have adequate knowledge, but who struggles to deploy that knowledge for patient care?" and "How can teachers effectively intervene?" This book explores these questions while providing insight and practical advice for clinical teachers and for program directors charged with introducing the subject of clinical reasoning into the curriculum for students and residents.

Jack Ende, MD, MACP
Philadelphia, 2015

Introduction/Preface

Robert L. Trowbridge Jr., MD, FACP
Joseph J. Rencic, MD, FACP
Steven J. Durning, MD, PhD, FACP

Physicians of the 21st century must possess abilities in a considerable number of wide-ranging and disparate domains of practice. Physicians must have a broad and deep knowledge of both basic and clinical sciences. They are required to have robust communication skills, including the ability both to speak the highly technical language of modern medicine and to explain complex and ambiguous concepts to patients. They need both to lead a team and to function within a team. Many must also possess highly developed technical and procedural abilities. Perhaps nothing is more central to the high-level functioning of the physician, however, than clinical reasoning.

Broadly defined, clinical reasoning may include nearly all of the cognitive tasks expected of a physician. Thus, everything from determining the best approach to screening for occult malignancy, to devising a primary disease prevention strategy for an individual patient, to evaluating a symptom or physical sign, to considering the best therapeutic plan for a patient falls within the realm of clinical reasoning. Those who think clinical reasoning cannot be explicitly taught may think the title of this book is presumptuous and that valuable books have been written with the focus on learning rather than teaching clinical reasoning (1). To this we respond that all teachers of medicine teach clinical reasoning whether intentionally or not and have been doing so for millennia. We believe that the theoretical and

empirical knowledge of cognition, education, and expertise have developed
to a degree that valuable constructs now exist to guide teachers of clinical
reasoning.

❖ Defining Clinical Reasoning

We define clinical reasoning as "the cognitive and noncognitive process by
which a health care professional consciously and unconsciously interacts
with the patient and environment to collect and interpret patient data,
weigh the benefits and risks of actions, and understand patient preferences to determine a working diagnostic and therapeutic management
plan whose purpose is to improve a patient's well-being." This definition
seeks to incorporate the modern understanding of reasoning, or thinking,
as both a conscious and subconscious process that is dramatically affected
by physical and environmental factors. It entails establishing both a diagnosis and a treatment plan that is specific to a patient's circumstances and
preferences.

❖ The Focus of This Book: Diagnostic Reasoning

For the purposes of the book, however, we have narrowed the focus of
clinical reasoning to establishing a diagnosis or *diagnostic reasoning*. We
chose to address only diagnostic reasoning for purposes of clarity and focus.
This aspect of clinical reasoning includes the processes used in collecting
and analyzing the information that contributes to the establishment of a
working diagnosis, acknowledging that it is not always practical or even
possible to make a diagnosis. A substantial portion of the diagnostic reasoning literature has emerged from the psychology, expertise, and education
literature, whereas therapeutic reasoning has traditionally been described
in the medical decision-making or decision analysis world with a strong
mathematical focus. Many excellent books have been written on this medical decision-making (2), and we did not wish to duplicate them. Although
we touch upon therapeutic reasoning and many of the suggestions made
can be applied to the teaching of therapeutic reasoning, this book's explicit
recommendations relate to the teaching of diagnostic reasoning.

❖ The Purpose and Contents of This Book

This book, written by experts in education, clinical reasoning, and
clinical medicine, aims to consolidate current knowledge regarding the
teaching and learning of clinical reasoning and to provide guidance on

how to enhance learners' and clinicians' clinical reasoning abilities. We approach this through a variety of lenses and from multiple perspectives. We acknowledge that much remains to be learned about how clinicians reason, how the process may fail, how to assess reasoning, and how best to foster this ability among both novices and experts. Given the current level of understanding, no gold standard for teaching clinical reasoning exists; therefore, the book provides a menu of options from which teachers may choose based on their goals.

The book begins with a general discussion of diagnosis in "Clinical Reasoning and Diagnostic Error." This establishes the importance of clinical reasoning in medicine and argues that teaching clinical reasoning should be central to medical education rather than a passive byproduct of clinical experience. This chapter also details the current rates of diagnostic failure and the impact of diagnostic error in medicine, including a discussion of the many factors that may contribute to suboptimal diagnostic performance.

We believe that understanding current theories of clinical reasoning is an important foundation on which to build. Chapter 2, "Theoretical Concepts to Consider in Providing Clinical Reasoning Instruction," provides this basis, discussing the current knowledge of the clinical reasoning process and how such an understanding can inform instruction in clinical reasoning. It stresses the concept of context specificity, which has important implications for the teaching of clinical reasoning.

Few published clinical reasoning curricula exist in undergraduate or graduate medical education, in part a result of the challenges of clinical reasoning assessment. Much of clinical reasoning teaching relies on the rather haphazard and unstandardized approach of simply providing medical students and residents with clinical experiences under the direction of a more experienced clinician. We believe a more standardized curricular approach is necessary given the recent advances in the science of clinical reasoning, recognizing that guided clinical experience is still the cornerstone of learning clinical reasoning. Chapter 3, "Developing a Curriculum in Clinical Reasoning," outlines several approaches to building a model of clinical reasoning instruction. It discusses the importance of grounding the curriculum in the theories described in the previous chapter and suggests content appropriate for different levels of learners. It additionally addresses several barriers to building a curriculum, including those generally inherent in the process as well as those specific to clinical reasoning.

Cognitive errors occur with remarkable frequency. Chapter 4, "Educational Approaches to Common Cognitive Errors," describes this phenomenon and outlines an approach teachers may take in speaking to such errors. This discussion highlights the concept of "diagnosing the learner." This "diagnosis" serves as the basis for choosing teaching methods to improve clinical reasoning going forward. Interventions that may be appropriate for specific levels of learners, both experienced and inexperienced, are additionally described.

Clinical reasoning is primarily taught at the bedside in the context of clinical care. Unfortunately, many clinician-educators may lack awareness of the educational techniques that can be used to teach clinical reasoning, even when they are clinical reasoning experts themselves. Chapter 5, "General Teaching Techniques," details many of these techniques, their theoretical basis, and their impact on learning clinical reasoning. The authors describe techniques that may apply to all levels of learners and specifically address the challenges the individual clinician may face in implementing these teaching practices.

The concept of "diagnosing the learner" is again addressed in Chapter 6, "Assessment of Clinical Reasoning." Assessment of the clinical reasoning process remains challenging because of our limited understanding of the process. In the past, assessment of clinical reasoning rested with clinical supervisors who may have evaluated learners solely on the basis of their diagnostic accuracy in a few cases. A more nuanced and detailed understanding of how clinical reasoning works, including the importance of context specificity, however, has led to the development of multiple methods of assessing clinical reasoning in both the classroom and the clinical setting. Although the most valid and reliable means of assessing clinical reasoning remains unclear, some progress has been made. This chapter delineates how a program of assessment many be implemented, as well as the details of the individual components of such a program.

As mentioned previously, many clinician-educators may have advanced clinical reasoning abilities but possess little knowledge of the theory, vocabulary, or tenets that underlie teaching clinical reasoning. To enhance the teaching of clinical reasoning, faculty need to understand the process better, especially as methods of learning and assessment evolve. Chapter 7, "Faculty Development and Dissemination," provides a blueprint for creating a faculty development program, describing practices for engaging the busy clinician-educator. The authors specifically address how these practices may apply to teaching the teachers about clinical reasoning, although the literature on this specific subject is remarkably limited.

In developing the faculty for teaching clinical reasoning, many may be interested in improving their own clinical reasoning yet have no clear means of doing so. Chapter 8, "Lifelong Learning in Clinical Reasoning," describes several approaches that individual clinicians may use to further their own capabilities. These practical techniques, grounded in deliberate practice, capitalize on many of the clinical opportunities for learning present in day-to-day clinical experience that may be implemented relatively easily.

At the other end of the continuum, struggling learners often fail to develop the expected level of clinical reasoning ability. Educators can be flummoxed on how to approach such learners, especially given that the process of arriving at a diagnosis is often opaque, rendering it difficult to ascertain the exact nature of the leaner's problems. Chapter 9, "Remediation of Clinical Reasoning," builds on the concepts presented in the chapters on cognitive errors and assessment and presents an approach to problems common to the struggling learner. This chapter provides specific suggestions for improving the learner's abilities by using several illustrative cases centered on aspects of clinical reasoning with which learners often struggle.

Although we now better understand how clinicians reason, there is much we do not know about teaching, assessing, and remediating clinical reasoning. Chapter 10, "Innovations and Future Directions," details several intriguing and innovative teaching and assessment strategies, while acknowledging that these methods require further exploration to advance our knowledge of clinical reasoning.

❖ Closing

With this book, we aim to help teachers at all levels of medical education and have attempted to describe teaching techniques that may be most beneficial for learners at differing levels of experience, specifically the preclinical student, the clinical student/resident, and the practicing clinician. Although we frequently refer to "learners," many of the teaching techniques described may be useful for clinicians at all levels of experience, including the seasoned clinician.

We also acknowledge some overlap among the chapters. Although we have strived to avoid unnecessary redundancy, key topics are mentioned several times in multiple chapters with the recognition that many readers may not read this book cover to cover. In view of this, each chapter also includes summative "Take-Home Points," and many of the chapters have practical "Teaching Tips" that emphasize the key content for busy clinician educators. A glossary of common terms is also included at the end of the text. Finally, the online component of the book available at www. acponline.org/teachingbooks contains considerable supplemental content. Included are examples of clinical reasoning curricula, practical teaching tips, the discussed assessment methods, and outlines for faculty development workshops.

Given the progress made in the understanding of clinical reasoning, we believe now is an excellent time to reflect on the current state of affairs and provide practical guidance to those who are required to practice and teach clinical reasoning every day. We recognize that there is likely no single "right" way to teach and learn clinical reasoning, but we hope this book will provide strategies already being used and encourage exploration of new methods in teaching and assessing clinical reasoning.

REFERENCES

1. **Kassirer J, Kopelman R, Wong J.** Learning Clinical Reasoning. 2nd ed. Baltimore, MD: Lippincott Williams & Wilkins; 2010.
2. **Sox H, Higgins M, Owens D.** Medical Decision Making. Hoboken, NJ: John Wiley and Sons; 2013.

1

Clinical Reasoning and Diagnostic Error

Robert L. Trowbridge Jr., MD, FACP
Mark L. Graber, MD, FACP

Rory Staunton was a 12-year-old boy from New York City who fell ill after sustaining a minor cut diving for a basketball. Just a few days after the seemingly inconsequential arm injury, Rory developed abdominal pain, fever, and vomiting. He was seen by both his pediatrician and emergency department staff, and he and his parents were told he had a common viral infection, which was rampant throughout the community at the time. He was treated supportively with fluids and pain relievers and sent home. Yet Rory had several factors that were discordant with the diagnosis of a viral infection, including abnormal vital signs, "blotchy" skin, and an elevated white blood cell count. The results of the blood test, however, were not available until after his discharge from the emergency department. Within days of release from the emergency department, he died of an overwhelming streptococcal infection (1).

The death of a 12-year-old boy who saw multiple physicians and other health care professionals raises a powerful question: "Why?" Why did all his physicians misdiagnose his infection before its progression to septic shock and death? Why did their clinical reasoning fail them as they attempted to make the diagnosis? At this point, the question, "Why is clinical reasoning important?" can be simply answered, "Because a patient's life may depend upon it." Although this story may seem sensational, morbidity and mortality caused by faulty clinical

---

KEY POINTS
- Diagnostic errors are common and result in substantial patient morbidity and mortality.
- Diagnostic errors often have multiple causes, with many having their origins in both systems and cognitive failures.
- Improvement in the clinical reasoning abilities of clinicians has the potential to limit diagnostic error and the harm incurred.

---

reasoning are not rare (2). Exploring the complexity of clinical reasoning provides some insight into the causes of such errors.

Indeed, perhaps no task of the practicing physician is more challenging than assigning a clinical diagnosis. The sheer number of diagnostic possibilities alone can make the process difficult for both experienced and novice clinicians; the International Classification of Diseases, 10th Revision, lists more than 12,000 discrete diagnoses, and new diseases are discovered every year (3). The volume of potential diagnoses, however, represents just a small aspect of the complexity of making a diagnosis. Much of the data necessary to make a correct diagnosis, for example, can be difficult to obtain. Taking an efficient and targeted history is a skill that can take years to master. Many of the most important findings on physical examination are technique dependent, such that only those who devote themselves to the craft become skilled enough to put trust in their findings (4, 5). Laboratory and imaging studies can be helpful, but they take time and come with myriad shortcomings. A test that is very useful for one disease, for example, may be near-useless for a closely related disorder. Furthermore, reconciling these multiple sources of data, which are often conflicting, can be tremendously difficult. The clinical examination, for instance, may strongly suggest one disorder, whereas the "confirmatory" imaging study suggests an altogether different process.

Simply integrating all of the above variables into the diagnostic process stretches the limits of human cognition. Making a diagnosis is further complicated by the high stakes of establishing the correct diagnosis because at the core of all this is the patient. Clinicians recognize the consequences a wrong or missed diagnosis can have for an individual and they feel the pressure. Without the correct diagnosis, treatment is uninformed and prognosis is unclear. Furthermore, clinicians may be subject to innumerable biases, unconscious predispositions, or preconceptions that influence thinking as they approach the patient. They may have positive or negative feelings toward specific patients or may be particularly wary of or sensitive to a certain disease, skewing the objectivity of the diagnostic process (6). All these factors render an already complicated process rife with potential for error and, more important, patient harm.

Given all these challenges, it is remarkable that physicians establish the correct diagnosis at the current level of accuracy, estimated to be in the range of 95% to 98% for physicians in the perceptual specialties (radiology, pathology, and dermatology) and over 85% for primary care specialties (2, 7–9). The question remains, however, can these rates be improved? If the overall error rate in the emergency department, medical and surgical wards, and primary care clinics is 10% to 15%, patients are being harmed from diagnostic error every day in the typical health care organization. Furthermore, the effect of even a single diagnostic error can be devastating, as demonstrated by the Rory Staunton case. With hindsight, it is easy to impugn the care that Staunton received, as may be done with many instances of faulty reasoning. Yet such errors are neither limited to low-performing physicians nor uncommon. All physicians, despite being talented, dedicated, and caring professionals, are subject to faulty reasoning (10, 11).

❖ Rationale for Teaching Clinical Reasoning

Given the centrality of clinical reasoning to the practice of medicine, the inherent difficulty of the reasoning process, and especially the current level of sub-optimal performance, it should be evident that clinical reasoning should be a major focus of medical education. Yet there is a relative dearth of formal instruction on the subject at both the undergraduate and graduate levels of medical education. Traditionally, the accrual of clinical experience under the tutelage of experienced mentors was believed sufficient to achieve competence in clinical reasoning. A shift toward concentrating on developing the critical thinking skills of learners was reflected in the wide adoption of the problem-based learning that occurred in the late 20th century (12–14). This method of education, however, has been largely scaled back because educational outcomes were disappointing (15). These results may have been in part secondary to the concept that achieving excellence in reasoning is context specific (i.e., performance depends on the clinical content as well as the environment and good performance in one situation is not necessarily "transferable" to other situations). Relatively few undergraduate schools have explicit curricula in clinical reasoning or faculty development programs that teach their faculty how to teach and assess clinical reasoning. Graduate medical education programs are similarly lacking in formal instruction in clinical reasoning. The Accreditation Council for Graduate Medical Education, with its shift to the "Milestones" paradigm, has the potential to shift significant attention to this domain, but these changes have yet to be realized (16).

By extension, and not surprisingly, few continuing medical education opportunities focus on improving the clinical reasoning skills of the practicing clinician. Journal-based clinical problem-solving cases and clinical problem-solving sessions at several national meetings center on this concept, but little else is available (17). This lack of emphasis on the clinical reasoning skills of faculty members clearly affects their ability to teach the subject themselves.

❖ The Case for Improving Clinical Reasoning: Diagnostic Error

To fully understand why the teaching of clinical reasoning is so important, the current limits of diagnostic accuracy, the frequency with which the correct diagnosis is identified in a timely fashion, must be discussed in greater detail. Several different definitions of diagnostic error have been advanced, all with subtle but important differences. The most straightforward definition describes diagnostic error as a situation in which the clinician had at his or her disposal all the information necessary to make the diagnosis but then made the diagnosis later (delayed diagnosis), made a different diagnosis (wrong diagnosis), or missed the diagnosis altogether (missed diagnosis) (7). This definition has the advantage of simplicity, but it requires a "gold standard" and does not take into account patient harm, as many would argue that a diagnostic error with no potential for patient harm is inconsequential. Another definition considers diagnostic error as a missed opportunity in the diagnostic process (18). This occurs when the correct diagnosis could have been made earlier on the basis of information available at the time or, at the very least, further evaluation should have been undertaken given the available information. A third definition views making a diagnosis as a function of a multifaceted and multidisciplinary process and errors as breakdowns anywhere in this complex and interwoven route (19). Each of these definitions have merit and make important distinctions, although all are based on the premise that the correct diagnosis could have been established earlier in the diagnostic process with the potential for improved patient outcomes.

The struggle in defining diagnostic error is mirrored by the difficulty in identifying such errors. Determining the presence of an error is a subjective judgment because the reviewer must ascertain whether the diagnosis "should" have been made (or at least tested for) on the basis of the information available at the time. Most of these errors are identified retrospectively, and such analysis is highly subject to hindsight bias (2). The reviewer usually knows that an error was made or that harm has occurred, making it difficult to objectively evaluate whether the diagnosis "should" have been made. It is also extraordinarily difficult to retrospectively recreate the true context of patient care in evaluating a diagnostic error. Thus, identifying both the error and the contributory causes is, at best, an inexact and subjective process.

Despite all of the difficulties in evaluating the diagnostic process, the effect of diagnostic errors on the healthcare system is undeniable. Most important, diagnostic breakdowns result in a remarkable degree of patient harm. Diagnostic errors result in an estimated 40,000 to 80,000 deaths annually in the United States alone (20, 21). Data from autopsy studies support the significant scope and effect of these errors, with 5% to 20% of postmortem studies revealing a lethal diagnosis that, had it been recognized and treated antemortem, may have averted patient death (22). Patient safety studies have revealed similar numbers; one showed that 17% of adverse events in hospitalized patients were secondary to diagnostic missteps (23).

Patient satisfaction is also remarkably affected by errors in the diagnostic process. It is extraordinarily difficult for patients to realize they have been undergoing treatment for a disorder they don't actually have or to recognize that a serious diagnosis could have been caught at an earlier and more treatable stage. Clinicians who are involved in diagnostic errors are also subject to psychological harm. Making a diagnosis is central to the physician's role in the care of patients, and accepting mistakes in this realm can be very difficult. This may be particularly true in the more cognitively based specialties, such as internal medicine and pediatrics, where "thinking is the procedure." Finally, despite the recognition that all clinicians make mistakes, recognizing that one's cognitive error resulted in significant patient harm can be devastating to an individual clinician.

The financial impact of diagnostic errors is also unmistakable. At the most basic level, diagnostic errors are cited as one of the top causes of tort claims in multiple patient populations. In fact, claims data show that the payout for diagnostic error exceeds that for surgical and medication errors, each of which has been a major focus of the patient safety movement (24, 25). Malpractice claims, however, represent but a small fraction of the financial cost of diagnostic error. The delayed recognition of serious diagnoses, for example, leads to significantly higher health care costs. A patient who is diagnosed with early-stage colon cancer and cured with surgery, for example, incurs much less cost than if the diagnosis is delayed until after metastases have developed. Furthermore, missed diagnoses may result in unnecessary and costly testing for an alternate diagnosis. A patient may present with clear symptoms of a viral upper respiratory tract infection, for example, but unnecessary testing is subsequently done for pulmonary embolism, perhaps because the clinician recently missed the diagnosis of pulmonary embolism in another patient and is overly sensitive to doing so again.

❖ Causes of Diagnostic Error

Given the complexity of the diagnostic process, it is not surprising that the causes of diagnostic error are multifactorial and difficult to ascertain. Several different classification schemes have been proposed, but all account for the fact that failures commonly occur at the level of both health care systems and human cognition. In fact, most errors are rooted in multiple causes; a study of errors in the internal medicine population, for example, found an average of 6 contributors to each event (2).

A wide variety of systems issues may result in or contribute to a diagnostic error (2, 7). Issues rooted at the organizational level are very common and often reflect difficulties with communication. A critical laboratory or imaging result, such as an elevated prostate-specific antigen level or abnormal mammogram, for example, may not be communicated to the ordering physician, resulting in an avoidable delay in the diagnosis of cancer. Clinicians may not be aware of critical policies or procedures, such as the need to obtain approval before a specialized laboratory test is run and without which the test is never completed. The balkanization of care between specialists and the inpatient and outpatient settings may also facilitate the loss of critical data when the patient moves from one care setting or clinician to another, resulting in delayed or missed diagnoses.

Organizational issues may also go beyond the realm of communication. The imaging services necessary to make an expedited diagnosis, such as magnetic resonance imaging for potential cord compression from epidural metastatic disease, for example, may not be available off-hours or on weekends, resulting in delays in time-critical diagnoses. Institutionally defined productivity concerns may also be a barrier to clinicians spending the necessary time with patients to obtain the proper history or perform an adequate physical examination. Similarly, external interference may occur, such as the insurance company that requires the completion of an onerous and opaque precertification process before referral to a specialist or an imaging test may be completed.

Less commonly, technical issues may result in diagnostic error. A blood chemistry machine, for example, may misread the serum calcium as normal when it is actually elevated, or a poorly calibrated glucometer may incorrectly show a patient to be hyperglycemic. Similarly, a faulty computed tomography machine may result in poor image quality, obscuring a diagnostic finding. Such technical failures, however, are much less frequent than organizational issues.

Although such systems-based errors are common, most errors also contain an element of faulty cognition on the part of the clinician. It is likely that improvements in clinical reasoning skill can prevent many such errors. Cognitive errors and their prevention should be a major focus of instruction in clinical reasoning (6, 26). It is also increasingly recognized that expertise in human factor interactions will be needed to understand the interplay between cognitive and systems-based issues. An example is an overwhelmed emergency physician working in a loud and understaffed department who misses the heart murmur in a patient whom he must examine in the hallway because no beds are available. This difficulty, however, should not preclude a careful consideration of how improved skills in clinical reasoning could have prevented such an error.

❖ Differentiation of Teaching Clinical Reasoning and Avoidance of Diagnostic Error

Distinguishing between the promotion of expert performance in clinical reasoning and the avoidance of diagnostic error is a valuable exercise. These concepts significantly overlap, and the differences are, in large part, a result of the differing origins of the two "fields." The academic treatment of clinical reasoning is strongly rooted in the educational, expertise, and psychology literature. These fields have provided the basis for much of our knowledge of the clinical reasoning process. In contrast, the more focused, specific, and relatively new principle of avoidance of diagnostic error has its origins in the patient safety movement. Although diagnostic error was not a focus of the original Institute of Medicine report that spurred international interest in patient safety, appreciation of the importance of diagnostic accuracy has increased dramatically over the past decade (27). The patient safety movement's work in reducing diagnostic error has concentrated on improving systems rather than the performance of the individual clinician, despite explicitly recognizing the critical importance of cognitive processes in diagnosis.

Although distinguishing cognitive from system-based elements simplifies the process of assigning the "root causes" of diagnostic error, this distinction is artificial and oversimplifies the true state of affairs. Many concepts that at first glance seem to involve just the cognitive performance of clinicians actually reside in both worlds. Decision-support resources are illustrative: These tools are a "systems" resource but are used to augment the cognitive processes of deriving an appropriate diagnosis. The distinction between systems and cognitive elements is better reconciled by the emergence of social cognitive theories, such as situativity and human factors research, both of which emphasize the impact of patient and environmental factors on clinician performance (28, 29). Thus, as advances in both fields continue, the distinction between the two will probably continue to diminish, perhaps completely. Even issues traditionally considered "systems issues," such as the erroneous reporting of a laboratory result on the basis of machine malfunction or the lack of availability of specialty testing in resource-poor settings, may be addressed in an expanded model of clinical reasoning, such as social cognitive theories.

❖ Barriers to Teaching Clinical Reasoning

Despite the centrality of clinical reasoning and avoidance of diagnostic error to the practice of medicine, there are significant barriers to incorporating explicit discussion of clinical reasoning into the curriculum of both graduate and undergraduate medical education. Primary among these barriers is lack of curricular time. Traditionally medical education has centered on the dissemination of facts, the sheer volume of which has expanded logarithmically over the past several decades. Competing with this conventional priority is the shift toward developing physician skills in multiple other domains that have not been considered in traditional curricula. Influential calls for expanding the skill sets of physicians have been made, with remarkable effect on medical education, as initiatives in shared decision-making, palliative care, geriatric care, and global health have all been advanced and championed over the past 10 years (30, 31). The addition of formal instruction in clinical reasoning will need to compete with these and other emerging educational priorities.

Another major barrier to the addition of clinical reasoning to the formal curriculum is a lack of consensus regarding the best means of teaching the ability to reason (14, 32). Despite the growth in interest in "how doctors think" and the progress reflected in the psychology, expertise, and educational literature, there has been relatively little rigorous investigation into how to effectively teach clinical reasoning. The beneficial effect of clinical experience and deliberate practice under the guidance of coaches and mentors, however, is clear and represents the means by which most practicing clinicians, at least in part, have acquired their own reasoning ability (14). Some thus argue that explicit instruction is not necessary and that it is sufficient to simply provide the opportunity for budding clinicians to obtain their "10,000 hours of experience" under the tutelage of experienced clinicians. Yet this argument ignores the random nature of experience, the lack of time for reflection-on-action, and the noncognitive and at times menial nature of much of a learner's or trainee's first "10,000 hours" of work, all of which lessen clinical reasoning development.

Even if we imagine that educational techniques proven to improve clinical reasoning are developed, the lack of faculty expertise in teaching clinical reasoning remains a significant barrier (33). Most faculty are not well versed in cognitive psychology and the nomenclature of the diagnostic process. Teaching the teachers how to teach a subject in which they themselves received little formal training may be challenging. This particular challenge may go beyond educators' inexperience with the underlying theory. Clinician-educators may resist teaching a subject closely tied to evidence-based medicine, a domain that has been derided as "cookbook medicine" and lacking a basis in the "art of medicine."

A final barrier to instituting more formal clinical reasoning instruction is the lack of clear means of assessing both the effectiveness of this instruction and the performance of the learners themselves (34). No gold standard exists for the assessment of the clinical reasoning process, and assessing only outcomes (e.g., diagnostic accuracy) limits the ability to provide feedback to the learner. Furthermore, because performance in clinical reasoning is context-specific, it is difficult to ascertain the overall clinical reasoning of an individual without extensive sampling in multiple contexts. Without robust assessment methods, it is difficult to provide feedback on performance to both programs and individuals. This clearly has important implications for educators as they try to devise and implement programs and techniques in clinical reasoning.

❖ The Future of Diagnosis

With the increasing recognition of the complexity of the diagnostic process and the limitations of human cognition, the way we view the diagnostic process may change significantly (19). Emphasis on the role of the clinical team in diagnosis will probably increase, with more specific and tangible participation of the patient in the process. There may be a shift away from the "master diagnostician" model and a movement toward clinicians as experts in integrating their clinical acumen with input from others and clinical support systems (35). Experience with atypical presentations of illnesses and uncommon diseases may be taught through simulation, replacing years of actual practice. Global health care costs and the development of even more sophisticated and expensive diagnostics will also force physicians to carefully consider the diagnostic evaluation and the best means of safely and efficiently establishing a diagnosis. These potential changes, however, far from mitigate the importance of an individual clinician being an expert in clinical reasoning. If anything, the individual clinician must be even more of an expert in how to reason clinically given the remarkable increase in available data and information.

Current training programs are focused appropriately on competency—acquiring a broad knowledge base, learning the art of the physical examination, and synthesizing information to derive appropriate diagnostic considerations. But competency is not enough; the quest to improve clinical reasoning demands that we also produce well-calibrated physicians who know when to slow down, ask for help, or defer making a diagnosis if need be.

At its most fundamental level, medicine is a conversation and a relationship between patient and clinician. Although systems changes and diagnostic aids are likely to effect improvements in diagnostic reliability, a clinician's ability to obtain the information at hand and reason through to a correct diagnosis will remain fundamental in defining what it means to be a clinician. It is the clear responsibility of medical educators to teach and nurture this ability among learners.

REFERENCES

1. **Dwyer J.** An infection, unnoticed, turns unstoppable. New York Times. 11 July 2012.
2. **Graber ML, Franklin N, Gordon R.** Diagnostic error in internal medicine. Arch Intern Med. 2005;165:1493-9.
3. International Classification of Diseases, 10th Revision (ICD-10-CM-PCS). Atlanta: Centers for Disease Control and Prevention; 2014.
4. **Verghese A, Charlton B, Cotter B, Kugler J.** A history of physical examination texts and the conception of bedside diagnosis. Trans Am Clin Climatol Assoc. 2011;122:290-311.
5. **Bordage G.** Where are the history and the physical? CMAJ. 1995;152:1595-8.
6. **Croskerry P.** The importance of cognitive errors in diagnosis and strategies to minimize them. Acad Med. 2003;78:775-80.
7. **Berner ES, Graber ML.** Overconfidence as a cause of diagnostic error in medicine. Am J Med. 2008;121(5 Suppl):S2-23.
8. **Berner ES, Miller RA, Graber ML.** Missed and delayed diagnoses in the ambulatory setting. Ann Intern Med. 2007;146:470; author reply 470-1.
9. **Graber ML.** The incidence of diagnostic error in medicine. BMJ Qual Saf. 2014;22 Suppl 2:ii21-ii27.
10. **Elstein A.** Clinical reasoning in medicine. In: Higgs J, ed. Clinical Reasoning in the Health Professions. Oxford: Butterworth-Heineman; 1995:49-59.
11. **Graber M, Gordon R, Franklin N.** Reducing diagnostic errors in medicine: what's the goal? Acad Med. 2002;77:981-92.
12. **Albanese MA, Mitchell S.** Problem-based learning: a review of literature on its outcomes and implementation issues. Acad Med. 1993;68:52-81.
13. **Koh GC, Khoo HE, Wong ML, Koh D.** The effects of problem-based learning during medical school on physician competency: a systematic review. CMAJ. 2008;178:34-41.
14. **Norman G.** Building on experience—the development of clinical reasoning. N Engl J Med. 2006;355:2251-2.

15. **Onyon C.** Problem-based learning: a review of the educational and psychological theory. Clin Teach. 2012;9:22-6.

16. **Swing SR, Beeson MS, Carraccio C, Coburn M, Iobst W, Selden NR, et al.** Educational milestone development in the first 7 specialties to enter the next accreditation system. J Grad Med Educ. 2013;5:98-106.

17. **Henderson M, Keenan C, Kohlwes J, Dhaliwal G.** Introducing exercises in clinical reasoning. J Gen Intern Med. 2010;25:9.

18. **Singh H, Meyer AN, Thomas EJ.** The frequency of diagnostic errors in outpatient care: estimations from three large observational studies involving US adult populations. BMJ Qual Saf. 2014. doi:10.1136/bmjqs-2013-002627.

19. **Schiff GD.** Diagnosis and diagnostic errors: time for a new paradigm. BMJ Qual Saf. 2014;23:1-3.

20. **Leape LL, Berwick DM, Bates DM.** Counting deaths due to medical errors-in reply. JAMA. 2002;288:2405.

21. **Newman-Toker DE, Pronovost PJ.** Diagnostic errors—the next frontier for patient safety. JAMA. 2009;301(10):1060-2.

22. **Shojania KG, Burton EC, McDonald KM, Goldman L.** The autopsy as an outcome and performance measure. Evid Rep Technol Assess (Summ). 2002;1-5.

23. **Brennan TA, Leape LL, Laird NM, Hebert L, Localio AR, Lawthers AG, et al.** Incidence of adverse events and negligence in hospitalized patients. Results of the Harvard Medical Practice Study I. N Engl J Med. 1991;324:370-6.

24. **Studdert DM, Mello MM, Gawande AA, Gandhi TK, Kachalia A, Yoon C, et al.** Claims, errors, and compensation payments in medical malpractice litigation. N Engl J Med. 2006; 354:2024-33.

25. **Weeks WB, Foster T, Wallace AE, Stalhandske E.** Tort claims analysis in the Veterans Health Administration for quality improvement. J Law Med Ethics. 2001;29:335-45.

26. **Trowbridge RL, Dhaliwal G, Cosby KS.** Educational agenda for diagnostic error reduction. BMJ Qual Saf. 2014;22 Suppl 2:ii28-ii32.

27. **Institute of Medicine.** To Err Is Human: Building a Safer Healthcare System. Washington, DC: Academy of Sciences; 1999.

28. **Durning SJ, Artino AR.** Situativity theory: a perspective on how participants and the environment can interact: AMEE guide no. 52. Med Teach. 2011;33:188-99.

29. **Henriksen K, Brady J.** The pursuit of better diagnostic performance: a human factors perspective. BMJ Qual Saf. 2013;22 Suppl 2:ii1-ii5.

30. **Horowitz R, Gramling R, Quill T.** Palliative care education in U.S. medical schools. Med Educ. 2014;48:59-66.

31. **Radwany SM, Stovsky EJ, Frate DM, Dieter K, Friebert S, Palmisano B, Sanders M.** A 4-year integrated curriculum in palliative care for medical undergraduates. Am J Hosp Palliat Care. 2011;28:528-35.

32. **Bowen JL.** Educational strategies to promote clinical diagnostic reasoning. N Engl J Med. 2006;355:2217-25.

33. **Eva KW.** What every teacher needs to know about clinical reasoning. Med Educ. 2005;39:98-106.

34. **Ilgen JS, Humbert AJ, Kuhn G, Hansen ML, Norman GR, Eva KW, et al.** Assessing diagnostic reasoning: a consensus statement summarizing theory, practice, and future needs. Acad Emerg Med. 2012;19:1454-61.

35. **Lucey CR.** Medical education: part of the problem and part of the solution. JAMA Intern Med. 2013;173:1639-43.

Theoretical Concepts to Consider in Providing Clinical Reasoning Instruction

Temple A. Ratcliffe, MD, FACP

Steven J. Durning, MD, PhD, FACP

S uccess in clinical reasoning is essential to a physician's performance. Although definitions and descriptions of clinical reasoning differ, they all converge on the idea that clinical reasoning entails the cognitive operations allowing clinicians to observe, collect, and analyze information, resulting in actions that take into account a patient's specific circumstances and preferences (1, 2). Any discussion of something as complex as clinical reasoning must start with definitions, distinctions, and theoretical concepts. Indeed, these important constructs represent major challenges for understanding "clinical reasoning," in part because our current conceptualization of clinical reasoning has emerged from many research fields and diverse perspectives. Numerous terms are used interchangeably to mean "clinical reasoning," even though many of these terms denote related but conceptually distinct phenomena.

In this chapter, we will briefly outline several theoretical concepts from a variety of fields to help the reader with teaching and studying clinical reasoning. This is not meant to be a comprehensive account, and as such we have chosen theoretical concepts that we believe best apply the theory, research, and practice of clinical reasoning today. We will begin with an overview of the history of clinical reasoning, highlighting major findings from several periods to help shape where we stand in our understanding of this complex phenomenon.

KEY POINTS

- Our understanding of clinical reasoning has been informed by theories from diverse fields, including psychology, expertise, and education, which can inform the teaching of clinical reasoning.
- Many scholars now view clinical reasoning as having both cognitive and noncognitive domains, as well as being a social as opposed to an individual construct.
- Context specificity refers to variation in physician performance when seeing 2 patients who present in an identical (or near-identical fashion) from a content perspective, which adds challenges to teaching clinical reasoning.
- Teaching institutions may need to reconfigure learning environments to maximize learner opportunities for deliberate practice.
- Dual process theory suggests that clinical reasoning curricula should focus on building both nonanalytic and analytic reasoning.

Next, we will address many theories, both cognitive and noncognitive, individual and social, as well as explore contemporary theoretical findings and challenges (such as the problem of context specificity). We will end with a brief summary and outline next steps for the field from our perspective. We also have included several practical examples throughout this chapter and encourage the reader to review Chapter 4 and Chapter 5 to explore the concepts in this chapter further.

❖ A Brief History of Clinical Reasoning

Over the past several decades, many approaches to clinical reasoning and its assessment (see Chapter 6) have been explored in parallel with contemporary prevailing hypotheses. Here we briefly outline highlights of these themes and the underlying theoretical perspectives that shaped each period.

The General Problem-Solving Era

In the 1960s, scholars believed that expertise in clinical reasoning meant that one was an expert in problem-solving, which could be measured as a distinct skill that was superior in experts as opposed to novices (3). This idea occurred in parallel with beliefs that were widespread in the educational literature. Clinical reasoning was believed to be a type of problem-solving, and problem-solving was considered a general teachable skill that would result in superior performance regardless of the specifics of a given version of the problem (e.g., an individual patient's disease presentation). Ultimately, this belief was demonstrated to be flawed.

For example, Patient Management Problems (4, 5), which were previously used in the United States to assess candidates for board certification, and other "long case" examinations demonstrated that a score derived from one problem, or case, did not necessarily predict performance on subsequent problems (6). In these Patient Management Problems, the reliability or reproducibility of performance for an individual between cases ranged from 0.1 to 0.3 (as a reference, the goal for a reliable test is at least 0.6 to 0.8) (6). In other words, the correlation between cases for an individual expert was low. In addition, the correlation between experts on the same case was also low. This variability in diagnostic performance from case to case helped to establish the concept of content specificity (i.e., that clinical performance is related to specific case content, such as the case's diagnosis). Indeed, we now understand that this variability in performance goes beyond the content of each case (context specificity builds on the concept of content specificity by explaining how factors in addition to the content of a case can affect diagnostic reasoning performance).

These findings were quite surprising at the time because problem-solving was felt to be a general skill that could be equally applied to different problems, or patient presentations. But upon reflection, is it surprising? Imagine challenging a physician who is widely considered to be an outstanding diagnostician, who therefore would be expected to possess exceptional general problem-solving skills, to diagnose not a patient but rather a car's mechanical problems. Clearly, content matters from a common sense standpoint. Beyond knowledge content, the outstanding physician's performance in a given situation may also vary on the basis of his or her experience and recent sleep patterns, as well as specific features of a patient's presentation—in other words, context matters (7, 8). Because of these observations, the idea that clinical reasoning was simply a general problem-solving ability, or trait, was abandoned.

Expertise as Knowledge Organization
Following the initial exploration (and subsequent demonstrated shortcomings) of Patient Management Problems and other evaluations, investigation of clinical reasoning assessment moved in a new direction. Instead of focusing on clinical reasoning ability as a skill or trait (i.e., a general problem-solving ability), researchers instead focused on knowledge acquisition and organization. Roughly in line with the emergence of the computer and

artificial intelligence, an information-processing model inspired by programming logic was applied to medical education. The goal was to provide a model of the clinical reasoning process to enhance our understanding of it (9). Information-processing theory led to work on knowledge organization (i.e., how knowledge is organized in memory) (10). Information-processing theory suggested that the more this knowledge resembled the orderly modeling of a computer program, the more it would result in efficient clinical reasoning and diagnostic success. This emerging theory also coincided with work on illness script theory (mental representations of the clinical symptoms and findings that can be seen with a given disease) (11) and cognitive load (like a computer, the brain has limits in its ability to attune to and process information) (3). In other words, information-processing theory as a construct coincided with multiple theories that built on knowledge representation in memory and the processes that could lead to enhancing acquisition, storage, and recall of knowledge in memory.

Thus, the focus moved from clinical reasoning as a teachable general skill to concentrating on the limits of working or short-term memory and examining processes that could lead to enhancing acquisition, storage, organization, and recall of knowledge in memory. Knowledge organization, or expertise conceived as acquiring and organizing a robust body of information and its interdigitation, became the prevailing framework for clinical reasoning assessment research (3). However, this focus on knowledge acquisition and organization does not readily explain the fundamental discovery of context specificity. If an individual had the knowledge and knowledge organization to answer one question on a specific symptom, finding, or disease, why did he or she fail to transfer that knowledge to a similar or even identical case? To answer this question, a new theoretical lens that could explain context specificity needed to be applied. Of note, despite these limitations with focusing on knowledge organization, the different information processing theories arguably remain the prevailing theoretical perspectives today.

Clinical Reasoning Expertise as a State: Context Specificity and Situativity Theory

Perhaps partly in response to difficulties stemming from the phenomenon of context specificity, researchers began looking beyond the confines of the individual problem solver's (or diagnostician's) brain to the environment, other participants (e.g., patients and their families) and his or her interactions within which a problem (or patient case) was being solved. Social cognitive theories, such as situativity, have emerged from this work. Situated cognition argues that cognition, or thinking, is situated (or located) in the specifics of a given encounter (12). It breaks down the encounter into several factors, including individuals (e.g., the patient, the physician, and other health care members) and the environment or system. This theory argues that these factors interact and that the outcome emerges (in this case diagnosis through clinical reasoning) as opposed to viewing reasoning as something that occurs solely in the physician's head. Because situated cognition (and other situativity theories) includes elements beyond case content, it offers a means of exploring context specificity. Using this situativity lens, work has also recently revisited the issue of expertise, not as a trait (expertise seen as a general "skill" within a field) but rather a state (dependent on the situation) (1). In other words, framing expertise as a state argues that expertise is specific to the patient, physician, and encounter environment factors (i.e., the specific situation). Situativity theories have transformed the traditional view of the cognitively isolated clinician into a clinician whose interactions with other health care providers, patients, and the environment profoundly affect his or her diagnostic ability.

❖ A Theoretical Perspective on Clinical Reasoning

We now explore specific cognitive theories that have shaped our approach to clinical reasoning. These theories have emerged from educational psychology, cognitive psychology, education, expertise, attention, and effort literature.

Expertise and Expert Performance

Several theoretical concepts of relevance to clinical reasoning have been derived from the expertise literature. One is the concept that expert performance is an adaptation—it is largely a matter of amassing considerable experience, knowledge, and mechanics that monitor and control cognitive processes to perform a limited set of activities efficiently and effectively (13). Further, expertise is inextricably tied to content knowledge in a domain. In other words, expert performance requires a rich content-specific knowledge base (as argued by information processing theory). This requirement has applicability to how we teach and assess medical students, residents, and even physicians in practice. From this view, knowledge-based examinations (such as the U.S. Medical Licensing Examination and specialty-specific examinations) have a continued role because they can and do correlate with clinical reasoning performance (14, 15). In other words, content-specific knowledge is necessary but not sufficient. So what else is needed? Deliberate practice provides one possible answer.

Deliberate practice theory argues that expert performance is the result of sustained (e.g., 10,000 or more hours) effortful engagement in component parts of an activity, which is at least initially performed under the guidance of a coach or mentor. This theory argues that expert performance in clinical reasoning emerges when one engages with the content(e.g., diagnosing and treating patients with the expected scope of conditions), with effort (e.g., deliberate versus simple observing), and under the direction of a coach (at least initially) who provides substantive feedback on the learner's performance. Deliberate practice as a means to acquire expert performance has been described in a variety of diverse fields, such as athletics, music, and chess (16).

What are the implications of deliberate practice theory on educating doctors-in-training? Table 2-1 outlines potential teaching implications for teaching clinical reasoning from the deliberate practice perspective as well as other theories discussed in this chapter. Clearly, students must deliberately practice component parts of clinical reasoning (e.g., history-taking, physical examination, laboratory interpretation) and incorporate these components into evaluating patients in clinical settings. They also require feedback on their performance from an experienced coach so they can improve their skills, although trainees may find this process challenging. There are no shortcuts to developing excellent clinical reasoning. So from the deliberate practice perspective of expertise, a vast amount of knowledge is necessary but not sufficient for expert performance. Knowledge, as well as practice (deliberate practice), is needed to achieve expert performance.

From the perspective of medical eduction, deliberate practice theory has several potential implications. From a macro view, its implications for undergraduate, graduate, and continuing medical education are potentially profound. For instance, work hour reforms in graduate medical education in the past decade have substantially altered both the time trainees spend with patients and the nature of these interactions. When viewed through the lens of deliberate practice, it is important to ask whether the consequences of these changes (e.g., decreased hours leading to both decreased patient exposures and truncated teaching time by faculty) are leading to less "coaching time" and subsequently less deliberate practice. On the other hand, the recent emphasis on providing longitudinal curricular experiences (e.g., longitudinal integrated clerkships) in medical school would be consistent with deliberate practice theory—larger gains are expected with a limited number of experienced coaches versus changing coaches every few weeks (17). As described above, on a more individualized level, deliberate practice theory has many implications for teaching in medicine (see Chapter 8 for additional practical details).

One of the central tenets of deliberative practice theory is effortful practice on component parts of an activity. The component parts of clinical

Table 2-1. Theories and Examples of Potential Clinical Reasoning Teaching Applications

Deliberate practice	• Longitudinal mentoring • Identification of which activities to practice (context-/situation-dependent) • Help in discriminating relevant from irrelevant findings for a diagnosis, differentiating typical from atypical presentations for a diagnosis • Emphasize common causes and big-picture concepts • Provision of frequent feedback to facilitate improvement with future practice
Knowledge organization (script theory)	• Compare-and-contrast assignments *How is diastolic dysfunction different from systolic heart failure?* • Create prototypic patient assignments *How would a patient with acute interstitial nephritis present?* • Change key features in presentation *How would this change the resident's differential diagnosis?* • Create algorithms/flowcharts • Think out loud
Dual process	• Explicit instruction on nonanalytic and analytic strategies • Encourage learners to use both analytic and nonanalytic thinking
Cognitive load	• Give learner time to think ○ Intentional pauses • Discuss essential concepts multiple times and via different ways • Return to same problem or diagnosis multiple times • Provide worked examples (e.g., "solved" cases) • Start with prototypes and gradually increase complexity • Gradually increase authenticity • Limit feedback (don't overwhelm learners)

Motivation and emotion (e.g., control value theory)	• Optimize learning environment
	  ○ Reduce burnout and sleep deprivation
	• Optimize engaging, relevant work activities
	  ○ Provide appropriate support
	  ○ Implement progressive independence (increasing responsibility)
	• Capitalize on emotion with learning
	  ○ Tell meaningful "story" (e.g., patients)
	• Encourage learners to commit to diagnosis and therapy
	  ○ Increase attention and enhance limbic valence

Situativity	• As an inclusive theory, all of the above recommendations would apply

reasoning, as alluded to above, are both myriad and not universally agreed upon. Yet medical educators agree on certain aspects of clinical reasoning as core components.

> **Example:** *When approaching an adult patient with a chief complaint of dyspnea and a history of heart failure, the proper performance and interpretation of the physical examination can be paramount to arriving at the correct diagnosis. Specifically, certain aspects of the physical examination (e.g., accurately assessing jugular venous pressure, assessing for hepatojugular reflux, or auscultating a third heart sound) are commonly difficult for a novice or intermediate learner yet are often key to making a correct diagnosis. By identifying these individual parts or, in this context, these subcomponents of the clinical reasoning process, resources can be channeled toward directed, specific effortful practice with feedback and coaching. In the setting of inpatient medicine, this may mean explicitly identifying one or more of these components as a specific goal to work on over the next 2 to 4 weeks. In this way, deliberate practice can allow the teacher to assist his or her learners with building a "toolbox" that will be useful with similar clinical problems in the future.*

Cognitive Theories

Dual Process Theory

Dual process theory refers to two (dual) processes that are used for reasoning. This theory has recently been popularized by the book *Thinking, Fast and Slow* by Daniel Kahneman. Kahneman applied dual process theory to economics (for which he won a Nobel Prize). Briefly, dual process theory argues that we have two processes: fast thinking and slow thinking. Fast thinking (or nonanalytic reasoning, also known as type I or system 1 thinking; these terms are interchangeable) is believed to be quick, subconscious, and typically effortless. This nonanalytic reasoning refers to pattern recognition (the proverbial diagnosis at a glance) as well as heuristics. Heuristics are cognitive shortcuts or rules of thumb that have become effortless (3, 18). The most straightforward examples of pattern recognition tend to be visual (and in the medical literature are often dermatologic), but pattern recognition can occur with inputs through any and all of our senses. An example of pattern recognition (nonanalytic reasoning) would be examining a patient with palpitations (a symptom that in isolation has a broad differential diagnosis) and immediately recognizing the cardinal features or pattern of Graves disease (e.g., palpitations along with exophthalmos, fine resting tremor, thyromegaly). Another example of this phenomenon might be the immediate, subconscious recognition of polydipsia and polyuria in an obese adult as being the result of type 2 diabetes mellitus. Effortlessly thinking of meningitis in a patient who presents with a fever, headache, and mental status changes or septic arthritis in a patient with fever and a single acutely swollen joint are examples of heuristics in action.

Slow or analytic thinking (also known as type II or system 2 thinking), on the other hand, is believed to be effortful and conscious. An example of analytic reasoning would be using a Bayesian approach to a patient presenting with a possible pulmonary embolism (i.e., estimating pretest probability with the Wells score prediction rule and then applying the likelihood ratio of a positive finding on computed tomographic angiography to determine post-test probability) or pausing to work through a patient's acid-base status (e.g., calculating an anion gap, performing Winter's formula, and calculating a delta-delta gap).

Dual process theory argues that both of these processes are used in clinical reasoning in varying proportions based on the specific nature of the task. Nonanalytic reasoning, in particular, frees up cognitive processing space within limited working memory. Expertise is likely due in part to the transition from analytic thinking to nonanalytic thinking. This transition is believed to require deliberate practice and, hence, provides an understanding of expertise as an adaptive phenomenon rather than a general skill (16). We will return to these concepts in more detail below.

Example: Conventional wisdom in teaching clinical reasoning used to be that novice learners would benefit more from reflection (preferential use of analytic reasoning) and "slowing down" to consider clinical problems more fully. The idea was that this approach had the potential to protect against biases, to which novices were more likely to succumb. However, research in this area has suggested that instructing learners to both search for patterns and reflect analytically (e.g., consider what aspects of a case don't fit the pattern) may be an optimal approach (19). Importantly, both nonanalytic and analytic thinking can lead to cognitive errors that are covered in detail in Chapter 4.

Cognitive Load Theory

Like dual process theory, cognitive load theory is an information processing theory, but it focuses on the nature of limited human cognitive architecture—the reproducible observation that short-term working memory can process only so many pieces of information at a given time (20). The tenets of cognitive load theory explain why your phone number is only 7 digits long, as studies have found that short-term working memory can only hold 7±2 or 4±2, depending on the field, pieces of information simultaneously. To overcome this limitation, memory "chunks" information into larger units (from semantic qualifiers and encapsulations to scripts, which we will discuss in more detail below) for easier storage and access. Chunking uses long-term working memory (LTWM), which, in contrast to short-term working memory, is believed to have endless capacity. This allows experienced clinicians to attune to more information during a given encounter and effectively and efficiently (and arguably elegantly) arrive at a diagnosis and therapy for a patient.

> ***Example:*** *Think again of the brain as a computer. Working memory is a processor with limited file capacity (e.g., RAM) at a given time (7±2). Each of these 7±2 files or documents could potentially have only 1 or 2 sentences of information or could represent entire chapters or books (through chunking and LTWM use). Regardless of whether there are a couple of sentences or a book for the document, it takes up the same amount of cognitive space/working memory/RAM because LTWM is believed to be endless in capacity. This helps explain how an astute attending physician can walk into a room and immediately recognize a complex diagnosis and be (elegantly) attuned to the patient's and family's needs—he or she is using a rich array of information per "document" or working memory space while not exceeding the limits of working memory. We will discuss knowledge organization, or "chunking," further in the next section.*

Encapsulations and Semantic Competence

The term *semantic qualifiers* refers to abstract, often binary terms that help narrow or specify the meaning of a symptom, sign, pathologic process, or disease to help to sort through, organize, and chunk patient information (21, 22). Effective use of semantic qualifiers has been labelled *semantic competence.*

> ***Example:*** *A 42-year-old man presenting with his third episode of sudden-onset stabbing chest pain worsened by deep inspiration in the last 2 years is described as "42-year-old man who presents with recurrent, acute pleuritic chest pain" (3 semantic qualifiers— recurrent, acute, and pleuritic—which clarify the character of the chest pain).*

Each term (chunk) can contain a large amount of information, and using semantic qualifiers may help learners build more clearly defined illness scripts (i.e., mental representations of a disease's "story" or the way it presents). Despite being consistent with the understanding of chunking, teaching students to use semantic qualifiers did not improve diagnostic accuracy in a study (23). This result suggested that detailed knowledge of the diagnoses associated with recognized semantic qualifiers, not just the ability to list them, is critical to making the correct diagnosis. Related to semantic qualifiers, encapsulations are compilations of a group of clinical symptoms and/or findings into a pathophysiologic concept or syndrome (24). For example, the term *congestive heart failure* encapsulates cardiac dysfunction characterized by symptoms and signs such as orthopnea, paroxysmal nocturnal dyspnea, jugular venous pressure elevation, and a third heart sound. An experienced clinician who has encapsulated a constellation of clinical findings into syndromes increases the availability of precious short-term working memory slots for other data. Both the formation of encapsulations and the use of semantic qualifiers are believed to be associated with chunking of knowledge. Although this is theoretical, educators should consider teaching these categories and terms because doing so may help learners form chunks. The highest form of a chunk is a script, which is a type of schema (Table 2-2).

Table 2-2. Different Levels of Chunking of Clinical Knowledge

Term	Definition	Examples
Semantic qualifier	Typically binary, abstract descriptor	Acute vs. chronic, mono vs. poly
Encapsulation	Underlying pathophysiologic mechanisms that may become part of schemas or illness scripts	Heart failure, sepsis, labeling pathophysiologic causes (e.g., ischemic, hemorrhagic)
Chunks	More generic term referring to the interdigitation of a collection of information or knowledge; chunks vary dramatically in size and organization and are affected by ongoing knowledge gains and experience	Vary in complexity from a semantic qualifier (e.g., acute vs. chronic) all the way to a well-formed illness script (i.e., an exemplar)
Schema	Larger, well-organized, defined chunks	What to expect when you enter a restaurant (e.g., waiter, paying a bill)
Illness script	An illness script is a specific type of schema (medical content)	Strep throat (exudative pharyngitis, fever, lymphadenopathy, and lack of cough)

Schemas and Script Theory
Schema are mental structures that help to organize and interpret information. They consist of large chunks of information, and in medicine we typically refer to them in the context of illness script theory. A diagnostic illness script (a type of schema) is believed to contain the range of representative symptoms and findings for a given diagnosis. Scripts are dynamic and are believed to be shaped by experience and continually refined throughout one's clinical practice.

Illness scripts are theorized to be used during clinical reasoning in the following manner. When a physician initially sees a patient, verbal and nonverbal cues immediately activate a (potential) variety of diagnostic illness scripts. This effortless (fast-thinking or nonanalytical) process is called *script activation*. (Note that script activation can also occur through effortful or analytic thinking.) In some cases, only one script is activated (as in the example of pericarditis in the pleuritic chest pain case), and in these cases, one may arrive at the correct diagnosis. In most other cases, multiple scripts are activated, and then theory holds that we choose the most likely diagnosis by effortfully comparing and contrasting alternative illness scripts (or at times non-effortfully) that were activated (*script confirmation*). Of course, we may not activate any scripts when we initially see a patient or may immediately exclude all of them, leading us to revert to solving the patient's diagnosis through alternative means other than scripts.

> ***Example:*** *Script theory has been used to provide a framework to "diagnose" learners' errors in clinical reasoning (25). By moving stepwise along the process of script activation, educators may be able to diagnose where their learners are having difficulties. While this approach may have some merit, the reader should recognize that most of the mental processes that take place with script theory are, in part, unconscious. Deconstructing a learner's clinical reasoning after the fact (i.e., after the learner presents the case) may lead to recall bias, and/or subconscious thought processes may not be accessible on recall. Therefore, deconstructing the process into discrete steps and diagnosing learners is an approximation of or model of the process. Please see Chapter 4 for a more detailed discussion.*

The Problem of Context Specificity
All of the theories discussed in detail so far are primarily solely individualistic, meaning that the emphasis is on the physician (decision-maker). While they provide many potentially useful strategies to help our learners, as we alluded to above, one problem in practice with these individual theories

is the phenomenon of context specificity (8). Context specificity has led to the emergence of several social theories in our field (and others) and an increased attention on the interactions among the patient, physician, and others, as well as the practice or setting and how it might affect a learner's clinical reasoning. Thus, the theories below emphasize not only the physician but also how the physician interacts with patients and their environment. From this viewpoint, teaching clinical reasoning should entail more than instruction of the learner—we should also pay attention to the team, the environment, and the interactions between participants in a situation in addition to the health care system and culture. We discuss this further in the following sections that pertain to social theories.

Noncognitive Theories

Relatively recent is the recognition that noncognitive personal attributes affect cognition. However, the categorization of attributes as cognitive and noncognitive is a simplification or categorization for research purposes and is not based on neurobiology. As an example of the power of emotion on memory (the prototypic noncognitive example), think about what you were doing on 9/11. You probably can state with clarity (like it happened yesterday) what you were doing and why. What were you doing at 9:03 a.m. yesterday? You probably will struggle with answering this with any specificity (incidentally, 9:03 is the time that the second plane crashed into the World Trade Center). Capitalizing on emotion can improve learning. It can also hinder learning and memory. Notably, implicit in deliberate practice is motivation—one will not engage in effortful practice for 10,000 hours to achieve expertise without significant motivation.

Control Value Theory

A leading theory on motivation and emotion is control value theory (26). This theory argues that our emotions, motivations, and activities affect our performance (in this case, clinical reasoning). There are both activating emotions (e.g., enjoyment) and inhibiting emotions (e.g., boredom or frustration). Notably, not all negative emotions inhibit learning. In fact, small amounts of negative emotions can actually improve performance as long as the learner is not overwhelmed (again demonstrating the interplay between these theories, in this case between control value theory and cognitive load theory). Control value theory incorporates three elements:
- **Motivational beliefs:** the value of the activity at hand (task value)
- **Self-efficacy:** confidence that you can do the task
- **Achievement goals:** mastery versus performance, with higher gains being associated with mastery goals than with trying to get an "A" (performance-based motivation)

The implications of control value theory include suggesting that educational environments should provide tasks that are authentic to maximize learner motivation and achievable, given the learner's current abilities, to foster a sense of self-efficacy. Furthermore, a teacher should tend to learners' emotions.

> *Example:* As opposed to discussing the signs and symptoms of heart failure with a ward team during walk or sit-down rounds, discussing and demonstrating at the bedside increase the authenticity of the task.

Situativity

Situativity (Table 2-3) refers to a group of social cognitive theories that incorporate the participants, the environment, and their interactions, as we have previously defined (12). One example of situativity is situated cognition, which breaks down an activity such as clinical reasoning into physician, patient, and environmental components as well as interactions among these components. The outcome (in this case clinical reasoning) is believed to emerge from these factors and their interactions. Another example of situativity, situated learning (which can be confused with

Table 2-3. Situativity versus Information Processing Theory

Theory	Clinical Reasoning Process	Implications
Situativity	Reasoning takes place as a dynamic interaction among the physician, the patient, and environmental factors	• Environmental factors, such as an electronic health record or appointment length, are not viewed as noise but as important to the clinical reasoning process • Interactions may be nonlinear; hence, small changes can produce large changes in results
Information processing theory	Reasoning is a cognitive process within a physician's head, and success is based on specific knowledge and its organization; the other participants and the environment or setting are largely considered to be "noise"	• Clinical reasoning takes place exclusively in the physician's mind; external factors are deemed less important • Assumes a fairly linear relationship between inputs and outputs

situated cognition), stresses participation in an activity and identity formation as learning versus acquisition of "static" facts. Identity is formed through legitimate peripheral participation (participating in the community with gradual increase in responsibilities and influence—an example being becoming a master tailor or a butcher; the tasks one performs increase as one gains experience and knowledge). Distributed cognition is a third theoretical perspective that relates to group thinking; the answer does not "sit" in the head of any one individual, and there are activities that require interactions with several participants to be successful (e.g., how a crew navigates a ship; indeed, this context is one of the activities where work in distributed cognition began). Situated learning shares features with our apprenticeship model to medicine and also suggests ways to improve our system (e.g., increasing responsibility with learner readiness), while the other 2 theories remind medical educators to pay attention to factors beyond the learner to teach clinical reasoning when teaching in clinical environments.

> **Example:** *Learners often use electronic resources during patient care activities. From a situated cognition perspective, these electronic resources are a valid way for learners to augment their clinical reasoning. Teaching points in this setting focus on the appropriate use of these resources (such as the type of resource using evidence-based medicine principles and the appropriate time and place to use these resources [e.g., not necessarily when taking the initial history and performing the physical examination]).*

Situation Awareness

Situation awareness is typically conceptualized as an up-to-date understanding of the world around the observer. Formally stated, situation awareness is defined as "the perception of the elements in the environment within a volume of space and time, the comprehension of their meaning, and the projection of their status in the near future" (16). Situation awareness can also inform decision-making and performance in the context of a medical encounter. Environmental features that affect how well individuals perform include the capability of the system to provide the needed information (e.g., limited time in busy practice), the design of the system interface that determines which information is available (e.g., availability of records), system complexity (e.g., number of patients, number of problems, support), the level of automization present in the system (e.g., support from the front desk and nurses and triage of appointments), participant stress, and workload. Furthermore, situation awareness includes many factors internal to participants, factors that affect performance in space and time. These include perceptual processing and limited attention, limited short-term working memory, expectation bias, and pattern-matching to existing schemas. Attention to these features, and how they might interact, has implications for research and teaching.

Individual versus Social Theories and Linearity

The social theories described above have multiple component parts that can and do interact in a cyclical nature, giving rise to the possibility of nonlinearity or results that may not approximate a straight line. Such an approach raises theoretical as well as assessment challenges as our current methods of assessment are heavily steeped in a psychometric world view, which assumes that the expected results do approximate a straight line. Please see Chapter 6 for a more in-depth discussion of assessment of clinical reasoning and its challenges.

Contemporary Theoretical Challenges

We have explored our current understanding of clinical reasoning through the lenses of diverse theoretical backgrounds, such as educational psychology, cognitive psychology, education, expertise, attention, and effort literature. Despite the progress made, several questions remain regarding our understanding of how to best apply these concepts to teaching early learners (e.g., medical students) and especially advanced learners (e.g., the effect of aging on the clinical reasoning process). Finally, while many of the theories focus on the individual and assume linear relationships between inputs and clinical reasoning outputs, other theories expand the focus beyond the individual (e.g., social cognitive theories) and place increased importance on the patient and the environment or the entirety of the context of the encounter, which allows for nonlinear assessment (see Chapter 6) and includes opportunities to enhance our understanding of context specificity. Social theories also call for teacher attention to individual, team, and environment or setting factors and their optimization to facilitate learning. In addition, these theories would suggest that clinical reasoning certification and its maintenance require more than tests of knowledge. Finally, the notion of nonlinearity and the problem of context specificity suggest that we should consider new approaches when exploring clinical reasoning from a research perspective, such as when designing studies and interpreting the results.

❖ Summary

Our intention in this chapter was to provide a brief primer on a sample of the diverse theoretical concepts that underlie our current understanding of the clinical reasoning process. Although it is apparent that numerous gaps remain in our collective understanding of the clinical reasoning process, it is also clear that progress into a more thorough understanding of this process is advancing.

REFERENCES

1. **Eva KW, Hatala RM, Leblanc VR, Brooks LR.** Teaching from the clinical reasoning literature: combined reasoning strategies help novice diagnosticians overcome misleading information. Med Ed. 2007;41:1152-8.
2. **Durning S, Artino AR Jr, Pangaro L, van der Vleuten CP, Schuwirth L.** Context and clinical reasoning: understanding the perspective of the expert's voice. Med Educ. 2011;45:927-38.
3. **Norman G.** Research in clinical reasoning: past history and current trends. Med Educ. 2005;39:418-27.
4. **McCarthy WH, Gonnella JS.** The simulated patient management problem: a technique for evaluating and teaching clinical competence. Br J Med Educ 1967;1:348-52.
5. **McGuire CH, Babbott D.** Simulation technique in the measurement of problem solving skills. J Educ Measurement. 1967;4:1-10.
6. **Elstein AS, Shulman LS, Sprafka SA.** Medical Problem Solving: An Analysis of Clinical Reasoning. Cambridge, MA: Harvard University Press; 1978.
7. **Eva KW.** On the generality of specificity. Med Educ. 2003;37:587–8.
8. **Eva KW, Neville AJ, Norman GR.** Exploring the etiology of content specificity: factors influencing analogic transfer and problem solving. Acad Med. 1998;73(10 Suppl):S1-5.
9. **Pauker SG, Gorry GA, Kassirer JP, Schwartz WB.** Towards the simulation of clinical cognition: taking the present illness by computer. Am J Med. 1976;60:981-96.
10. **Bordage G.** Elaborated knowledge: a key to successful diagnostic thinking. Acad Med. 1994;69:883-5.
11. **Charlin B, Tardif J, Boshuizen HP.** Scripts and medical diagnostic knowledge: theory and applications for clinical reasoning instruction and research. Acad Med. 2000;75: 182-90.
12. **Durning SJ, Artino AR.** Situativity theory: a perspective on how participants and the environment can interact: AMEE guide no. 52. Med Teach. 2011;33:188-99.
13. **Feltovich PJ, Prietula MJ, Ericsson KA.** Studies of expertise from psychological perspectives. In: Ericsson KA, Charness N, Feltovich P, Hoffman RR, eds. Cambridge Handbook of Expertise and Expert Performance. New York: Cambridge University Press; 2006:41-67.
14. **Reed DA, West CP, Holmboe ES, Halvorsen AJ, Lipner RS, Jacobs C, McDonald FS.** Relationship of electronic medical knowledge resource use and practice characteristics with internal medicine maintenance of certification examination scores. J Gen Intern Med. 2012;27:917-23.
15. **Norcini JJ, Boulet JR, Opalek A, Dauphinee WD.** The relationship between licensing examination performance and the outcomes of care by international medical school graduates. Acad Med. 2014;89:1157-62.
16. **Ericsson KA, Charness N, Feltovich P, Hoffman RR, eds.** The Cambridge Handbook of Expertise and Expert Performance. New York: Cambridge University Press; 2006.
17. **Hirsh DA, Ogur B, Thibault GE, Cox M.** "Continuity" as an organizing principle for clinical education reform. N Engl J Med. 2007;356:858-66.

18. **Kahneman D.** Thinking, Fast And Slow. New York: Farrar, Straus and Giroux; 2011.
19. **Norman GR, Eva KW.** Diagnostic error and clinical reasoning. Med Educ. 2010; 44:94-100.
20. **Van Merrienboer J, Sweller J.** Cognitive load theory and complex learning: recent developments and future directions. Educ Psychol Rev. 2005;17:147-77.
21. **Bordage G, Lemieux M.** Semantic structures and diagnostic thinking of experts and novices. Acad Med. 1991;65:S70-2.
22. **Bordage G.** Elaborated knowledge: a key to successful diagnostic thinking. Acad Med 1994;69:883–5.
23. **Nendaz MR, Bordage G.** Promoting diagnostic problem representation. Med Educ. 2002;36:760-6.
24. **Schmidt HG, Rikers RM.** How expertise develops in medicine: knowledge encapsulation and illness script formation. Med Educ. 2007;41:1133-9.
25. **Bowen JL.** Educational strategies to promote clinical diagnostic reasoning. N Engl J Med. 2006;355:2217-25.
26. **Artino AR, La Rochelle JS, Durning SJ.** Second-year medical students' motivational beliefs, emotions, and achievement. Med Educ. 2010;44:1203-12.

3

Developing a Curriculum in Clinical Reasoning

Joseph Rencic, MD, FACP
Robert L. Trowbridge Jr., MD, FACP
Steven J. Durning, MD, PhD, FACP

To develop a curriculum in clinical reasoning, the term *clinical reasoning* must first be defined because descriptions of this term vary in the literature. Considered broadly, clinical reasoning may include disparate topics, such as deciding whether to screen for prostate cancer using shared decision-making (i.e., a form of diagnostic reasoning) and taking into account a patient's comorbid conditions and specific genetic and immunologic markers to decide upon the most appropriate treatment regimen for breast cancer (i.e., a form of therapeutic reasoning). It may also include complex mathematical modeling of clinical questions and even cost-effectiveness analysis of potential screening or treatment options (e.g., forms of diagnostic and therapeutic reasoning). This book, however, focuses on the process of making a diagnosis (diagnostic reasoning). This process involves synthesizing the patient history, physical examination, and laboratory and imaging results, as well as response to therapy and time course, with the goal of establishing a diagnosis. Although principles of diagnostic reasoning and clinical decision-making overlap, the differences between these approaches warrant separation. Diagnostic reasoning includes all steps up to and including the diagnosis (i.e., the specific process of establishing a diagnosis), while clinical decision-making typically emphasizes the decision step.

KEY POINTS

- Development of a local curriculum in clinical reasoning can elevate the field to that of a foundational "basic science" while also ensuring that clinical reasoning is emphasized throughout the educational continuum.
- Curriculum development should be steeped in the theory of clinical reasoning, including information processing theory and social cognitive theory.
- Using a systematic approach (e.g. Kern's 6-step model to curriculum development) can increase the likelihood of curricular success.
- A curriculum in clinical reasoning should start early in the education of medical learners, gradually increasing in complexity with increasing clinical experience.
- Curricula should include both explicit instruction in the process of clinical reasoning and guided clinical experiences.

Historically, teaching clinical reasoning has differed from describing ways to avoid diagnostic error. These differences are in large part secondary to the origins of each of these fields: Clinical reasoning is centered on the psychology, education, and expertise literature, whereas the study of diagnostic error originated largely in the more recent patient safety movement. Reducing diagnostic error has typically focused on factors outside of individual diagnostic performance, especially systems-based influences (e.g., the availability of necessary testing and the timely and correct reporting of laboratory results). This difference, however, is lessened by the increasing appreciation of the effect of the surroundings (e.g., system-based influences) on clinical reasoning. Social cognitive theories, such as situativity, and constructivism have introduced this appreciation. This intertwining of context and cognition is an important concept and may eventually result in further "merging" of the fields of diagnostic error and clinical reasoning. Thus, many of the concepts integral to a curriculum in clinical reasoning may also improve diagnostic reliability and decrease diagnostic error.

❖ Defining Curriculum

Definitions of *curriculum* derive from the varied backgrounds and perspectives of educators. Practically, we define *curriculum* as the formal educational content, structure, and processes developed to enable students to perform at a competent level for a given stage of training. This definition excludes the informal or "hidden" curriculum, which is beyond the scope of this chapter but clearly must be accounted for to achieve the desired outcomes. The term *curriculum* is derived from the Latin *currere*, meaning "race." Thus, literally speaking, curriculum is the race that learners run with the hope that through teaching, assessment, and feedback they will meet the educational goals and objectives.

The goal of both medical education and curriculum is to promote the progressive independence of learners whereby they no longer need the teacher to "take care of" the content, in this case, patients. With regard to a clinical reasoning curriculum, the goal is to foster and facilitate the gradual independence of learners under more authentic circumstances so that they can take care of patients with less supervision over time. The goal of undergraduate medical education is to prepare for graduate medical education, and the goal of graduate medical education is to prepare independent practice. This notion is derived from Vygotsky's "zone of proximal development" and the educational concept of allowing the scaffolding (or educational support) to be dismantled over time (1).

An institution's philosophy of learning and teaching profoundly shapes the structure and processes used to create its clinical reasoning curriculum. Hence, a one-size-fits-all approach is not possible. However, we believe that certain core clinical reasoning content should be considered in all clinical reasoning curricula, as described later in this chapter. As with all curricular development, goals and objectives and the methods by which these will be assessed must be clearly defined. Additionally, it is important to recognize that assessment drives learning, so even the best curriculum is likely to fail if the assessment system is poorly designed.

❖ Philosophical Approaches to Curriculum

A teacher's curricular approach reflects, explicitly or implicitly, his or her own perception and values. There are many ways to approach this activity, which we will briefly describe: behavioralist, systematic, and humanistic. Each has its advantages and disadvantages, and the best approach (or a combination thereof) depends on how the curriculum designer envisions success.

A behavioralist approach is based on principles of behavioralism whereby the learner is typically expected to demonstrate a series of observable actions (e.g., knowledge, skills, and/or attitudes) upon completing the unit, course, clerkship, residency, or fellowship rotation or continuing professional development activity (2). It typically involves creating goals and objectives (behaviors to be demonstrated), as well as a step-by-step approach, a blueprint, and educational outcomes. It arguably is both the oldest and the most common approach used in medical schools and residencies in the United States. Aspects of behavioralism are also re-emerging in popularity with the recent emphasis on competency-based medical education, milestones, and entrustable professional activities (3).

The systematic approach is often called *curriculum engineering* (2). This approach includes the planning of the curriculum, the broader curriculum aspects (e.g., design, implementation, and evaluation), and the curriculum components (e.g., subjects, lesson plans, overall curriculum plans). It is based on systems theory and also stresses the interrelatedness of the component parts of the curriculum. Examples of the systems approach include total quality management and RAND's Planning, Programming, and Budgeting System (2). In this case, the system is the curriculum and its various parts. A systems approach to curriculum planning would ensure that the design, execution, and evaluation have a quality assurance plan. Kern's 6-step model provides a valuable practical framework for a systems approach to curriculum development (Box 3-1) (4), which can be used for designing a curriculum in clinical reasoning. Each step informs the next steps in this model, and the steps are meant to be cyclical in nature.

The humanistic approach considers the learner as a whole (5). The goal is not just cognitive elements, such as those emphasized in the

---

Box 3-1. Kern's 6-Step Model for a Systems Approach to Curriculum Development

1. Problem identification and general needs assessment (e.g., proficiency in selected topics)
2. Needs assessment for targeted learners (e.g., differences between the ideal and actual characteristics of the learners)
3. Goals and objectives (what the curriculum hopes to achieve will direct the choice of curricular content and assignments as well as suggest which learning methods to choose)
4. Educational strategies (specific material and methods or ways in which to present the content [e.g., small vs. large group; classroom vs. clinic; problem-based vs. case-based vs. team-based learning])
5. Implementation (identify needed resources, such as personnel, time, space, funding, communication; may choose a pilot phase prior to full implementation)
6. Evaluation and feedback (e.g., guides successive cycles)

behavioralist and systematic approaches, but also the social and cultural aspects of the learner. This approach gained momentum with the emergence of humanistic psychology and its emphasis on domains such as value, ego, and self-actualization (5). Activities may include group projects, games, field trips, and tutoring activities. A humanistic perspective to curriculum planning would also include attending to the "hidden curriculum" and ensuring emotional readiness for activities that are meaningfully constructed to help trainees learn (5).

❖ Fundamental Considerations in Clinical Reasoning Curriculum Design

Two fundamental questions need to be addressed in developing a curriculum on teaching clinical reasoning. These include the following: "Can clinical reasoning be taught?" and, if so, "What is the most effective and efficient approach?" In response to the former, we reply, "Can you teach a child to distinguish a dog from a cat?" Few would argue the contrary. Little effort is required to recognize the similarity of this teaching to the process of teaching a student to distinguish heart failure from pneumonia (i.e., nonanalytic diagnostic clinical reasoning). Likewise, most would agree that a student can be taught how to estimate the pretest odds of a disease and multiply them by a likelihood ratio to obtain a post-test probability (a form of analytic diagnostic reasoning).

In answering the first question affirmatively, we now face the more challenging quandary of how to teach clinical reasoning. We believe that educational theories (see Chapter 2) provide useful answers to this question in several ways. First, they provide a substantial body of empirical evidence from a variety of fields on which to structure learner education. Second, they provide a "lens" for assessing success as educational theory typically provides predictions regarding what one would expect with its formal use. Third, using educational theory orients the curriculum designer to viewing curriculum in clinical reasoning as scholarship and, as such, provides a greater opportunity for collecting data that may be generalizable to others in the scientific community. We thus believe that the concepts of and distinctions between information processing theory (e.g., dual process theory) and social cognitive theories (e.g., situativity), as discussed in detail in Chapter 2, can inform the curriculum designer.

Information processing theories focus on the acquisition and organization of knowledge in the learner (6). These theories emphasize reading and remembering facts that can be recalled when necessary. Because these theories emphasize acquisition, areas such as the authenticity of how the content is delivered (e.g., a paper case versus a standardized patient encounter) or the class size (e.g., large versus small group) are given less attention. In addition, with the emphasis on the individual learner, little attention is typically given to aspects such as working in teams or the environment for learning and performance (e.g., a clinic, ward, or classroom). On the other hand, social cognitive theories (e.g., situativity) endorse the importance of knowledge acquisition and organization but also emphasize the inclusion of the system (environment), other participants (e.g., other students and/or the patient), and their interactions (6). Information processing focuses on the individual learner and considers the other participants and the environment as noise; in contrast, situativity sees these other elements as important components for teaching clinical reasoning and its performance. In general, curriculum designers are probably biased toward information processing theory, but we believe an understanding of social cognitive theories can allow for curricula that customize the environment to maximize learning experiences.

For example, designing a small teaching session for a clinical reasoning course from a social cognitive perspective would view not only the content (e.g., syllabus, other readings, and teaching points for a session) as important but also learner goals and motivation, authenticity of materials, group size, educational setting, and student team dynamics.

As another example, in designing a clinical reasoning block in graduate medical education, a social cognitive perspective would also consider components such as fatigue, burnout, team dynamics, time for the session, and immediate relevance of the material in addition to content. Indeed, situativity can assist with identifying the root cause of curricular outcomes that are not consistent with expectations, which we discuss below.

❖ Teaching Dual Process Theory

Dual process theory, a form of information processing theory, can inform educators how to teach as well as assess clinical reasoning. The brain uses fast (nonanalytic) and slow (analytic) thinking/reasoning to solve problems and make decisions (7). A clinician who makes a snap diagnosis of shingles when seeing a patient with a dermatomal vesicular rash is using nonanalytic reasoning (e.g., pattern recognition). Nonanalytic reasoning is often based on mental representations of disease presentations (i.e., illness scripts or stories of diseases), which are used as the template for categorizing the patient's presentation. Curricula centered on the importance of illness scripts stress comparison and contrast of diseases in the differential diagnosis to determine defining and discriminating features of those diseases. These curricula have also included teaching semantic qualifiers (i.e., words that qualify the meaning of a symptom, such as *acute* or *recurrent*), which can significantly affect the differential diagnosis (e.g., acute vs. chronic cough) (8). The evidence that teaching these methods improves diagnostic performance is limited but is based on neuroscience and our understanding of how knowledge is organized (9).

The experienced physician is believed to typically use nonanalytic reasoning when encountering common diagnoses in her or his practice. The question then becomes, 'How does one develop nonanalytic reasoning or pattern recognition abilities?' This may emerge from both regular associations and explicit instruction. Our brains are constantly making associations or connections, and this is one reason for the difference between teaching and learning—much is learned without formal teaching, such as language acquisition in babies. Furthermore, evidence exists that teaching nonanalytic reasoning helps learners across the educational continuum (10).

Discussion of analytical reasoning approaches should also be included in a clinical reasoning curriculum. Strategies of analytic thinking include Bayesian reasoning, hypothetico-deductive reasoning, evidence-based medicine, rule-out/worst-case scenario, key feature approach, and meta-cognitive monitoring (e.g., thinking about one's thinking). Teaching analytic reasoning is important not only because it is a precursor to nonanalytic thinking (we automate slow thinking over time if we repeat it multiple times) but also because sequentially combining nonanalytic with analytic reasoning may reduce clinician error in complex cases (11). We would thus recommend that both analytic and nonanalytic reasoning strategies be incorporated into clinical reasoning curricula, regardless of the level of the learner. Before describing these approaches, however, we consider the challenges in designing clinical reasoning curriculum.

❖ Specific Challenges in Developing Clinical Reasoning Curriculum

The broad and fundamental nature of clinical reasoning in medical training means that it is housed nowhere but should be taught everywhere. To avoid making clinical reasoning an "orphan," we believe that curriculum designers should treat clinical reasoning as a "foundational science" like anatomy and physiology. It should be explicitly integrated into various courses throughout each year of medical school and residency training in a developmental fashion. Defining clinical reasoning as a core theme within the curriculum serves as one practical solution to this dilemma. Curricular designers can then systematically identify areas where clinical reasoning content can be integrated into the curriculum. Unfortunately, implementing a clinical reasoning curriculum faces many specific challenges (Table 3-1).

Table 3-1. Challenges to Curriculum Development

Challenges	Potential solutions
No evidence-based gold standard for design	• Use psychology, expertise, education, and other literature as foundations to build curriculum • Use multiple teaching strategies • See Chapter 5 on teaching techniques
Vast scope	• Emphasize intermediate steps to the diagnosis • Focus on key core of symptoms and diseases • Build a standardized virtual national/international simulation curriculum of multiple cases for common and uncommon diagnoses and typical and typical presentations
Domain-specific knowledge is essential	• Develop biomedical knowledge (e.g., anatomy, pathophysiology) • Encourage illness script development (e.g., classic prototypes, then atypical presentations) • Teach schema (e.g., algorithms) for approaching common symptoms • Teach analytic reasoning strategies (e.g., Bayesian reasoning, thresholds) • Encourage use of both nonanalytic and analytic reasoning • See Chapter 5 on teaching techniques and on Chapter 4 on approaches to cognitive errors
Complicated nature	• Design developmentally (teach basic component skills first, then integrate into whole) • Attend to emotion, identity formation, and progressive independence of the learner
Lack of a longitudinal, curricular home	• Create a clinical reasoning "theme" throughout all levels of education (preclinical, clinical, continuing education)
Lack of core faculty	• Develop faculty • See Chapter 7 on faculty development
No gold standard for assessing the process of clinical reasoning	• Continue research to enhance understanding of the process • See Chapter 6 on assessment

Several of these barriers deserve specific mention. The vast scope and domain-specific nature of clinical reasoning, for example, makes curriculum development a daunting task. Focusing on typical presentations of common diseases (e.g., Clerkship Directors in Internal Medicine and

Society of General Internal Medicine core clerkship training problems) (12) in the preclinical years helps students build illness scripts. Subsequently, learners can advance to illness scripts of atypical presentations of common diseases and typical presentations of uncommon diseases in clinical years of medical school and residency. In addition, teaching approaches and constructs for specific problems (e.g., use of a prerenal, intrarenal, and postrenal scheme to approach acute kidney injury) can be a valuable exercise. Similarly, Van Merrienböer and colleagues suggest that complicated abilities like clinical reasoning can be taught by teaching component tasks separately and subsequently integrating these components over time to enhance whole-task (clinical reasoning) performance (13). Within clinical reasoning, component parts include history-taking, physical examination, building a problem representation, generating hypotheses, and confirming hypotheses.

Faculty development (see Chapter 7) poses the typical challenges. However, an advantage is that nearly all physician faculty perform or have performed clinical reasoning. Instructing a core group of a faculty to teach the key aspects of the curriculum reduces time and resource utilization. In addition, stressing "think aloud" teaching strategies for all faculty and encouraging learners to ask questions about faculty's clinical reasoning may be helpful. Finally, as mentioned previously and acceding to the role that assessment plays in driving teaching, assessment forms that require faculty to describe a learner's clinical reasoning ability emphasize the importance of clinical reasoning to both leaners and faculty.

The evidence base for clinical reasoning curricula is primarily limited to learner satisfaction, but these interventions have been limited in scope and design. They provide limited guidance to curricular designers as a result (14–16). Nevertheless, applying principles derived from the education, expertise, and psychology literature as further described in later chapters can help in curricular design.

❖ Curricular Structure and Content

Some of the key questions to ask in developing a curriculum on clinical reasoning include the following:

1. Should clinical reasoning be taught in a stand-alone course, integrated into multiple courses, or both?
2. When should a clinical reasoning curriculum start and where should it continue?
3. What kind of instructional formats and teaching methods should be used? Classroom? Online? Bedside teaching? Small group discussions?

4. How should the curriculum be evaluated?

5. What are the faculty development needs?

Scant evidence in the literature supports specific answers to these questions, but several recommendations can be made on the basis of the underlying theories of education and clinical reasoning. Perhaps most important, the structure and content of a curriculum in clinical reasoning will vary according to the experience of the specific group of target learners. The approach to teaching clinical reasoning to first- or second-year medical students, for example, may be very different from the tack taken with experienced clinicians as part of a continuing medical education activity. This distinction is further amplified by the acknowledgment that much clinical reasoning is context specific. In addition, as learners become more experienced, their needs may shift. Thus, curricular flexibility to allow each learner to develop at her own pace may be as important as as, if not more important than, any other aspect of the curriculum, especially for more experienced learners (see the section on microanalytic techniques in Chapter 10). Despite this limitation, however, we believe it is possible to outline curricular components that are appropriate for each level of learner. Below are a series of recommendations for curricular design, segregated by level of learner.

Preclinical Medical Education

Several guiding principles should be considered in teaching clinical reasoning to preclinical students (Box 3-2). First, because of the relative lack of clinical experience among medical students, especially in those in the very early stages of their education, we believe a progressive approach is most appropriate: starting with straightforward presentations of common diseases and eventually progressing to complex presentations of atypical diseases. Emphasizing the importance of learning prototypical presentations of common diseases early in the educational continuum builds the

---

Box 3-2. Suggested Principles for Teaching Preclinical Students

1. Begin with typical presentations of common diseases and gradually increase complexity.

2. Explicitly discuss clinical reasoning processes during clinical case discussions, including integration with basic science content.

3. Discuss the basics of cognitive psychology, drawing parallels to everyday nonclinical decision-making.

foundation for the development of the learners' pattern recognition abilities. This can be accomplished in many ways, including case discussions, patient presentations, paper cases, and even real patients. Specific clinical content may also be introduced into basic science courses to allow students to participate in case-based discussions of specific presentations. Although high-fidelity simulations are very engaging and stimulating, we believe at this stage the exposure to straightforward content matters more than the manner in which it is delivered. Indeed, complicated forms of delivery may negatively affect performance and learning because of increased cognitive load (17). Studies are now exploring importance of the authenticity of instructional content (e.g., paper case versus live patient with the same condition). There are many reasons that authenticity may be important, including the complexity of the information (element interactivity) and motivation. To date, however, studies focusing on cognitive outcomes have not demonstrated an effect of authenticity of instructional materials in medical students. The curricular designer should thus be mindful of costs and benefits, goals and objectives, learner readiness, and desired outcomes when considering the authenticity of instructional materials in clinical reasoning curricula (18).

Second, incorporating discussion of clinical reasoning concepts, such as our understanding of theory and errors, in the classroom or other learning settings may be a successful means of teaching about the process itself. Even in the setting of clinical inexperience, many topics central to the clinical reasoning process may be taught. For students in the first 2 years of the traditional basic science–oriented medical school curriculum, the lack of clinical experience may initially limit the use of a case-based approach; however, cases can be integrated into curricular topics being covered in other parts of the curriculum. When students are immersed in a course centered on the anatomy, physiology, and pathophysiology of the heart, for example, cases centered on cardiac disease can be used to demonstrate basic reasoning techniques. As such, discussion of a patient presenting with chest pain in the context of a cardiac course may introduce the analytical reasoning concepts of "worst-case scenario" medicine and thresholds for testing by teaching students to always consider "can't miss" diagnoses and the rationale for this approach. Using this tactic, one that combines teaching clinical content with teaching clinical reasoning, may also promote buy-in from students. Some students may be reluctant to spend time learning about reasoning techniques, despite their clinical applicability, when no specific identifiable section on exams covers this content.

Finally, clinical reasoning shares many similarities with the decision-making that everyone does in everyday life, and these parallels may be exploited to educational benefit in demonstrating the clinical reasoning process. Thus, the basic tenets of the education, expertise, and psychology literature may be taught in a manner that draws connections to the clinical setting without requiring clinical expertise to understand. The lay popularity of books such as Daniel Kahneman's *Thinking, Fast and Slow* and Malcolm Gladwell's *Blink: The Power of Thinking Without Thinking* (7, 19), both of which discuss many topics germane to clinical reasoning, are testament to this concept.

Content
Using a progressive approach to the curriculum (i.e., a spiral curriculum) allows the introduction of clinical reasoning concepts with progressively more complexity in clinical material and clinical reasoning content. On the initial pass, basic clinical content may be introduced in conjunction with simple clinical reasoning concepts, with increase in complexity in both areas with subsequent encounters. As experience with the clinical reasoning process grows, concepts demonstrated with one area of clinical content may be reinforced in other clinical areas. More complex and nuanced clinical content, such as the atypical presentations of common diseases and the prototypical presentations of less common diseases, may be introduced concurrently.

No matter the means of instruction used, concepts of cognitive psychology and clinical reasoning appropriate to discuss early in medical education include the following:
- The dual process model of thinking and specific strategies used with each mode
- The role and potential shortcomings of heuristics
- The effect of bias on the reliability of decisions
- Bayesian reasoning and analysis
- Use of thresholds to test and treat in decision-making
- Script theory and problem representation

Methods
The overall structure of the local undergraduate curriculum is a major factor in determining the most appropriate approach to integrating a clinical reasoning curriculum, but multiple methods may be used to implement such a curriculum. Lectures on the important concepts of clinical reasoning may play a role, but small group discussions, including case-based discussions as described above, would seem most likely to be effective. The presence of faculty guides to help students to work through the clinical content and to explain and demonstrate the clinical reasoning content can be very helpful. Specific teaching tips for use in this setting are presented in Box 3-3. Verbal and written reflections requiring deconstruction of the

Box 3-3. Practical Tips for Teaching Preclinical Students With Case-based Discussions

1. Establish and emphasize the key teaching points for each case to ensure consistency of content.
2. Encourage students to develop diagnostic problem lists, including pertinent symptoms, physical findings, and laboratory data, for each case.
3. Encourage students to generate a prioritized differential diagnoses, including "can't miss" diagnoses, and record on board.
4. Stress the benefit of combining nonanalytic with analytic reasoning serially to improve diagnostic accuracy.
5. Probe students about how changing clinical elements may alter the differential diagnosis, emphasizing the importance of key clinical data.
6. Model clinical reasoning; think out loud and demonstrate clinical reasoning.
7. Focus on classic disease and syndrome associations.
8. Teach and reinforce the syndrome before the diagnosis (e.g., exudative pleural effusion before effusion secondary to lung cancer; obstructive renal failure before prostate cancer causing obstruction).
9. Help learners prepare for an encounter by reviewing the approach and differential diagnosis for the chief complaint; allow pauses for critical thinking and reflection after the encounter.
10. Encourage students to compare and contrast related diagnoses; identify key discriminating factors, especially epidemiology and risk factors.
11. Require students to commit to gestalt or evidence-based (e.g., prediction rule) pretest probability estimates by weighing clinical findings (using likelihood ratios when possible) to defend their diagnostic decisions.
12. Reinforce the importance of context (e.g., an afebrile immunosuppressed patient may still have infection).

diagnostic process, including reflection on videos or the learner's own clinical experiences, may also be an effective technique.

Overall, implementing such a curriculum early in the education of medical learners can ensure that students enter their clinical experiences with a strong understanding of the clinical reasoning process, serving as the foundation for the development of their own clinical reasoning abilities. The students can develop a vocabulary with which to speak "the language of diagnosis." This may occur in much the same way that a pharmacology course prepares students for the clinical use of medications, with the resultant elevation of clinical reasoning to a foundational "basic science" similar to anatomy, physiology, and histology. We have included a sample syllabus for an 18-month curriculum on clinical reasoning that follows the above principles (www.acponline.org/teachingbooks).

Clinical Medical Education

Learners at the clinical medical education level (clinical medical students and residents) have substantially more clinical experience, and the goal of the teaching at this level should shift to consolidating knowledge of the clinical reasoning process and reflecting on their own clinical reasoning. Accumulating clinical experience may be the most important aspect of the process at this stage because it continues to strengthen and expand the learner's base of illness scripts on which to draw. The teaching process may incorporate more advanced clinical knowledge, such as atypical presentations of common diseases and acknowledging the likelihood ratios for key findings. It may also include instruction on how to account for conflicting information and extraneous data, as well as strategies for dealing with the difficulties encountered in collecting the necessary data.

Much of the teaching at this level is done in the context of providing clinical care. This setting has the advantage of being centered on real patients and thus forces the teachers and learners to deal with the often ambiguous and nuanced presentations of disease and the difficulties inherent to collecting the necessary data. It also further emphasizes the need to be aware of the systems in medicine and their effect on both individual cognition and the diagnostic process as a whole. Social cognitive models would also emphasize the need for progressive independence and identify formation of the learner, as well as optimizing the learning environment (20). The advantage of such teaching being based in the workplace may be countered by the concurrent need to provide excellent care for patients. These "service" obligations on the part of both learners and teachers, and the time they require, may limit the ability to establish a formal curriculum in clinical reasoning.

Although likely to be effective, embedding such teaching in the clinical setting can be challenging, especially because students are often dispersed across a wide range of specialties and even geographic locations. Case discussions led by specifically trained clinician-educators who are also well versed in clinical reasoning may solve this problem (21). Such an initiative may require significant faculty development but is likely to reinforce and further develop the clinical reasoning abilities learned at an early stage. As learners become more sophisticated, further discussion regarding errors and the role of systems in diagnosis is also appropriate because learners will have the necessary experience to understand these more advanced and nuanced concepts.

There are several other means of instituting curricula in clinical reasoning at this level (Box 3-4). The importance of having a clinical guide in the form of an experienced faculty member is worth emphasizing. Even at the level of a single interaction, such a teacher may help to create context and help to define the importance of a specific clinical encounter. Emphasis, for example, may thus be placed on the challenges of deciding when to evaluate a patient for potential pulmonary embolism, a common clinical scenario, rather than focusing on rare "zebra" disorders, even when the latter may be particularly meaningful to residents because of their experiences. Perhaps the most effective, if unproven, means of guiding these learners is to provide a faculty guide or coach who works with a specific learner over an extended period. This apprenticeship, or coaching model, effective in many other fields, provides an educator with the continuity of exposure to develop a clear and strong understanding of the clinical reasoning abilities of a specific learner. Although logistically difficult, this is an educationally worthy goal and allows for the identification

---

Box 3-4. Methods for Introducing a Clinical Reasoning Curriculum in the Clinical Setting

1. Provide learners with longitudinal mentors to enhance continuity of education.
2. Track learner experiences via patient logs to ensure wide breadth of clinical exposure.
3. Increase exposure to patients with undifferentiated presentations and symptoms rather than patients with diseases.
4. Emphasize building knowledge of atypical presentations of common diseases and typical presentations of uncommon diseases.
5. Introduce concept of diagnostic error and causes with learner reflection on personal experiences.
6. Promote focus on both the clinical reasoning process and outcome (i.e., diagnosis) at established conferences, such as "morning report" and morbidity and mortality conferences.

and needed practice (e.g., deliberate practice) of trainee-specific needs in clinical reasoning.

Given the importance of seeing as many patients and patient presentations as possible in the development of clinical reasoning abilities, programs can aspire to both keep track of the learners' clinical experiences and provide individual feedback on these experiences. Many medical schools now require students to keep track of all the patients they encounter to ensure they are receiving a broad-based clinical education. Graduate medical education programs may institute a similar program, tracking the clinical experiences of its learners to ensure exposure to a wide variety of clinical presentations and diseases. When a learner is lacking in a particular area, steps could be taken to fill the gaps, perhaps via schedule adjustments or targeted clinical activity. Ideally this could be linked to individual feedback from faculty with expertise in clinical reasoning, although this may be difficult to achieve.

Clinical activity may also be structured to ensure exposure to "undifferentiated" patients and to encourage learners to propose, if not direct, the diagnostic evaluation of such patients. The recent emphasis on patient safety, with the resultant increase in clinical supervision of residents, however, may limit the independence of residents and inadvertently inhibit their development. Similarly, limitation of duty hours may truncate the volume of clinical experiences to which residents are exposed, further restraining their development. Structuring programs to increase exposure to "diagnostic opportunities" and training faculty in methods of supervision that allow for progressive independence in the diagnostic process are important solutions to this potential problem.

Introducing a formal curriculum on how the diagnostic process may fail and diagnostic errors occur is also appropriate at the clinical level (22, 23). Learners have sufficient clinical experience such that they have committed errors in reasoning or witnessed them and thus have a rich blend of experiences to draw upon. The discussion of common biases and the effect of systems on diagnosis are among many topics the discussion of which can be enriched by learners' reflections on clinical experiences.

If nothing else, clinical programs can work to ensure that specific emphasis is placed on the diagnostic process. Case discussions such as "morning report" and morbidity and mortality conferences, which often play a major role in residency programs, can be structured around diagnosis and the reasoning process (21). Core clinical reasoning content can also be reinforced during the regular didactic sessions that most residency programs require. Programs may similarly ensure that faculty are well versed in teaching techniques that are likely to promote the development of clinical reasoning (and that are more comprehensively discussed in Chapter 5).

Table 3-2. Shift in Instructional Themes in Teaching Clinical Reasoning

Preclinical Medical Education	Clinical Medical Education
Classroom learning; often paper or computer-based cases	Patient-based; workplace learning
Straightforward clinical content (typical presentations of common disorders)	Advanced and nuanced clinical content (atypical presentations of common disorders; rare disorders)
Small-group learning (learners more likely to be closely clustered at same level of inexperience)	Individualized instruction and feedback (learners with more widely varying levels of experience and abilities)
Avoidance of topics requiring experience to fully appreciate, such as diagnostic error and role of systems in diagnosis	Introduction of more-nuanced topics in which teaching is enhanced by clinical experience (e.g., diagnostic error and role of systems in diagnosis)

Overall, there are important shifts in the instructional themes regarding clinical reasoning as the learner gains clinical experience and progresses from the preclinical undergraduate to the clinical educational level. As shown in Table 3-2, there is a shift toward working in the more authentic clinical setting, more personalized instruction, and coverage of more nuanced topics that require some degree of personal experience to fully understand. These shifts, although important, are gradual and should not be considered to be absolute. An experienced resident, for example, may still learn from a low-fidelity paper case just as a preclinical student may learn from a live patient.

Continuing Medical Education

Conceptualizing a curriculum in clinical reasoning for the practicing physician is perhaps most difficult. Although medical and specialty board licensing agencies have numerous requirements for maintaining certification, educational requisites vary significantly among them. Many clinicians lack the time or inclination to participate in significant educational initiatives, but there are several means of structuring a curriculum to engage practicing physicians.

Faculty development for clinician educators centered on the basics of script theory may help teachers refine their teaching on the topic. Similarly, teaching educators about dual process theory and other basic tenets of "how doctors think" may help inform both their own practice and their teaching of clinical reasoning (see Chapter 7). A situativity approach can incorporate the role of the patient, their family members, the environment, the system, and other health care workers into the clinical reasoning process, providing a more elaborate model to help "diagnose" and "treat" the patient and help to improve understanding of problems such as context specificity.

Other discrete topics, especially those that until recently were absent from most undergraduate medical curricula, may also be of value not just to clinician educators but to all practicing physicians. The concepts of bias, affective error, and heuristics may all be introduced via didactics or, more appropriately, interactive workshops. In addition, finding way to promote diagnostic closure and feedback on diagnostic performance may be invaluable in improving diagnostic performance.

Finally, involving practicing clinicians in the teaching of clinical reasoning may help improve their own abilities in clinical reasoning; growing evidence suggests that teaching is an important deliberate practice activity (24). Reflective exercises, including those with learners, may be a particularly effective means of prompting frank consideration of one's reasoning abilities. Additional ways to improve clinical reasoning abilities in practicing physicians are presented in Chapter 8.

❖ Challenges in the Evaluation of Curriculum

Curriculum evaluation is critical in determining the successes and failures of educational strategies. The evaluation of a clinical reasoning curriculum poses particular challenges because it encompasses the entire curriculum (whether at the undergraduate or graduate medical education level) and the true measure of success is the individual reasoning abilities of the learners. A social cognitive approach such as situativity can be helpful in exploring why curricular outcomes were or were not achieved. Situativity provides an inclusive model, with multiple factors and interactions (see Chapter 2) to help a designer with determining reasons for successes or failures that may not be evident otherwise. However, as described in Chapter 6, numerous challenges exist in assessing clinical reasoning. If we cannot assess clinical reasoning ability well, then gauging the success of a curriculum is difficult. Despite this significant challenge, institutions can still evaluate key components of their clinical reasoning curriculum that may provide a sense of efficacy of the program, especially if a multimodality assessment program is used.

Multiple outcomes may be studied in attempting to determine the success of a program. Of note, the assessment may be targeted both to the steps of clinical reasoning and to whether learners can come up with the "correct" answer in a given situation. Evaluation, for example, may include measurement of learner ability to identify the key discriminatory findings for a specific patient presentation, to properly interpret how a test result affects the likelihood of a specific disease, and to construct a diagnostic summary statement that includes all of the key elements of a patient presentation. It may also include the ability to construct an appropriately detailed and prioritized differential diagnosis. Attempts may also be made to determine the ability of learners to arrive at the correct diagnosis, and this may be done in the classroom setting via paper cases, the simulation laboratory via observed structured teaching encounters, and simulated cases. Other potential outcomes include learner satisfaction and knowledge gains, as assessed via traditional testing methods.

Although much of this evaluation may be done in the classroom and via various forms of simulation, completing evaluation in the setting with the closest approximation of the clinical arena is most desirable. Even the most advanced simulation, for example, is unlikely to truly incorporate all of the unpredictable and unforeseen variables that may affect clinical reasoning abilities in "real life." For reasons described previously and in Chapter 6, however, authentic workplace assessment of clinical reasoning and thus, by extension, the effectiveness of a curriculum in clinical reasoning may be complex logistically and difficult to standardize. Furthermore, the context specificity of clinical reasoning ability may necessitate a very large "sample" of reasoning behavior in order to reliably reflect ability.

Although desirable, randomized experimental designs to evaluate curriculum are resource intensive and methodologically challenging. Other, more practical designs include knowledge pre-/post-tests and the use of historical controls in the instance of a new curriculum. The quality improvement Plan-Do-Study-Act (PDSA) model is another practical alternative. Existing structures for collecting data and evaluating courses and curriculum (e.g., curriculum committees, medical education representative councils) should be used when available. This may be another role for social cognitive approaches, such as situativity, as a more inclusive view of the curricula is used than with traditional information processing approaches that emphasize the learner's acquisition.

REFERENCES

1. **Chaiklin S.** The zone of proximal development in Vygotsky's analysis of learning and instruction. In: Kozulin A, Gindis B, Ageyev V, Miller S, eds. Vygotsky's Educational Theory and Practice in Cultural Context. Cambridge: Cambridge University Press; 2003;39-64.
2. **Ornstein A, Hunkins F.** Curriculum: Foundations, Principles, and Issues. 6th ed. Harlow: Pearson Education; 2013.

3. **ten Cate O.** Entrustability of professional activities and competency-based training. Med Educ. 2005;39:1176-7.

4. **Kern D, Thomas P, Hughes M.** Curriculum Development for Medical Education—A Six-Step Approach. 2nd ed. Baltimore: Johns Hopkins University Press; 2009.

5. **Onstein A, Levine D.** Foundations of Education. 10th ed. Boston: Houghton Mifflin; 2008.

6. **Durning SJ, Artino AR.** Situativity theory: a perspective on how participants and the environment can interact: AMEE guide no. 52. Med Teach. 2011;33:188-99.

7. **Kahneman D.** Thinking, Fast and Slow. New York: Farrar, Straus and Giroux; 2011.

8. **Bordage G.** Elaborated knowledge: a key to successful diagnostic thinking. Acad Med. 1994;69:883-5.

9. **Nendaz MR, Bordage G.** Promoting diagnostic problem representation. Med Educ. 2002; 36:760-6.

10. **Eva KW.** What every teacher needs to know about clinical reasoning. Med Educ. 2005; 39:98-106.

11. **Mamede S, Schmidt HG, Rikers RM, Custers EJ, Splinter TA, van Saase JL.** Conscious thought beats deliberation without attention in diagnostic decision-making: at least when you are an expert. Psychol Res. 2010;74:586-92.

12. **DeFer T, Fazio S.** Core Medicine Clerkship Curriculum Guide. Vol. 2014. Alexandria, VA: Alliance for Academic Internal Medicine; 2006.

13. **Merrienböer JV, Kirschner P.** Ten Steps to Complex Learning: A Systematic Approach to a Four Component Instructional Design. 2nd ed. New York: Routledge; 2013.

14. **Gay S, Bartlett M, McKinley R.** Teaching clinical reasoning to medical students. Clin Teach. 2013;10:308-12.

15. **Jacobson K, Fisher DL, Hoffman K, Tsoulas KD.** Integrated cases section: a course designed to promote clinical reasoning in year 2 medical students. Teach Learn Med. 2010;22:312-6.

16. **Norman G, Sherbino J, Dore K, et al.** The etiology of diagnostic errors: a controlled trial of system 1 versus system 2 reasoning. Acad Med. 2014;89:277-84.

17. **van Merrienboer JJ, Sweller J.** Cognitive load theory in health professional education: design principles and strategies. Med Educ. 2010;44:85-93.

18. **Durning SJ, LaRochelle J, Pangaro L, et al.** Does the authenticity of preclinical teaching format affect subsequent clinical clerkship outcomes? A prospective randomized cross-over trial. Teach Learn Med. 2013;24:177-82.

19. **Gladwell M.** Blink: The Power of Thinking Without Thinking. New York: Little, Brown; 2005.

20. **Lave J, Wenger E.** Situated Learning. Legitimate Peripheral Participation. Cambridge: University of Cambridge Press; 1991.

21. **Kassirer JP.** Teaching clinical reasoning: case-based and coached. Acad Med. 2010;85:1118-24.

22. **Ogdie AR, Reilly JB, Pang WG, et al.** Seen through their eyes: residents' reflections on the cognitive and contextual components of diagnostic errors in medicine. Acad Med. 2012;87:1361-7.

23. **Reilly JB, Ogdie AR, Von Feldt JM, Myers JS.** Teaching about how doctors think: a longitudinal curriculum in cognitive bias and diagnostic error for residents. BMJ Qual Saf. 2013;22:1044-50.

24. **Durning SJ, Ratcliffe T, Artino AR Jr**, et al. How is clinical reasoning developed, maintained, and objectively assessed? Views from expert internists and internal medicine interns. J Contin Educ Health Prof. 2013;33:215-23.

4

Educational Approaches to Common Cognitive Errors

James B. Reilly, MD, MS, FACP

The rate of diagnostic errors can vary widely across medical specialties (1–3). They are common and costly, occurring approximately 15% of the time in internal medicine and accounting for a disproportionate amount of morbidity, mortality, and malpractice claims compared to most other categories of medical errors (4, 5). Until recently, medical education has focused on systems as the most significant and proximal cause of medical error (6). Yet in the face of new research on the topic, medical educators and patient safety practitioners have placed a renewed focus on diagnostic errors (2, 7–9). This has led to an acknowledgment that cognitive processes, which are at the root of a substantial proportion of diagnostic errors (10), drive medical errors in addition to systems issues, such as test availability and laboratory error. Cognitive errors are often multifactorial, highly subjective and imprecise, difficult to analyze, and impossible to separate from the systems-based and environmental contexts in which they occur. They can be the result of pervasive, subconscious processes in the minds of clinicians of all levels of skill and experience, making them difficult to detect and modify. However, advances in cognitive psychology have provided insight into these ubiquitous processes, making the mysteries of improving clinical reasoning more accessible to clinicians and teachers alike.

KEY POINTS

- Cognitive errors are prevalent, complex, highly subjective, and extremely difficult to identify and analyze. They are becoming increasingly recognized as a driver of medical errors, but interventions shown to reduce their occurrence are scarce.
- Instructors should recognize that cognitive errors can occur at any step in the diagnostic process, including inadequate knowledge, poor data collection or organization, faulty synthesis, biased thinking, and influences from the external environment and system. A systematic but individualized approach must be taken to be able to identify all faulty cognition at play in a given error.
- For the individual clinician, building knowledge and knowledge organization are important means of reducing diagnostic error.
- Several cognitive techniques have the potential to improve diagnostic performance in both learners and practicing physicians and deserve further study in realistic clinical environments.

CHALLENGES

- The subjective, personal nature of cognitive errors has left the medical community slow to recognize and hesitant to call attention to these events, perhaps out of fear of stigmatizing those involved.
- Clinical learners place great emphasis on speed as a marker of expertise and may be overconfident despite owning repositories of illness scripts that still require development.
- Analysis of cognitive error is always subject to hindsight bias, sometimes making it extremely difficult to determine whether an error definitely occurred and especially whether it was preventable.
- Research is needed to prove the efficacy of cognitive strategies for reducing error.
- Forced cognitive strategies may be viewed as unnecessary or inefficient by learners and physicians, limiting their adoption and incorporation into daily practice.

In this chapter, we discuss approaches to the analysis of diagnostic errors and teaching about the avoidance (or perhaps, more accurately, mitigation) of cognitive bias, perhaps the most inaccessible aspect of the diagnostic process. Although we frequently refer to "the learner" throughout this chapter, many of the concepts presented apply to clinicians at all levels of experience, from the preclinical medical student to the seasoned faculty member.

❖ Diagnosing the Error

Identifying cognitive errors is difficult for many reasons. While diagnostic errors are increasingly recognized as a significant source of preventable morbidity and mortality, cognitive contributions to diagnostic error still remain unclear (11). Flawed diagnostic reasoning often eludes the conventional approaches that capture medical errors. Cognitive errors may be infrequently reported because of limited understanding of clinical reasoning processes or a tendency to focus on identifying and reporting systems errors. Furthermore, the personal nature of some cognitive errors may dissuade those who commit or witness an error from reporting it. At times, individuals may not bring cognitive errors to light in order to spare themselves or colleagues from the potential for embarrassment, shame, or fears of disciplinary action. Last, and perhaps most important, recognition and discussion of errors in diagnostic clinical reasoning are typically inferred from behaviors. Even the individual who makes an error may be able to rationalize his or her behavior, yet many of the decisions made are based on subconscious cognitive processes. Accurate re-creation of the clinical scenario and individual thought process is, unfortunately, often impossible. Further, knowing the outcome is likely to influence one's perceptions of past events, making it even less clear what individuals involved knew (or could have known) at the time. This phenomenon, known as *hindsight bias*, is omnipresent and nearly impossible to measure (12). As a result, discussion of the effectiveness of techniques to identify, analyze, and prevent cognitive errors, although necessary and appropriate, will remain speculative.

A multiplicity of potential causes of error should be acknowledged and sought for during any error analysis (see Chapter 1). A thorough systems evaluation and an appreciation of the context of the error are also the first steps in the approach to analyzing a cognitive error because the medical literature emphasizes that systems and cognitive factors often co-occur and contribute to errors (10). Other factors, such as the environmental and personal factors among team members or patients, also contribute by making cognitive processing more difficult or creating a situation where biases become more likely (13).

Careful elucidation of these contextual factors will always facilitate effective cognitive analysis. This can be done one of several ways. Interviews of all members of the health care team in the context of a root cause analysis, with construction of a fishbone diagram that outlines both cognitive and systems factors, has been described (Figure 4-1) (14). Alternatively, individual recall and reflection with a single teacher or small group, either verbally (15) or through narrative writing (the process of reflecting upon and writing about one's thoughts and impressions of an encounter or experience) (13), is a potentially fruitful approach to clarifying the various factors contributing to an error.

The Role of Bias in Cognitive Errors

According to the dual process theory of decision-making (see Chapter 2), clinicians make decisions by using two types of processes: nonanalytic processing (also called *intuitive* or *system 1 reasoning*), and analytic processing (also called *system 2 reasoning*) (16, 17). Nonanalytic thinking provides a highly efficient, rapid approach to decision-making that allows busy clinicians to cope with the enormous complexity of clinical medicine while maintaining speed and a high level of accuracy. Experienced clinicians spend up to an estimated 95% of their time making decisions using these intuitive processes (18). The speed of nonanalytic reasoning relies in part on heuristics that generally tilt the odds of success in the clinician's favor when the clinician is facing a decision. Heuristics are mental shortcuts that allow a rapid response to information and often result in an appropriate result; when they fail, however, they are often called *cognitive biases*.

Dozens of these heuristics have been described in great detail in the medical literature (12, 19). The most prevalent of these have particular implications for learners who are still developing expertise in clinical reasoning (13, 20–22), although these biases can affect physicians at all levels. While often unavoidable and generally useful, biases have the potential to lead clinicians down the wrong diagnostic path. However, because heuristics often lead to correct diagnoses, clinicians may not appreciate their potential negative effects or when they might actually contribute to a diagnostic error. Below, we briefly describe a few commonly encountered biases in medical education and the aspects of the diagnostic process in which they might have an effect. Table 4-1 describes these common biases. None of these biases are mutually exclusive, and multiple biases can be present in a given situation.

The literature on cognitive error focuses a great deal on heuristics and biases without commenting on another significant cause of cognitive error: inadequate knowledge and/or knowledge organization. The expertise literature highlights these factors as a key to successful performance

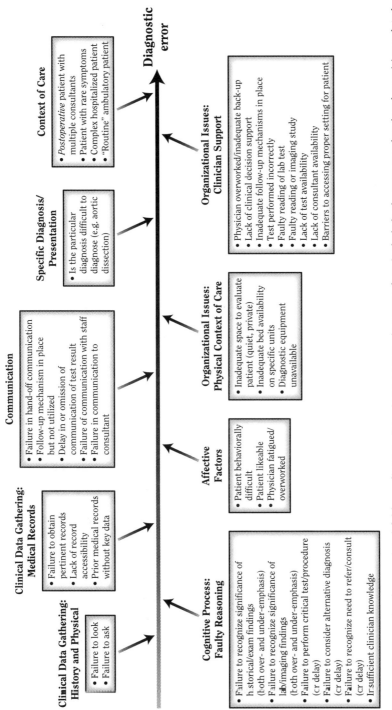

Figure 4-1 Example of a completed fishbone diagram. By using a systematic approach to include both systems-related and cognition-related causes, a fishbone diagram illustrates specific opportunities for improvement while demonstrating the complex causes for potential errors in diagnosis.

Table 4-1. Common Biases and Definitions

Bias	Definition
Affective	Also called *visceral bias*; emotional influences can induce thinking errors, including the feelings physicians have about their patients, both positive or negative
Anchoring	Narrow focus on a single feature in a patient's presentation to support a diagnostic hypothesis, even if other concurrent features or subsequent information refutes the hypothesis
Availability	The tendency to think that things that come to mind immediately are more likely or more common
Blind obedience	Inappropriate deference to the recommendations of authority, either by direct superiors or by "expert" consultants, even in the absence of a sound rationale
Confirmation	The tendency to search for evidence to support an initial diagnostic impression, and the tendency not to search for, or even to ignore, evidence that refutes it
Diagnostic momentum	The tendency of a diagnostic label to become propagated by multiple intermediaries (patients, physicians, nurses, other team members) over time; what might have begun as a possible "working diagnosis" becomes "definite"
Framing effect	The susceptibility of diagnosticians to be disproportionately influenced by how a problem is described, by whom it is described, or even the environment where an encounter takes place
Hindsight bias	Knowing the outcome of an event influences the perception and memory of what actually might have occurred; in analyzing diagnostic errors, this can compromise learning by creating illusions of the participants' cognitive abilities, with potential for both underestimation and overestimation of what the participants knew (or could have known)
Overconfidence	The tendency to think one knows more than one does, especially in physicians who might place faith in opinions without gathering the necessary supporting evidence
Premature closure	Making a diagnosis before it has been fully verified

because broad knowledge and highly integrated networks of knowledge organization are clearly necessary if not sufficient for diagnostic accuracy. Many errors may appear to be related to biases when in fact the basis for them could reside in limited knowledge. Inadequate knowledge and knowledge organization can lead to inadequate or faulty data collection, problem representation, and illness script selection. A clinician, for example, may be unaware a disease may present in a certain manner and thus not ask the necessary questions. It is valuable to keep this in mind as we explore the more common biases below.

Anchoring/Premature Closure

Perhaps the most common cognitive mistake in the diagnostic process is the decision (usually a subconscious one) to complete the process before arriving at the correct answer. Experts also may call this *premature closure* of the diagnostic process. Because most definitions of diagnostic error specify that a correct diagnosis actually "existed," and an opportunity to make an accurate diagnosis was present but missed, in theory all cognitive errors of diagnosis are secondary to the result of premature closure and failing to open one's mind to considering or reconsidering the correct diagnosis. Some have taken to using the term *anchoring* synonymously with *premature closure,* and it may be acceptable to use these terms interchangeably in some situations. However, if one thinks of premature closure as a broader sine qua non for diagnostic errors, adding greater specificity to the term *anchoring* facilitates a more nuanced discussion, but one that can cause confusion. One way to distinguish between the two would be to specifically define anchoring as premature closure that occurs particularly early in the diagnostic process, an inflexible position adopted based on one's initial diagnostic impression that does not acknowledge or incorporate data that come after the diagnostic decision, even data that refute the initial impression. An additional use of the term, and perhaps the use most directly tied to the medical literature, is a narrow focus on a single aspect of the patient's presentation, or one specific diagnostic test, on which one bases the entire clinical impression, without incorporating all data—especially data that might contradict the thing on which the clinician is "anchored" (12). Failing to diagnose clinically evident congestive heart failure because of a normal B-type natriuretic peptide level is an example of this.

Availability Bias

The availability bias is based on an assumption that things should be considered more likely if they are more easily remembered. For busy clinicians, availability bias generally comes from seeing higher volumes of common diseases in the course of patient care. An example is to assume that in January, in the middle of flu season, the acute onset of fever, myalgia, malaise, dyspnea, and cough represents influenza and not decompensated heart failure from bacterial endocarditis and mitral valve failure. A specific, memorable case may also skew overall impressions of disease prevalence. For example, a clinician who missed a fatal pulmonary embolus, or encountered a rare disease such as familial Mediterranean fever, is likely to consider both these diagnoses to be more prevalent than they actually are. For the less experienced clinician, susceptibility to this bias might also spring from the preclinical curriculum, where rarer diseases can be discussed in great detail because of their unique clinical-pathological correlation in driving home an important learning point, or as an element of preparing for standardized examinations.

Framing Effect and the Concept of Diagnostic Momentum
How clinicians and learners formulate their diagnostic impressions can be strongly influenced by the way a problem is described and the environment in which it takes place (e.g., how it is framed). For example, in a primary care office one might be less likely to consider a diagnosis of acute coronary syndrome for chest pain than if the same patient was being seen in the emergency department. Or in the teaching environment, attending physicians hearing patient presentations are likely to be influenced not only by how a learner presents the case but also by their impression of whether the learner is reliable. On the other side, when less confident learners receive information from their attendings, these opinions are likely to hold a great deal of weight. In this age of increased "handoffs," opinions of one's colleagues might also matter as much as what information is actually exchanged.

Patients who are discussed as having a "diagnosis" are likely to carry that diagnosis forward in the mind of the health care team, whether that diagnosis was more of a preliminary, working diagnosis or just a hypothesis yet to be tested. This "diagnostic momentum" can have significant implications for patient care, especially in electronic health records, where progress notes might have a high degree of templating or cut-and-paste shortcuts in the name of efficiency, carrying unsubstantiated diagnoses forward as if they had been verified.

Affective Bias (Visceral Bias)
Emotions are widely acknowledged to affect cognitive processes such as clinical reasoning, and these visceral or affective biases have been described in the medical literature (15, 23). The emotions that patients elicit in clinicians (both positive and negative) have the potential to affect every

cognitive component of the diagnostic process. Additionally, fatigue, stress, and other external factors can affect how much emotion influences one's cognition. A body of literature on how emotions bias decision-making in medicine is growing (15, 23–27).

Overconfidence
Overconfidence is one of the more commonly encountered biases in medical decision-making, especially in situations of complexity and uncertainty. It is well described that physicians' initial diagnostic impressions in patients presenting with nonspecific symptoms, as is often the case in emergency medicine and internal medicine, are unreliable (28, 29). Yet confidence remains high even in "difficult" cases, which highlights the poor abilities of physicians in the domain of self-assessment (30).

Blind Obedience
Alternatively, learners who might not have confidence in their own abilities may express overconfidence in laboratory, radiographic or other studies, or especially superiors and "expert" consultants. This phenomenon can be called *blind obedience*. Learners exhibiting this trait may feel in need of greater guidance (i.e., they are less confident in themselves) and be less likely to question or challenge suggestions or advice from a supervisor or expert consultant. It may also potentially lead to excessive ordering of laboratory and imaging studies.

Cognitive Errors
The biases described above can exert effects anywhere in the process of collecting and synthesizing information; such effects highlight the importance of diagnosing a cognitive error by examining each step of the diagnostic process and understanding that this is not a linear process (Figure 4-2) (31).

Medical Knowledge and the Importance of Illness Scripts
In the preclinical stages of medical training, early learners work to integrate basic science principles into an understanding of clinical physiology and pathophysiology, applying clinical prototypes to represent a disease. Early on, these illness scripts tend to consist of common presentations of common diseases and a representation of preclinical didactic instruction. One's repertoire expands and evolves over time as informed by clinical experiences, continued accumulation of knowledge, and reflection. Especially in early learners, current opinion seems to be that one's ability to generate appropriate differential diagnoses from nonanalytic reasoning is likely limited to the existing repository of illness scripts.

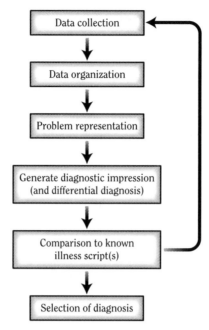

Figure 4-2 Steps where cognitive errors can occur.

Those with larger repositories of illness scripts, particularly experienced physicians, might be more likely to arrive at the right diagnosis because the diagnosis is more likely to correspond to a script in that collection. However, especially in those who have limited clinical experiences, these scripts might be rigid, narrowly defined, or possibly incorrect. Rarer diseases, and common diseases that are presenting in an unusual way, will present particular diagnostic challenges for those who have integrated a limited number of illness scripts or those whose illness scripts have been formed inaccurately or incompletely.

Inadequate or Faulty Data Collection
An accurate diagnosis depends on the formation of an organized clinical database that contains all necessary information. A clinician's ability to create this database depends on the clinical skills of history-taking, physical examination, review of medical records, and prior diagnostic testing. Moreover, it is essential to recognize that the actual questions asked, and perhaps their specific order, examination maneuvers performed, and/or the areas of past records reviewed, depend on the initial differential diagnosis even as they inform its development. Throughout the patient encounter (and often before), cognitive biases and the clinician's repository of illness scripts inform the collection of this database by influencing what questions are and are not asked and what physical examination is performed.

For example, the busy resident who receives an admitted patient described as having heart failure by a colleague in the emergency department may be the victim of a framing effect as well as diagnostic momentum. As a result of confirmation bias, the resident might ask the patient only about heart failure symptoms, neglecting to ask questions about symptoms or risk factors for other diseases that might present similarly, such as chronic obstructive pulmonary disease, as a challenge to the diagnostic hypothesis. Biased cognition has an effect throughout the entire patient encounter (31), and this is why faulty data collection is not always due to poor execution of clinical skills. Finally, and importantly, incomplete or disorganized medical records are a common source of frustration and inaccuracy for clinicians attempting to make a diagnosis (32).

Faulty Synthesis

An ongoing aspect of the diagnostic process consists of synthesizing a clinical impression from the data gathered. Errors in synthesis can be from faulty problem representation, faulty interpretation of the data, and/or faulty script selection.

Problem representation depends on the clinician's ability to translate the patient's historical data, physical examination, and diagnostic data into an accurate set of descriptors that summarize the case. Prioritizing the importance of data (and eliminating unimportant data) hones this collection into a summary statement, often called the *one-liner*, at the end of an oral presentation or written note. This statement should be considered a pivotal "deliverable" from the learner's clinical encounter, and from it may spring possibilities for diagnostic hypothesis generation. Faulty problem representation, from inaccurate assignment and prioritization of descriptors, can have important implications for generating an accurate differential diagnosis. Misinterpreting a chronic illness as acute, de-emphasizing critical attributes in favor of emphasizing nonspecific or misleading ones, or over- and underspecification are all examples of ways that learners can fail to properly represent the problem. This is an especially pertinent problem for novice learners who will have difficulty differentiating the "red herrings" from the critical data.

Once an appropriate representation of the problem is generated, errors can still occur. These errors can be difficult to recognize and difficult to address. The explanation for this may not be so simple as failing to recall the best "match" from a mental repository of illness scripts to match the perfectly represented problem or the clinician not having the appropriate illness script in his or her repertoire. Additional testing, for example, may be necessary to confirm or refute the diagnostic hypotheses. Test selection at any given time is based on the clinical impression to that point.

While it is possible that learners may order the wrong test because they are already heading down the wrong path, flaws in Bayesian decision-making (such as inaccuracies in estimating pretest probability, faulty selection of tests, and translation of the above into an inaccurate post-test probability for a given condition) may instead occur. Failure to confirm an initial diagnostic impression with the appropriate test may be more frequent than initially apparent, and external pressures, including time pressures, combined with cognitive biases, can force the clinician's hand into a premature closure of the diagnostic process (13). This is why in discussion of the choice of the final diagnosis, the clinician-learner should be asked to justify the decision with supportive data, the thought process, and the reasons for choosing particular tests, as well as to describe as much about the external context of the case as possible.

Overall, in "diagnosing" an error, a systematic approach should be used because several factors contribute to most diagnostic errors, both from within the clinician's thinking (or the team's thinking in many cases) and from the contextual environment or the system, combining to create the ultimate result (10). The examiner may put himself or herself in the clinician's shoes, seeking to discover what about the case stimulated the clinician to think the way he or she did, and why that line of thinking made sense at the time. Ultimately, however, to define a diagnosis as an error, there should be confidence that all the information necessary to make the diagnosis was available (or could have been tested for) at the time of the encounter. As we have said before, because retrospective analysis of these occurrences probably lends itself to hindsight bias, it might be impossible in many cases to have confidence to apply the term "error." Re-creating the context of the actual event is impossible, but even when it is unclear whether an individual or team is actually at fault, defining a diagnostic error as a "missed opportunity," as some have done (33), may still facilitate learning from a suboptimal outcome without assigning responsibility for the event. Finally, diagnostic errors can be classified as failure to reach a diagnosis at all, selection of the wrong diagnosis, an avoidable delay in making the appropriate diagnosis (again acknowledging the subjective nature of determining this), or perhaps even a breakdown in the appropriate diagnostic process (e.g., getting to the right answer by the wrong route).

❖ Diagnosing the Learner

An individualized approach to any cognitive error is critical. A potentially helpful approach for identifying the learner's mistakes, especially if they involve cognitive missteps, is the technique Croskerry calls the *cognitive autopsy* (15). In this exercise, one asks the learner to walk the teacher through his or her memories of the entire case, perhaps guided by the patient's chart to "stimulate recall" of important factors (34). The learner should describe as much as possible, including interactions with the patient, other members of the health care team, all ambient and external conditions, and especially the emotions and thought processes of the learner during the encounter, even from the beginning of the day if necessary. Although likely to be biased, these recollections can help explain the learner's impressions of the case at the time and the reasons for what the learner thought and did. Instructors may find it useful to corroborate or flesh out details afterward by interviewing other members of the team (or even the patient), but it is important that the learner not discuss the case with other team members in advance to avoid undue influence in perceptions. See Box 4-1 for a listing of situations where biases may be especially prevalent.

Next, we describe common issues stratified by learner level, based on educational theory and our own experiences. However, these tendencies are not necessarily pathognomonic for a certain level of experience.

Box 4-1. Situations Where Biases May Contribute to Error

- ► Handoffs
  - • Change of shift
  - • Transfer between units
  - • Intra-facility transfers
- ► Time pressures
  - • High patient volume
  - • Distractions or interruptions
- ► Individual physician factors
  - • Fatigue or sleep deprivation
  - • Individual stress
  - • Cognitively overextended
- ► Patient factors
  - • Uncooperative/difficult patient
  - • Bad reputation
  - • Countertransference/stereotyping
  - • Complex illness
- ► Team factors
  - • Hierarchy
  - • Specialty service (as opposed to generalist)
  - • "Group think"

In reviewing errors, one should proceed systematically and avoid making assumptions, remembering that initial impressions of the nature of the error are hypotheses to be tested to identify the faulty cognitive steps at play. Only then can one construct an appropriate plan for instruction and, if deemed necessary, remediation for those who need more intensive coaching. Please note that Chapter 6 provides a detailed approach for assessment for each component of the diagnostic process. For those who desire more intensive techniques for the learner who may be in need of remediation, see Chapter 9. As this chapter concludes we offer several possible techniques for mitigating the effects of cognitive biases that may affect all steps of the diagnostic process.

Issues That May Be Specific to Learner Level

Preclinical Medical Education

Diagnostic reasoning in medical students is often limited by gaps in basic medical knowledge, history and physical examination skills, and/or data organization. Medical students, especially early in their careers, also have a limited number of illness scripts, and these illness scripts may be incomplete or inaccurate. Students are accustomed to generating prototypes using the most common presentations of the most common diagnoses, but many patient presentations reflect less common features of a common diagnosis or an uncommon diagnosis. As such, much of the time medical students may not be able to "match" the patient's presentation to a pre-formed illness script, forcing them to perform analytic reasoning (system 2 reasoning) to identify the diagnosis. Because of the highly energy-intensive nature of the process, spending too much time using analytic reasoning can easily lead to cognitive overload, hindering the student's ability to proceed with forming a diagnostic impression. This, over time, can also lead to frustration for early learners, who may feel behind the rest of the team. The team is generally composed of more advanced learners, who, because they might be using nonanalytic reasoning, appear to be expending much less effort. Anticipating that medical students may aspire to "efficiency"—as for them speed in diagnosis is often viewed as the primary manifestation of expertise—will aid in properly diagnosing and advising them. It is important to point out that with greater experience, the repository of illness scripts will naturally grow. Challenging the student to generate a "gut" impression is very helpful for development of reasoning and is especially helpful in assessing the learner (35). However, in instructing students one can also promote the use of the analytic "double-check" (21, 36). This process can help ensure that corners are not cut and that proper reflection on the diagnosis is performed (while being sure not to create the impression that using nonanalytic reasoning is "bad"). This should ensure that the illness script formed from the encounter is accurate and adaptable. Indeed, the carefully applied double-check" has been proposed as the marker of true clinical expertise (37).

However, while undergraduate medical learners certainly should continue to expand their medical knowledge and their repository of illness scripts, today's medical students (and, at this point, most residents as well), are accustomed to being awash in data as a result of having grown up in the digital age. Most medical students will not be able to recall a time when the Internet (and search engines such as Google) did not exist. However, despite facility in accessing data, today's learners may still struggle prioritizing and synthesizing information into logical clinical impressions or questions. This is essential to keep in mind while instructing the medical student. These learners have grown up craving and expecting immediate feedback and are likely to be frustrated with advice to "read more" and "see more patients" without a suggested framework or approach. They may need to hear not just what their teachers know but, more important, how they think (38). Demonstrating one's thinking within the framework of a team environment can thus be an effective means of instruction. For example, as an instructors walk novices through their immediate impressions from key data, as well as their analytic thought process on rounds, this process can easily serve as the valuable analytic double-check" for the team, who may have made the diagnosis using largely intuitive processes. Encouraging the development of a gut impression but actually assigning the double-check as the student's "job" for team-based rounds can be very effective in ensuring the student's autonomy and contribution to the team while still working on development of their foundational skills.

Clinical Medical Education
Advanced medical students and residents have usually formulated a larger repertoire of illness scripts, especially by the end of the intern year, and during the later years of training these learners are flexing their intuitive muscles while developing their decision-making skills. Advanced learners have developed clinical skills of history-taking and physical examination and should be well versed in the routines of patient care. With each day, advanced learners spend more of their clinical lives using nonanalytic reasoning, gaining efficiency and confidence. However, while these learners may hold a robust formulary of illness scripts, they probably have not yet seen many atypical presentations of common diseases. As a result the illness scripts they have may be relatively underdeveloped, a realization that the learner may not make because of a high level of confidence. Because "common things are common," learners may still be right quite often

when using their relatively unrefined nonanalytic processes, further reinforcing a confidence that may be inappropriately high.

In clinical medical education, instructors can capitalize on the fact that learners take a great deal of responsibility for the outcomes of their patients and for their own learning. Especially when an error has clear adverse effects for patients, residents have the opportunity to demonstrate the ability and the willingness to reflect on their own thinking, recognize flawed cognitive patterns in both themselves and others, and devise strategies to avoid similar mistakes moving forward (13). The instructor can facilitate this reflection by supporting the learner, destigmatizing the error in the context of known fields (such as cognitive psychology), highlighting the contextual contributions to the error, and providing other learning materials (such as simulation) or other case-based modules where learners can identify and discuss flawed thinking patterns in other clinicians. This may be much easier to do within the context of training than with practicing physicians, where both formative and summative feedback is expected as part of training. In addition to looking retrospectively, trainees can be encouraged to artificially gain additional clinical "experience" in other ways; these approaches include adding hypothetical complexity to relatively straightforward cases, a technique called *progressive problem solving*, and simulation. These approaches are discussed in detail in Chapter 8. Forcing the learner in clinical education to make a commitment, tying an emotional valence to an outcome of a given case or teaching exercise, can increase the proportion of learning that is experiential. Doing this may therefore decrease the amount of exposure that may be necessary to form proper diagnostic habits.

Continuing Medical Education
Continuing medical education is probably the most difficult realm in which to improve performance in diagnostic reasoning. Practicing physicians have the most illness scripts of all levels of learners and also have more incentives to perform efficiently than do others. These gains in efficiency could come at the expense of accuracy. Furthermore, specialization or focused clinical experience will galvanize commonly encountered illness scripts, while others outside of one's specialty are likely to atrophy without the clinician's knowledge. For these reasons, physicians who have completed training may be just as prone to cognitive bias and overconfidence as anyone. Experienced clinicians, working independently in busy clinical environments, may also be in a system that "sanctions" them from receiving feedback on patient outcomes (39). This makes them less able to recalibrate and maintain their thinking processes than trainees, who are always performing their work under close supervision.

However, getting feedback may be the most effective way that an active practitioner can learn. Continuing to grow as an experienced clinician is about continuing to develop better habits, which may be very hard to do without great effort and constant feedback. Working with a clinical mentor or "coach" who can help identify specific areas of weakness while also suggesting means of improvement also has terrific, if unproven, potential, although the logistics of such an approach can be daunting. For the individual looking to improve one's own clinical habits, Chapter 8 provides a practical framework with which clinicians can continue their own education in this area.

❖ Specific Techniques to Remedy Cognitive Errors

Building and Strengthening Illness Scripts
Given the amount of time we spend using nonanalytic reasoning (system 1), and the power that it has, building a comprehensive repository of illness scripts will definitely reduce the opportunities for cognitive diagnostic errors. As stated before, nonanalytic, intuitive thinking enables clinicians to deal with the complexities and uncertainties of medical diagnosis in a way that maintains a high degree of accuracy and efficiency. This great benefit is worthy of considerable effort from both the learner and the teacher when teaching clinical reasoning. A robust foundation of illness scripts, formed through expansive medical knowledge, combined with practical clinical experience, is a true path to gaining expertise, maximizing the impact of the nonanalytic approach to clinical decision-making.

Are Cognitive Forcing Strategies Necessary?
Despite the power of nonanalytic reasoning, its limitations have also been described. It is our opinion, supported by some evidence, that analytic cognitive strategies have the potential to complement nonanalytic thinking (11). The subconscious nature of most nonanalytic thinking, and the combination of learners' incompletely formed intuition with their tendency towards overconfidence, makes them generally poor at recognizing these crucial moments and responding to them in real time. Therefore, we feel that other habits and cognitive aids are likely necessary to provide additional support in helping the busy clinician focus on the appropriate "slow down" times and spend the remainder of the time trusting intuition. These strategies may be considered time-consuming and require effort because they are usually pushing intuitive clinicians and learners from nonanalytic reasoning to a combination of nonanalytic and analytic means of thinking. This may not always be advantageous for any busy practitioner who

---

Box 4-2. Four Basic Questions to Screen for Risk of Cognitive Bias

▶ What else could this be?
▶ What finding doesn't fit with my diagnosis?
▶ Could there be multiple processes going on at once?
▶ Is there any other reason I need to slow down?

---

may be living in the nonanalytic mode up to 95% of the time (26); moreover, forcing one to perpetually slow down may also cause undue cognitive and emotional stress for minimal gains in diagnostic accuracy. It has been suggested that the trick to gaining diagnostic mastery, as written by many experts, is to figure out when it is most important to proceed cautiously; in other words, learning to slow down only when it's necessary (Box 4-2) (37). Sequentially combining nonanalytic with analytic reasoning improves diagnostic accuracy only in low-fidelity simulations (i.e., paper cases). However, we feel that using some or all of these habitual strategies can help clinicians double-check their intuition, increase accuracy without being overly time-consuming, and help clinicians expand and refine their illness scripts in the course of their regular work.

Raising Awareness of Cognitive Bias and Dual Processing
Given the profound influence that the dual process model and biases appear to have on clinical decision-making, especially in diagnosis, it follows that raising awareness of the model and educating clinician-learners on cognitive biases "primes the pump" for incorporation of other cognitive strategies to improve performance. Instruction from fields such as cognitive psychology can be of great interest to clinical learners, and clinical learners have been shown capable of understanding the dual process model and using its tenets in clinical problem-solving (40). While instruction on the dual process model alone has not been shown to decrease actual incidence of diagnostic errors, it has been effective in high-fidelity simulated clinical scenarios (41). Greater awareness of one's thinking probably has great potential to inform the development of better diagnostic habits, either alone or by establishing a foundation of thought that facilitates the adoption of any of the techniques discussed in the following sections. It is quite unlikely that education on the dual-process model alone will lead to fewer diagnostic errors, but the greatest value in stimulating learners to build this theoretical foundation is that it improves understanding of the rationale for some of the following strategies and facilitates their adoption.

Metacognition and Reflective Practice

Metacognition, or the act of "thinking about one's thinking and feelings," has potential to mitigate diagnostic errors, both by allowing the learner to develop insight and awareness of one's own thought patterns and by practically providing a double-check to catch potentially biased thinking. Further, habitual metacognition may also be useful as a reflective exercise for learning, both in successful and unsuccessful diagnoses.

Learners can also be trained to routinely support an initial "gut" impression with a more analytic second pass. In complex diagnostic tasks, such as reading an electrocardiogram, novice learners who are trained to double-check their initial intuitive impression with a structured, analytic approach are more accurate in studies (41–43). A 2-pass diagnostic approach in which a clinician specifically articulates data to support the initial impression may reduce biased decision-making.

Learners who wish to build diagnostic skills and mitigate bias this way might practice by performing a structured reflection. In this technique, when presented with a case, learners could list their suggestion for the most likely diagnosis, naming facets of the case that supported their working diagnosis, as well as those whose presence argues against that diagnosis. After repeating this process for several possibilities on the differential diagnosis, learners are prepared to proceed with a diagnostic plan, as well as a structured approach to respond to additional diagnostic information that may confirm the initial impression or lead them to choose a different diagnosis. In studies of clinical learners, using the structured reflection approach has actually improved diagnostic performance, even in cases that are encountered later (36). There is further evidence that this approach is especially useful when initial presentations are nonspecific or contain discordant information (44). Learners may find this double-check to be unnecessary while introducing inefficiency; this is a powerful deterrent for students who might wish to emulate more senior members of the team, who appear to be moving much faster (likely because of their expertise). Clinical teachers should be prepared for this eventuality and not shy away from slowing down learners who do not support their impression with clinical data. When it comes to choosing a diagnosis, especially in learners, pushing to explain why a diagnosis is likely—not just saying what the diagnosis is—might make it more likely that the diagnosis will turn out to be correct.

Metacognition and Affective De-biasing

Metacognition also has the potential to reduce errors through the acknowledgement of affective influences on one's thinking. Physicians are humans and as much as anyone are subject to good and bad moods, fatigue, sleep deprivation, ambient stress, and even emotions driven by interactions with patients and countertransference. How physicians feel while taking care of patients, either in general or specifically about their patients, may affect their diagnostic performance. Physicians might be trained to recognize when they are in a situation where the risks for affective bias and other cognitive errors are high. These situations, such as a fatigued state, periods of high workload intensity, periods of personal stress, or general low mood, can have real effects on one's thinking (15, 23). Although not shown to directly reduce errors, teaching learners to reflect and anticipate their own tendencies to respond to these different ambient stressors, individual mood cycles, and specific patient attributes may help them recognize when a stressful or emotional situation places learners at risk for faulty cognition during the diagnostic process. While Box 4-1 suggests several common scenarios in which affective biases may occur, the instructor can encourage learners to acknowledge that these responses are unique to the individual and the specific scenario and are not one-size-fits-all.

Teaching Better Thinking: How to Foster
Intuition/Nonanalytic Reasoning

With the development of expertise comes the increasing acquisition of experience and more robust, accurate diagnostic intuition (i.e., nonanalytic reasoning or system 1 reasoning). This nonanalytic reasoning remains the foundation for diagnostic prowess and clinical teachers are obligated to assist learners with the calibration of their intuitive compass. A few potential strategies described in the literature (45) can help learners gain expertise and accuracy with using nonanalytic clinical reasoning. One strategy is to train learners' minds to prepare for the unanticipated or the unexpected, by mapping out contingency scenarios or an algorithmic approach to adjusting the diagnostic and treatment plan based on the patient's initial response to a treatment. This technique, called *progressive problem solving,* has been well described in high-performing diagnosticians as a means of continually honing diagnostic intuition (46, 47).

Ensuring feedback on patient outcomes is another way for both beginning and advanced learners to continue to refine diagnostic thinking. Teachers should follow up on patient outcomes after a transfer of care or the end of a clinical rotation and continually empower learners to follow up on those patients themselves.

Finally, new developments in simulation offer many opportunities for learners to develop (and receive feedback on) their clinical reasoning. Simulated experience outside of patient care is a valuable way for learners to galvanize their nonanalytic reasoning with positive feedback, make appropriate adjustments in response to constructive feedback, and incorporate new approaches into their diagnostic style using a technique that is more experiential and therefore possibly more likely to be retained. These and other techniques to improve nonanalytic reasoning are covered in greater detail in Chapter 8.

Making Thinking Easier: Reducing Reliance on Memory

Reducing reliance on memory is also an important means of reducing cognitive errors. Systematic checklists, in the form of mnemonic devices (like MUDPILES for the elevated anion gap metabolic acidosis) and written checklists for differential diagnoses for common symptoms (48, 49) or even for skill-based clinical tasks (50, 51) have high degree of potential. In fact, use of checklists actually increases accuracy in reading electrocardiograms—both for experienced clinicians and even more so for learners (52). In addition, technology-based clinical decision support (such as computer-based differential diagnosis generators) may assisting experienced clinicians and learners alike as an analytic double-check for the initial, intuitive impression. Rational use of these resources, as well as improved design and increased use of electronic health records, can continue to enhance how both learners and experienced clinicians think (53).

Systems Awareness and Error Analysis

While systems-based errors are a focus in an earlier chapter of this book (Chapter 1), recognition of the complex interplay between individuals and the system during the entire diagnostic process should inform all performance and discussion of the diagnostic process. Perhaps an even more important reason for learners to become comfortable with a systems approach to error is that it fosters openness, and even desire, to discuss diagnostic errors openly (13) and the development of strong interventions to assist diagnostic thinking within a culture of continuous improvement. Treating diagnosis as a process similar to all other processes, comprising both individual and system-based components, facilitates this approach by reducing, and ideally removing, the individual stigma often associated with these errors. This can create a psychologically safe environment to discuss all errors, including cognitive errors that may previously have been unrecognized.

There are several potential approaches to analyzing cognitive errors. As outlined earlier, the cognitive autopsy as described by Croskerry is a great framework on which to reconstruct a diagnostic error in order to identify flawed thinking. While this exercise could be as simple as a relaxed discussion between the learner and a single teacher, reviewing the case as a chart-stimulated recall, or even as a narrative writing exercise (13) shows promise as well. This can be an individual assignment or an entrée to a small peer group discussion, depending on the situation. At the conclusion of the discussion, construction of a diagram to organize the contributions of both cognitive, systems, and contextual components, once they are identified, can demonstrate the complexity of these errors for learners and facilitate the incorporation of teaching points.

The fishbone diagram, traditionally a tool used in industry to analyze systems-based errors (54), serves as a framework to organize a review of these complex events, It has been used both for education and root cause analysis of diagnostic errors (14, 55). Teaching learners to construct a fishbone diagram, using a systematic approach, that includes both systems-related and cognition-related causes, will illustrate specific opportunities for improvement while demonstrating just how complex these errors frequently are (see Figure 4-1 and online content for examples of completed fishbones). As part of a systematic approach to diagnostic error, these analyses might also be presented and discussed in program-wide, departmental, or broader institutional venues, such as morbidity and mortality conference, to demonstrate not only the faulty cognitive processes but also how systems imperfections may have exerted a negative influence on individual or team cognition, and can offer myriad opportunities to identify potential improvements and further develop a culture of good diagnostic habits.

Admitting Mistakes

Acknowledging one's faults as an attending and modeling a robust approach to one's own cognitive errors could be a potentially powerful tool for those with and without learners. Thinking through a shared diagnostic error with the team, or recounting a past personal error with learners, has great potential for learning and can also go a long way to establish trust. Acknowledging uncertainty and the imperfect science of diagnosis will do much to allow learners to explore their own thought processes in a psychologically safe environment and will maximize the learning value of any error analysis. Learners at both the undergraduate and graduate levels can reflect and learn from errors they were involved in and recognize flawed thought processes in themselves.

❖ Summary

Cognitive errors are believed to be prevalent, pervasive, and under-recognized but are at the core of the diagnostic process. Despite limited empirical evidence that teaching techniques translate into improved patient outcomes, these techniques are likely to help learners develop improved diagnostic habits, a benefit that is likely borne out over the longer term of one's career outside of the scope of any single study (Box 4-3). Most clinical

Box 4-3. Teaching Techniques to Avoid Cognitive Errors

▶ Improving data collection
▶ Building and strengthening repository of illness scripts
  • Promote knowledge of atypical presentations of disease
  • Symptom-based Reading
  • Case reports (e.g., *NEJM* series)
  • Flash cards
▶ Raising awareness of dual processing cognition
  • Reduce personal stigma of cognitive errors
  • Facilitate adoption of other techniques
▶ Metacognition: "thinking about your thinking"
  • Cognitive forcing strategies
    ○ Structured reflection
    ○ "Two-pass" diagnostic approach
  • Know one's favored biases
  • Acknowledge emotions
    ○ Due to external demands
    ○ Due to internal stresses
    ○ Stemming from patient interactions (counter-transference)
▶ Fostering better intuition
  • Bayesian reasoning
  • Progressive problem solving
  • Giving feedback
  • Simulation
▶ Reducing reliance on memory
  • Checklists
  • Mnemonics
  • Clinical references (e.g., ACP Smart Medicine modules)
  • Differential diagnosis tools
  • Clinical decision support (e.g., through EHR)
▶ Systems thinking
  • Understanding how systems affect thinking
  • Recognizing and compensating for system flaws
  • Openness to discussing error
  • Analysis of errors
    ○ Due to external demands
    ○ "Cognitive autopsy" (chart-stimulated recall and narrative writing)
    ○ Root cause analysis (e.g., fishbone diagram)
    ○ Morbidity and mortality conference

studies of these techniques were performed in controlled experiments on early medical learners and, rarely, more seasoned clinicians. These techniques harbor great potential for improving diagnostic habits, and more study is required in real-life clinical settings.

REFERENCES

1. **Lee CS, Nagy PG, Weaver SJ, Newman-Toker DE.** Cognitive and system factors contributing to diagnostic errors in radiology. AJR Am J Roentgenol. 2013;201:611-7.
2. **Graber ML, Wachter RM, Cassel CK.** Bringing diagnosis into the quality and safety equations. JAMA. 2012;308:1211-2.
3. **Raab SS, Grzybicki DM, Janosky JE, Zarbo RJ, Meier FA, Jensen C, et al.** Clinical impact and frequency of anatomic pathology errors in cancer diagnoses. Cancer. 2005;104:2205-13.
4. **Saber Tehrani AS, Lee H, Mathews SC, Shore A, Makary MA, Pronovost PJ, et al.** 25-Year summary of US malpractice claims for diagnostic errors 1986-2010: an analysis from the National Practitioner Data Bank. BMJ Qual Saf. 2013;22:672-80.
5. **James JT.** A new, evidence-based estimate of patient harms associated with hospital care. J Patient Saf. 2013;9:122-8.
6. **Kohn LT, Corrigan J, Donaldson MS.** To Err Is Human: Building a Safer Health System. Washington, DC: National Academy Press; 2000.
7. **Wachter RM.** Why diagnostic errors don't get any respect—and what can be done about them. Health Aff (Millwood). 2010;29:1605-10.
8. **Myers JS, VonFeldt JM.** Diagnostic errors and patient safety. JAMA. 2009;302:258-9; author reply 9-60.
9. **Newman-Toker DE, Pronovost PJ.** Diagnostic errors—the next frontier for patient safety. JAMA. 2009;301:1060-2.
10. **Graber ML, Franklin N, Gordon R.** Diagnostic error in internal medicine. Arch Intern Med. 2005;165:1493-9.
11. **Graber ML, Kissam S, Payne VL, Meyer AN, Sorensen A, Lenfestey N, et al.** Cognitive interventions to reduce diagnostic error: a narrative review. BMJ Qual Saf. 2012;21:535-57.
12. **Croskerry P.** The importance of cognitive errors in diagnosis and strategies to minimize them. Acad Med. 2003;78:775-80.
13. **Ogdie AR, Reilly JB, Pang WG, Keddem S, Barg FK, Von Feldt JM, et al.** Seen through their eyes: residents' reflections on the cognitive and contextual components of diagnostic errors in medicine. Acad Med. 2012;87(10):1361-7.
14. **Reilly JB, Myers JS, Salvador D, Trowbridge RL.** Use of a novel, modified fishbone diagram to analyze diagnostic errors. Diagnosis. 2014;1:167-71.
15. **Croskerry P.** Diagnostic failure: a cognitive and affective approach and methodology. In: Henriksen K, Battles JB, Marks ES, Lewin DI, eds. Advances in Patient Safety: From Research to Implementation (Volume 2: Concepts and Methodology). Rockville, MD: Agency for Healthcare Research and Quality; 2005.
16. **Croskerry P.** Clinical cognition and diagnostic error: applications of a dual process model of reasoning. Adv Health Sci Educ Theory Pract. 2009;14 Suppl 1:27-35.
17. **Norman G.** Dual processing and diagnostic errors. Adv Health Sci Educ Theory Pract. 2009;14 Suppl 1:37-49.

18. **Croskerry P.** Bias: a normal operating characteristic of the diagnosing brain. Diagnosis. 2014;1:23-7.

19. **Jenicek M.** Medical Error and Harm: Understanding, Prevention, and Control. New York: Productivity Press/CRC Press; 2010.

20. **Berner ES, Graber ML.** Overconfidence as a cause of diagnostic error in medicine. Am J Med. 2008;121(5 Suppl):S2-23.

21. **Mamede S, van Gog T, van den Berge K, Rikers RM, van Saase JL, van Guldener C, et al.** Effect of availability bias and reflective reasoning on diagnostic accuracy among internal medicine residents. JAMA. 2010;304:1198-203.

22. **Kostopoulou O, Russo JE, Keenan G, Delaney BC, Douiri A.** Information distortion in physicians' diagnostic judgments. Med Decis Making. 2012;32:831-9.

23. **Croskerry P, Abbass AA, Wu AW.** How doctors feel: affective issues in patients' safety. Lancet. 2008;372:1205-6.

24. **Croskerry P, Singhal G, Mamede S.** Cognitive debiasing 2: impediments to and strategies for change. BMJ Qual Saf. 2013;22 Suppl 2:ii65-ii72.

25. **Ofri D.** What Doctors Feel: How Emotions Affect the Practice of Medicine. Boston: Beacon Press; 2014.

26. **Croskerry P, Singhal G, Mamede S.** Cognitive debiasing 1: origins of bias and theory of debiasing. BMJ Qual Saf. 2013;22 Suppl 2:ii58-ii64.

27. **Croskerry P, Abbass A, Wu AW.** Emotional influences in patient safety. J Patient Saf. 2010;6:199-205.

28. **Hertwig R, Meier N, Nickel C, Zimmermann PC, Ackermann S, Woike JK, et al.** Correlates of diagnostic accuracy in patients with nonspecific complaints. Med Decis Making. 2013;33:533-43.

29. **Meyer AN, Payne VL, Meeks DW, Rao R, Singh H.** Physicians' diagnostic accuracy, confidence, and resource requests: a vignette study. JAMA Intern Med. 2013;173:1952-8.

30. **Cavalcanti RB, Sibbald M.** Am I right when I am sure? Data consistency influences the relationship between diagnostic accuracy and certainty. Acad Med. 2014;89:107-13.

31. **Zwaan L, Thijs A, Wagner C, van der Wal G, Timmermans DR.** Relating faults in diagnostic reasoning with diagnostic errors and patient harm. Acad Med. 2012;87:149-56.

32. **Hartzband P, Groopman J.** Off the record—avoiding the pitfalls of going electronic. N Engl J Med. 2008;358:1656-8.

33. **Singh H, Giardina TD, Meyer AN, Forjuoh SN, Reis MD, Thomas EJ.** Types and origins of diagnostic errors in primary care settings. JAMA Intern Med. 2013;173:418-25.

34. **Schipper S, Ross S.** Structured teaching and assessment: a new chart-stimulated recall worksheet for family medicine residents. Can Fam Physician. 2010;56:958-9, e352-4.

35. **Ilgen JS, Bowen JL, McIntyre LA, Banh KV, Barnes D, Coates WC, et al.** Comparing diagnostic performance and the utility of clinical vignette-based assessment under testing conditions designed to encourage either automatic or analytic thought. Acad Med. 2013;88:1545-51.

36. **Mamede S, van Gog T, Sampaio AM, de Faria RM, Maria JP, Schmidt HG.** How can students' diagnostic competence benefit most from practice with clinical cases? The effects of structured reflection on future diagnosis of the same and novel diseases. Acad Med. 2014;89:121-7.

37. **Moulton CA, Regehr G, Mylopoulos M, MacRae HM.** Slowing down when you should: a new model of expert judgment. Acad Med. 2007;82(10 Suppl):S109-16.

38. **Roberts DH, Newman LR, Schwartzstein RM.** Twelve tips for facilitating Millennials' learning. Med Teach. 2012;34:274-8.

39. **Croskerry P.** The feedback sanction. Acad Emerg Med. 2000;7:1232-8.

40. **Reilly JB, Ogdie AR, Von Feldt JM, Myers JS.** Teaching about how doctors think: a longitudinal curriculum in cognitive bias and diagnostic error for residents. BMJ Qual Saf. 2013;22:1044-50.

41. **Sibbald M, McKinney J, Cavalcanti RB, Yu E, Wood DA, Nair P, et al.** Cardiac examination and the effect of dual-processing instruction in a cardiopulmonary simulator. Adv Health Sci Educ Theory Pract. 2013;18:497-508.

42. **Eva KW, Hatala RM, Leblanc VR, Brooks LR.** Teaching from the clinical reasoning literature: combined reasoning strategies help novice diagnosticians overcome misleading information. Med Educ. 2007;41:1152-8.

43. **Ark TK, Brooks LR, Eva KW.** The benefits of flexibility: the pedagogical value of instructions to adopt multifaceted diagnostic reasoning strategies. Med Educ. 2007;41:281-7.

44. **Coderre S, Wright B, McLaughlin K.** To think is good: querying an initial hypothesis reduces diagnostic error in medical students. Acad Med. 2010;85:1125-9.

45. **Trowbridge RL, Dhaliwal G, Cosby KS.** Educational agenda for diagnostic error reduction. BMJ Qual Saf. 2013;22 Suppl 2:ii28-ii32.

46. **Mylopoulos M, Lohfeld L, Norman GR, Dhaliwal G, Eva KW.** Renowned physicians' perceptions of expert diagnostic practice. Acad Med. 2012;87:1413-7.

47. **Sargeant J, Mann K, Sinclair D, Ferrier S, Muirhead P, van der Vleuten C, et al.** Learning in practice: experiences and perceptions of high-scoring physicians. Acad Med. 2006;81:655-60.

48. **Ely JW, Graber ML, Croskerry P.** Checklists to reduce diagnostic errors. Acad Med. 2011;86:307-13.

49. **Gawande A.** The Checklist Manifesto: How to Get Things Right. New York: Metropolitan Books; 2011.

50. **Sibbald M, de Bruin AB, van Merrienboer JJ.** Checklists improve experts' diagnostic decisions. Med Educ. 2013;47:301-8.

51. **Sibbald M, de Bruin AB, Cavalcanti RB, van Merrienboer JJ.** Do you have to re-examine to reconsider your diagnosis? Checklists and cardiac exam. BMJ Qual Saf. 2013;22:333-8.

52. **Sibbald M, De Bruin AB, van Merrienboer JJ.** Finding and fixing mistakes: do checklists work for clinicians with different levels of experience? Adv Health Sci Educ Theory Pract. 2014;19:43-51.

53. **Henriksen K, Brady J.** The pursuit of better diagnostic performance: a human factors perspective. BMJ Qual Saf. 2013;22 Suppl 2:ii1-ii5.

54. **Gupta P, Varkey P.** Developing a tool for assessing competency in root cause analysis. Jt Comm J Qual Patient Saf. 2009;35:36-42.

55. **Giardina TD, King BJ, Ignaczak AP, Paull DE, Hoeksema L, Mills PD, et al.** Root cause analysis reports help identify common factors in delayed diagnosis and treatment of outpatients. Health Aff (Millwood). 2013;32:1368-75.

5

General Teaching Techniques

Cynthia H. Ledford, MD, FACP

L. James Nixon, MD, MHPE

❖ Overview

Physicians are assumed to be experts in clinical reasoning. Unfortunately, there is no clear best practice to guide the teaching of this complex cognitive process. The lack of a "gold standard" for teaching clinical reasoning likely relates to our limited ability to assess clinical reasoning expertise (see Chapter 6). Without a clear best practice, conceptual frameworks of clinical reasoning and practical wisdom provide the best guidance for one's teaching.

Before talking about how to teach clinical reasoning, however, one should consider the challenges one might face.

❖ Challenges to Teaching Clinical Reasoning

We have categorized challenges in teaching clinical reasoning into 3 broad areas: the content itself, the learning environment, and the teacher.

The content itself presents a challenge because diagnostic reasoning is a complex ability with multiple components that a clinician must adapt to a large variety of different patients, clinical settings, and problem types. Whether clinical reasoning is modeled by the teacher or observed in the learner, it is often subconscious. Those doing the reasoning may not truly know why they make a specific decision,

KEY POINTS

- Explicitly discuss the clinical reasoning process with learners.
- Assess and adapt to the reasoning level of a learner:
  - Start with simple, typical presentations of common problems, progressively increasing case complexity
  - Over time, provide less structure and more independence
  - Recognize that teaching clinical reasoning is not amenable to a one-size-fits-all approach
- Role model and foster self-regulation.

although typically one can rationalize it after the fact. Thus, teachers of clinical reasoning face a difficult task: comparing and contrasting learners' words with their decisions and actions to obtain a full picture of their clinical reasoning ability.

The learning environment presents many challenges. For example, the traditional 2+2 structure (i.e., 2 preclinical years followed by 2 clinical years) used by many medical schools often separates knowledge acquisition from knowledge application. This separation may hinder application of what is learned from the preclinical to the clinical setting. Students may need to "relearn" or re-organize their preclinical knowledge to enable them to use it effectively in clinical environments. In addition, the types of patient symptoms and diseases that learners will see in the clinical setting are random and often unpredictable. The opportunity to "practice" clinical reasoning deliberately (e.g., work-up several patients with vasculitis to strengthen practical knowledge about these conditions) may not therefore arise because of this randomness unless explicitly planned. Further, even when a diverse patient mix is present, practice of diagnostic reasoning may be limited because patients have already been worked-up (1). Another environmental barrier is the lack of longitudinal follow-up with patients, which limits the opportunity for learners to get feedback regarding the diagnostic accuracy and effectiveness of their clinical reasoning. Finally, with physicians-in-training, the fast pace of clinical workflow and frequent handoffs further compound these challenges (2).

The teacher, and his or her expertise, can create barriers. The ability to teach clinical reasoning is related and, yet, somewhat independent of expertise as a diagnostician (3). An expert diagnostician may use nonanalytic reasoning (pattern recognition) when making a diagnosis, a reasoning process that is often not readily available to introspection. Some attending physicians may have difficulty explaining the rationale for their decisions

Table 5-1. Challenges and Barriers to Teaching Clinical Reasoning

Content factors	• Diagnostic reasoning is a complex ability with multiple components • Clinical reasoning is often tacit, inferred from decisions or actions
Environmental factors	• The 2 + 2 student curriculum may hinder knowledge transfer to the clinical context • Opportunities for clinical reasoning practice are limited by the randomness of exposures to different disease types • Practice of diagnostic reasoning is difficult when patients are already "worked-up" • A lack of longitudinal follow-up with patients limits natural feedback about reasoning success • Clinical care can be fast paced and associated with frequent transitions of care (handoffs)
Teacher or expert physician factors	• Lack of awareness of one's own reasoning processes • Limited knowledge of general clinical reasoning principles • Limited time to directly observe and assess learners' clinical skills • Difficulty providing specific, meaningful feedback on clinical reasonings

to learners who have less knowledge and experience with which to apply nonanalytic reasoning (4). Additionally, an expert clinician may have limited knowledge of general clinical reasoning principles, limiting one's ability to provide specific or meaningful feedback (Table 5-1).

This chapter briefly summarizes the conceptual frameworks that the authors have found to be most useful in guiding teaching, followed by a discussion of teaching methods and a guide on how to adapt teaching.

❖ Conceptual Frameworks

Several conceptual frameworks are useful in guiding different approaches to teaching clinical reasoning (see Chapter 2 for details). These include:
- Information processing theory
  - ▫ Dual process theory
  - ▫ Cognitive load theory
- Deliberate practice theory
- Self-regulated learning theory

Here we describe the relevance of each of these briefly.

Information Processing Theory

Much of our understanding about the way clinicians make diagnoses falls within the broad category of information processing theory. This overarching theory (or family of theories) is based on the principle that humans process information from the environment in a manner similar to that of a computer analyzing information (5). The theory emphasizes 1) attention needed to bring in new information, 2) the use of working memory (short-term memory) to manipulate and analyze information, and 3) storage of information in long-term memory for later use. Dual process theory and cognitive load theory are two examples of information processing theories and are ways of understanding clinical reasoning.

Dual process theory describes 2 main ways in which humans are believed to process information (Table 5-2). Nonanalytic reasoning is subconscious, largely automatic, and fast. One nonanalytic problem-solving strategy is pattern recognition, the method by which one rapidly compares incoming information with prototypes that are stored in long-term memory. In medicine, these prototypes and exemplars are often called *illness scripts*, or mental constructs of disease manifestations (6). Nonanalytic reasoning tends to be used more by clinicians who have acquired greater experience with a specific problem, when knowledge is organized into illness scripts, which can be used for pattern recognition (7). Heuristics, or mental shortcuts, also often fall within the realm of nonanalytic reasoning. These mental shortcuts can be seen as an adaptive process that helps one overcome the limited processing capacity of the human brain (7).

Analytic reasoning, in contrast, is typically conscious, purposeful, effortful, and slow. Various analytic problem-solving strategies have been described, including hypothetico-deductive and scheme-inductive reasoning. Diagnostic decision-making can also be approached analytically using a probabilistic approach termed *Bayesian reasoning*. Many teaching methods target different aspects of the slow and analytical clinical problem-solving, described in more detail in the next section. Both nonanalytical

Table 5-2. Dual Process Theory

Nonanalytic Reasoning	Analytic Reasoning
Automatic	Effortful
Involuntary	Deliberative
Emotional	Logical
Executes skilled responses and generates "intuition" with minimal effort	Requires attention, self- control and time

and analytical reasoning processes are believed to depend heavily on knowledge and its organization, including connections between clinical observations and foundational science concepts.

Cognitive load theory helps to understand how many discrete units of information we can handle in short-term (working) memory when trying to solve a problem. The average person can retain 7±2 units of information in this short-term memory (5). Thus, when solving a clinical problem, the number of clinical features that one can consider simultaneously is limited. An important aspect of acquiring expertise in clinical problem-solving involves the ability to take many different features (fever or hypothermia, hypotension, tachycardia, hyperventilation, altered mental status, warm or cool extremities) and group, or "chunk," them into a single unit (septic shock) and thus free up working memory to consider other bits of information. Chunking, as described above, is also sometimes termed *processing* of clinical information and results in encapsulation of facts. The expert clinician is more able to chunk data, allowing him or her to simultaneously consider more clinical features in order to arrive at a solution; while the cognitive load limitations remain the same as in the nonexpert, expert clinicians can often process information with less working memory effort because of this chunking or bundling of information.

Deliberate Practice Theory
Ericsson's theory of deliberate practice highlights the contributions of experience, coaching, and effortful practice (see Chapter 2 and Chapter 8 for more details). This theory states that one develops expertise through engagement in intense practice of specific aspects of an activity with full concentration. Studies have shown that motivation, timely feedback, and coaching are all important for effective deliberate practice. Deliberate practice provides a rationale for the use of virtual patients, computer case simulations, and other opportunities to practice solving problems, as a way to develop expert performance in diagnostic reasoning.

Self-regulated Learning Theory
Self-regulated learning is a social cognitive theory that highlights the importance of goal setting, motivation, and reflection (Box 5-1). A key aspect of self-regulated learning describes a three-phase feedback cycle of learning: In the forethought (preparation) phase, the learner analyzes the intended task, sets goals, anticipates the outcome, and assigns value of the task. During the performance phase, the learner is occupied by self-monitoring and focus on the task. In the final phase of self-reflection, one engages in self-evaluation and causal attribution of success or failure.

Box 5-1. Self-Regulated Learning Theory

- Forethought
  - Analyze and value task
  - Set goal
  - Anticipate outcome
- Performance
  - Monitor self
  - Focus on task
- Reflection
  - Evaluate performance
  - Attribute cause for success or failure

From these diverse conceptual theories, different approaches to teaching clinical reasoning have arisen. Several general tactics and specific teaching methods and tools are discussed in detail, followed by a guide on how to adapt or select from these methods.

❖ General Teaching Tactics

Before detailing specific teaching methods or tools, it is worth highlighting some general recommendations in teaching clinical reasoning. Most of these recommendations derive directly from the conceptual frameworks described previously. Some evidence supports them, although some recommendations draw primarily on the experience and observations of expert teachers. We describe them by theory, citing evidence where available.

Information Processing

Knowledge Organization
The clinical reasoning literature suggests that knowledge and knowledge organization are critical to expert performance in clinical reasoning. Knowledge organization refers to how information is arranged and integrated in the memory. Advanced modes of knowledge organization help the clinician to efficiently and effectively access the stored information. One recommendation based on this premise, albeit a daunting one, is "Know as much medicine as possible." Students should appreciate that vast knowledge and strong knowledge organization are the foundation for expertise in clinical reasoning. Beyond knowledge, students need to become facile with both nonanalytic and analytic reasoning so that they can be as flexible as needed for a given diagnostic problem (8, 9).

Tactics to Build Nonanalytical Skills

The most common form of nonanalytic reasoning is pattern recognition. To support development of pattern recognition, information processing theory suggests that students should store knowledge as disease prototypes that are organized as **illness scripts** (Box 5-2) (6). The concept of scripts was initially derived from psychology literature on schema- cognitive frameworks that provide a "script" for how to act or behave in a specific environment. In medicine, the concept was appropriated to describe the way diseases are expected to behave (i.e., the story of a disease). At its core, an illness script consists of epidemiology/risk factors, pathophysiology, and clinical manifestations (e.g., time course, symptoms, signs, and findings). Teachers can encourage students to use the structure of an illness script to organize newly acquired knowledge of diseases. Early in development of knowledge structures, we recommend a focus on typical presentations of common diseases in courses in such areas as pathophysiology. Exposure to these typical disease exemplars allows students to begin developing their "library" of illness scripts. Learners can use a compare-and-contrast approach to further organize and connect knowledge of related diseases (10). With increasing experience, clinicians further elaborate illness scripts, including alternative presentations and atypical features (Table 5-3).

Tactics That Build Analytical Skills

Analytical reasoning involves a systematic and deliberate approach to collecting and interpreting information and often involves applying knowledge based on learned rules; the analytical approach tends to be used by clinicians when time permits, stakes are high, or situations are complex or when faced by ambiguity or uncertainty (11). Two approaches to analytical thinking are hypothetico-deduction and scheme induction. **Hypothetico-deduction** involves generating a list of possible diagnoses and testing each against the clinical presentation of a patient, in a manner sometimes termed *backward reasoning*. **Scheme induction** describes a systematic

---

Box 5-2. Organize Knowledge About Diseases Into Illness Scripts

- Who gets it: epidemiology and risk factors
- How it presents with respect to time: temporal pattern (i.e., onset, duration, constant/intermittent, and pattern of progression)
- How it presents with respect to key features: symptoms and physical examination findings

Table 5-3. Example of Compare-and-Contrast Grid for Diseases Causing Polyarthritis

Disease	Who Gets It (Epidemiology and Risk Factors)	How It Presents With Respect to Time	Clinical Manifestations on Presentation
Rheumatoid arthritis	Women (younger or older ages); men (older) Ratio of women to men, 2–3:1 Most present between ages 40 and 75 y	Typically gradual onset, insidious and chronic (years, at least >6 weeks)	Inflammation of joints (red, warm, swollen, painful) Involvement of small joints of hands and feet; sometimes involves larger joints (wrists, knees, shoulders, cervical spine), but *not* lumbar or thoracic spine Morning stiffness (>30–60 min to resume full activity after prolonged rest) Extra-articular manifestations uncommon at presentation Exam with synovitis, later joint deformation with subluxations
Systemic lupus erythematosus	Typically women, ages 20–45 y Risk factors include African American ethnicity and countries with indigenous African population, family history,	Can present acutely or more insidiously; can be persistent and progressive or intermittent with flares	Migratory, symmetric joint pain and swelling with mild inflammatory changes (tender, swollen PIP) Extra-articular manifestations common (malar rash, mucocutaneous ulcers, alopecia, fatigue, fever, cardiopulmonary or renal involvement) Exam without joint deformity
Osteoarthritis	Common, especially if age >60 y; affects most people to some extent by age 70 y Risk factors are obesity, trauma, and overuse (sports or work-related) Ratio men: women, 1:1, equally; men may develop earlier	Chronic, progressive; can have acute flares	Typically not inflammatory Pain worse with movement or activity, improved by rest and simple analgesics "Gel effect": short-term stiffness after short periods of inactivity Reduced range of movement on examination Joint deformation with bony changes

PIP = proximal interphalangeal joint.

application of rules to narrow the differential diagnosis of a symptom, sign, or laboratory finding that is observed.

The provision of schema for common symptoms can provide learners with a guide to limit the differential diagnoses to be considered, mirroring the mental shortcuts used by more experienced clinicians. In addition, this use of reasoning rules can reduce a student's cognitive load, guiding students in how to purposefully chunk or process clinical information in useful ways. Diagnostic schemas are described further in the scaffolding section of this chapter.

> **Example:** *To diagnose the cause of anemia, first identify whether the anemia is microcytic, normocytic, or macrocytic.*

Causal reasoning is another potentially valuable form of analytical reasoning. Students likely learn by connecting science knowledge (e.g., pathophysiology) to their clinical observations and diagnostic reasoning processes in order to further enrich their knowledge organization (12). Teachers can encourage these connections by use of this causal reasoning, an approach that involves making inferences between clinical variables and underlying associated pathophysiology of the disease state (13, 14).

> **Example:** *Nephrotic syndrome: Kidney "leaks" protein into the urine → low serum protein → fluid flow into the tissues → low plasma volume → sodium retention by the kidneys → water retention (isotonic) by the kidney → edema*

The basis for using causal reasoning in education is strong. Experts often make accurate clinical decisions without obvious use of biomedical knowledge, at least as demonstrated by the think-aloud method (15, 16). However, there is reason to believe that as clinicians work through cases, particularly complex cases, they are activating biomedical knowledge, even if it is not readily apparent to the clinician (17, 18). Additionally, students who are taught to integrate science with what they are learning clinically have greater diagnostic accuracy after a 1-week delay (12). From a knowledge organization perspective, students can use the pathophysiologic basis of a disease to provide structure to learning clinical features, beyond rote memorization of a random assortment of signs and symptoms.

The more connected knowledge becomes, the more coherent with clinical features, the longer it is retained (12).

Problem Lists

Clinical reasoning involves multiple components; one component, perhaps the simplest and earliest described, is the identification and labeling

> ### Box 5-3. Features of Effective Problem Lists
> 1. Use precise language
> 2. Update and modify over time
> 3. Prioritize
> 4. Make associations between problems

of a patient's medical problems. The problem list, described by Lawrence Weed, was proposed as a framework for summarizing the state of a patient's health in written documentation (19, 20). He elaborated on the importance of accurately labeling problems, as precisely and specifically as possible, without prematurely closing on a single diagnosis, until the diagnosis was assured. Problem lists evolve as the clinical course and new information dictates. The problem list was proposed as a central framework for articulating a dynamic assessment. Problem lists may be helpful in identifying and tracking the pieces of the diagnostic puzzle to be solved. They can promote prioritization of the key issues to be addressed, and they may reinforce the importance of analysis to learners who rely primarily on pattern recognition. They also ensure that problems are tracked and not lost in the chaos of clinical care. The use of problem lists may be disadvantageous if they fragment the patient's overall presentation to such an extent that the "big picture" is lost (Box 5-3).

The following vignette displays how a problem list may evolve over time as clinical information accumulates, the patient is diagnosed and treated, and the clinical course emerges (21).

A patient presents to the emergency department after awakening with severe substernal chest pressure of 20 minutes' duration, associated with diaphoresis and shortness of breath.

Problems: *Chest pain, acute, anginal; suggestive of acute coronary syndrome*

Then, an electrocardiogram demonstrates ST-segment elevations in leads V1 to V4. Troponin I levels are elevated.

Problems: *Acute anterior ST-segment elevation myocardial infarction (MI)*

The patient undergoes cardiac catheterization and subsequent percutaneous coronary angioplasty of the left anterior descending artery. He experiences nonsustained ventricular tachycardia. An echocardiogram demonstrates an ejection fraction of 40%.

Problems: Anterior ST-segment elevation MI, ventricular tachycardia, likely due to MI, and ischemic cardiomyopathy, with mild systolic heart failure (new diagnosis).

Problem Representations and Summary Statements

Diagnostic reasoning is a matching exercise, where the clinician attempts to match the patient's presenting signs, symptoms, and other findings with a disease to allow for appropriate treatment. As discussed previously, this may occur via both nonanalytical reasoning (e.g., pattern recognition) and analytical reasoning (e.g., hypothetico-deductive reasoning). In the diagnostic literature, the description of the patient's presentation is called the **problem representation**. The summary statement (or problem representation) is related to problem lists in that they both capture key aspects of the clinical data (Box 5-4). Problem representations should include only aspects of a patient's presentation that are most germane to diagnosing and managing the acute concerns. For a patient presenting with headache and mental status changes, for example, a prior diagnosis of cholelithiasis would not be included on the problem representation but may belong on a problem list. Conversely, epidemiologic data are often included on a problem representation but not on a problem list; the epidemiologic data are included in a summary statement (problem representation) to capture attributes of the patient that make him uniquely at risk for potential diagnoses. That a patient is a 52-year-old man is not a "problem," for example, but is important in understanding the patient's risk for causes of chest pain.

To teach students problem representation, start by describing its 3 critical components: clinical context, temporal pattern, and the key clinical symptoms and examination findings that relate to the presenting symptoms. The clinician defines the clinical context (i.e., the patient's age or any sex, ethnic/racial, or geographic predispositions for diseases that might present with this problem) plus risk factors that may be discerned from a patient's past, social, family and/or medication history. In addition, the clinician clarifies the temporal pattern (i.e., the time course for development

---

Box 5-4. Use Summary Statements

Summary statements utilize:
- Illness script frameworks
- Epidemiology/risk factors
- Key features characterized by semantic qualifiers, especially their temporal pattern
- Medical terminology (instead of precise language)

of the patient's symptoms). This temporal pattern is often a key driver of the differential; patterns may involve suddenness of onset, duration, constancy versus intermittency, and stability versus progression. The final component of the problem representation is the identification of the key symptoms and examination findings, as well as laboratory and radiologic results. Some of these findings can be categorized as defining or discriminating. Defining features have high sensitivity (i.e., if absent, they significantly lower the likelihood of disease). For example, in a case where pneumonia is the leading diagnosis among a differential diagnosis of pulmonary embolism and heart failure, the presence of fever becomes a key feature that makes heart failure highly unlikely but has little impact on the probability of pulmonary embolism.

Problem representations come to life in **summary statements**. They are the "one-sentence summary" of a case and are presented during the "assessment" part of a presentation (i.e., the "A" of a SOAP [subjective, objective, assessment, and plan] note). Learners' summary statements can provide insight into how they interpret and synthesize pieces of clinical information within the context of the individual patient. These statements are a powerful way to determine whether a learner understands what elements of the patient's story really matter. Teachers should ask learners critical questions about the inclusion, exclusion, and/or prioritization of the clinical data within the summary statement. To support knowledge structures that may mimic those of an expert clinician, a well-structured summary statement should include the 3 components of the problem representation described previously (key epidemiology, temporal pattern, and key features) (Box 5-4). The purpose of this structure is to enhance a student's ability to match the patient's problem with the correct diagnosis.

Examples of summary statements:

"Mr. Smith is a 64-year-old man with ischemic cardiomyopathy who presents with a 2-day history of gradual-onset, worsening dyspnea on exertion and findings of hypoxia, bilateral crackles, elevated jugular venous pressure, and lower-extremity edema."

"Ms. Jones is a 33-year-old woman, with a history of heavy alcohol use and nonsteroidal pain medication use, who presents with 2 days of severe, burning, midepigastric abdominal pain and now 2 hours of melena. Her examination is remarkable for hemodynamic instability (pulse 110, blood pressure 88/55) soft, non-tender abdomen with normal bowel sounds, no organomegaly or jaundice, and normal rectal exam, with positive stool heme testing."

A well-structured summary statement should enable the listener/reader to fully understand the problem and independently arrive at the accurate differential diagnosis. Attention to the language used in the summary statement can provide a window into how the learner is thinking; particular attention should be paid to how the learner transforms language and uses semantic qualifiers (i.e., adjectives that categorize a presentation such as acute vs. chronic and progressive vs. intermittent). Summary statements from more advanced learners tend to demonstrate both of these characteristics (Table 5-4) (22, 23).

Bayesian Reasoning

Bayesian reasoning is another analytical approach, one that focuses on the logic of diagnostic decision-making. This approach is based on a mathematical framework that one can use to model reasoning by transforming pretest probability into post-test probability through the concept of a Bayes factor, the likelihood ratio (LR) (24). The LR is perhaps the most

Table 5-4. Summary Statements/Problem Representation

Component to Evaluate	Definition
Narrows differential diagnosis	Appropriately narrows the differential diagnoses by including the following: who this patient is, how he or she is presenting with respect to time, and the key features with which he or she is presenting
Transforms	Enhances meaning of statement by expressing key findings of case in qualified medical terminology and/or synthesizing details into unifying medical concepts
	Replacing lay language (e.g., *swelling*) and or discrete data (heart rate, 180 beats/min; sodium, 125 mEq/dL) with more precise and meaningful medical terminology (*edema, tachycardia, hyponatremia*)
	Combines constellation of findings into a syndrome (shortness of breath, rales, lower-extremity edema, elevated JVP, $S_3 \rightarrow$ volume overload or heart failure); may or may not use semantic qualifiers to do this
Semantic qualifiers	Qualitative terms, more abstract than the patient's actual signs or symptoms, often are binary in nature: e.g., onset over 3–4 mo is gradual (and not sudden), right and left or unilateral (and not bilateral); intermittent vs. constant; stable vs. progressive

Data obtained from reference 23. JVP = jugular venous pressure; S_3 = third heart sound.

Table 5-5. Likelihood Ratios Simplified

Likelihood Ratio	Change in Probability, %	Test Utility
≥10	+45	Strong
~5	+30	Moderate
~2	+15	Weak
~0.5	−15	Weak
~0.2	−30	Moderate
≤0.1	−45	Strong

Adapted from reference 25.

important concept. It provides an objective measure of the value of a test (e.g., historical, examination, laboratory, or radiologic finding).

McGee has developed a rough guide to probability changes based on LR values when the pretest probability is between 10% and 90% (Table 5-5) (25).

A useful Bayesian question for students is, "What positive test is better for ruling in the disease: egophony for pneumonia or nuclear stress test for coronary artery disease?" For students who may think only laboratory or radiologic studies matter, to learn that egophony has a better positive LR (5.5) than does a nuclear stress test (approximately 4) can be a powerful message. In addition, the LR gives a sense of the absolute value of a test in a given context. The fact that a nuclear stress test is only a moderately useful test surprises learners because most think a positive stress test result "rules in" coronary artery disease. Students who learn about LRs may become more efficient in their work-ups when they focus on performing or ordering moderate or strong tests. Teachers should stress that LRs are better than positive predictive values (i.e., the likelihood that the patient has a disease given a positive test result) or negative predictive values (i.e., the likelihood that the patient does not have a disease given a negative test result) in clinical settings because LRs are independent of prevalence. LRs can be applied directly to the patient at the bedside whatever the context and patient characteristics.

LRs present only part of the Bayesian story. The other aspect relates to pretest probability. The reason why many clinicians and teachers avoid Bayesian calculations relates to the challenge of estimating pretest probability for the individual patient (26). When prediction rules are available (e.g., Well's score), this estimate is readily determined. However, in the absence of prediction rules, novice clinicians may feel they are just "making up a number" and don't feel like it adds anything to their diagnostic reasoning. That may be true, but it is vital to realize that all experienced clinicians do this intuitively; this is an important part of developing one's clinical judgment. It is only a small step to do this explicitly. Pretest probability estimates can be done imprecisely at first (e.g., 20%, 50%, or 80% probability of disease). The power of such a step is that it can make this judgment more explicit, thereby accessible to analytic reasoning (e.g., "Just guessing, I would say the probability of gout is 50%. Why? Well I base that on . . ."). Furthermore, in the current information technology milieu, data on incidence of diseases in specific clinical settings (e.g., incidence of vasovagal causes of syncope in emergency department patients) are often readily discovered, allowing for potentially more accurate pretest probability estimates. We should stress that we do not recommend a Bayesian approach for every clinical encounter but rather primarily for challenging cases or high-stakes decisions, in which analytic reasoning may enhance the diagnostic evaluation (27).

For learners who are not averse to Bayes theorem, a teacher can role model or assign Bayesian calculations (i.e., Bayes theorem: pretest odds × likelihood ratio = post-test odds). Most learners and clinicians prefer probability to odds. Online calculators (e.g., http://easycalculation.com/statistics/post-test-probability.php) and nomograms allow for the use of probability, making these calculations more accessible. Estimating a decision threshold can help determine whether a diagnostic test is of high value in the context of deciding whether to test further or treat. For those who prefer to avoid the math, a qualitative approach to Bayes theory in clinical practice has also been described (28).

> **Example:** *A clinician estimates the pretest probability for small bowel obstruction, based on the clinical history and examination, to be approximately 50% (pretest odds, 50:50) for her patient. She considers ordering computed tomography (CT) to aid in diagnosing a small bowel obstruction; CT has positive and negative LRs of 2 and 0.5, respectively. With this information she calculates the probability of bowel obstruction as 34% (post-test odds, 1:2) given a negative CT result and 67% (post-test odds, 2:1) if the CT result is positive. She realizes that the CT result would not change her management and decides that in this situation, the CT does not add value. The test is not ordered.*

"From Problem List to Illness Script"

In the presentation titled "From Problem List to Illness Script," Catherine Lucey described a structure for a case-based conference for residents in internal medicine, a 3-step approach that incorporates several of the general tactics above (29). The result is a prioritized differential diagnosis that can then be used to drive the plan to diagnose and to treat a patient. A case is presented as the stimulus for discussion. The 3 steps are used to process information from the case, allowing learners to more slowly and analytically think through a difficult or unfamiliar patient problem. In step 1, problems are explicitly identified and processed (i.e., described with precise medical terminology; see discussion of problem list and problem representation above). Sets of problems on the list can be processed in sum or chunked into common medical syndromes, such as shock or dehydration. After reduction and prioritization, the problem list is used in step 2 to form a summary statement that represents the patient's illness script. Step 2's one-line summary documents the learners' understanding of the patient's problem and context (see discussion of problem representation and summary statement above). The use of the illness script framework organizes clinical information in a way that allows comparison with disease illness scripts. In step 3, the quality of the match between the patient's problem representation and various disease illness scripts is used to estimate the relative likelihood of each disease considered, with adjustments based on disease prevalence (6). During step 3, learners are forced to focus and categorize the considered diagnoses as most likely, less likely, and unlikely. Generally, learners should consider at least 3 possibilities, but usually no more than 5 to 8. The stepwise approach can be used to diagnose the learner, identifying whether reasoning errors are related to incomplete gathering of patient information, poor processing of clinical information, lack of knowledge about diseases, or difficulty matching patient information to disease knowledge (Table 5-6) (29).

Table 5-6. Problem List to Illness Script Schema

Step 1: Problem List	Step 2: Patient Illness Script (Summary Statement)	Step 3: Prioritized Differential Diagnoses
1. Process to medical terminology, descriptively and summatively 2. Remove duplications 3. Eliminate problems that are "due to" other problems 4. Remove uninformative, nonspecific markers of illness 5. Place in order of priority	1. Who? (Key and relevant risk factors or epidemiology) 2. Temporal pattern? (Onset, duration, pattern over time) 3. Synthesized syndrome statement	1. Compare/contrast the problem representation of the patient by using disease illness scripts 2. Use degree of pattern match and prevalence of disease to estimate likelihood

Data obtained from reference 29.

The 3-step "problem list to illness script" structure has since been adapted for use with learners of all levels and to other health professionals, and from use with real patient cases during case conferences for residents and clinical students to simulated patients.

Combining Fast and Slow Thinking
Expert clinicians navigate between non-analytic and analytic thinking as the need arises; evidence suggests that combining these two modes of reasoning (e.g, pattern recognition with an analytic double-check) may increase accuracy in diagnosis (9, 27). This type of strategy has been termed a **forced cognitive strategy**, a form of metacognition or thinking about one's thinking. As a teaching tactic, learners who arrive at a diagnosis through nonanalytical means can be asked a simple question, such as "But what if it is not?" or "What else might it be?" to prompt a check on reasoning. This tactic may also be useful when used as a self-regulatory measure (see discussion of self-regulated learning below).

Deliberate Practice
Clinicians and learners striving for expert performance in clinical reasoning can take deliberate steps to practice and maintain this complex ability (for details, see Chapter 8). Learners can identify areas for improvement through self-reflection or feedback and then deliberately practice on that area with further feedback. Learners should also be encouraged to gather their own information and arrive at an independent assessment and plan as if they were independently responsible for the patient's care. Similar practice can also be achieved through simulated cases. Teachers can identify opportunities for focused practice targeting work on physical diagnosis or other diagnostic skills. Practicing clinicians can commit to clinical judgment by attempting to predict diagnostic test results as a way of honing one's skills.

> ***Examples:*** *A clinician sees a patient whose rash he is unable to identify. He decides to practice from images, diagnosing one unknown dermatologic image every day for 4 months. A third-year student practices identifying unknown heart sounds on a high-fidelity simulator.*

Self-Regulated Learning
All learners and clinicians can practice self-regulated learning, by incorporating forethought, performance monitoring, and self-reflection, into their routines (Box 5-5). Some practical questions that might be used to help learners reflect on common pitfalls of reasoning appear in Box 5-6 (30–32).

Box 5-5. Foster Motivation and Reflection

- Commit to most likely diagnosis, even when uncertain
- Try to predict diagnostic test results
- Analyze and reflect on successes and failures in clinical reasoning

---

A reasonable way to first introduce these questions is to suggest a "diagnostic timeout" (32).

A natural place for this to occur is at the end of a clinical presentation, particularly when the learner has given what is believed to be the diagnosis, without an associated differential. In the clinical setting, this diagnostic timeout can be framed in the context of patient safety, similar to the procedural timeout with which many health care teams are familiar.

Bias and Error

Bias and error can be explored to increase self-awareness and reflection. As learners increase their use of nonanalytic reasoning, they may come to appreciate how heuristics, as mental shortcuts, sometimes mislead. Common heuristics and biases that are encountered in medical decision-making include the availability heuristic, anchoring effect, confirmation bias, affective bias, and representativeness heuristic (7, 32). These are discussed in more detail in Chapter 4. Because heuristics are unconscious and involuntary, some may argue that understanding the possible errors and biases does not prevent occurrence (7). Helping learners understand the strengths and weaknesses of the use of nonanalytical reasoning, however, should help them identify instances in which more analytic reasoning may be needed (33). Additionally, giving learners general guidelines about

---

Box 5-6. Questions to Prompt Reflection

1. What else could it be?
2. Is there anything that doesn't fit?
3. What can't we explain?
4. What are you most worried about?
5. How does this patient make you feel?
6. Is it possible the patient has more than 1 problem?
7. Why?

Data obtained from reference 32.

---

situations in which errors are more likely to occur (sleep-deprived, hurried, stressed) may help them to be more aware of when they may want to use forced cognitive strategies to avoid heuristics and bias. Unfortunately, simply telling learners to pay attention for challenging cases is not likely a good warning because physicians are not always accurate at gauging the difficulty of a case (34). With appropriate guidance, error and bias awareness may be useful to help foster self-regulation (Table 5-7).

> ***Example:*** *A learner seeing a new patient with cough plans to review the differential diagnosis for cough before entering the room and to ask hypothesis-driven questions (i.e., questions used to confirm or exclude the differential diagnosis) during the interview. Afterwards, she reflects on whether this approach was beneficial.*

❖ Specific Teaching Tools and Methods

Several teaching methods can be used to develop learners' clinical reasoning. In the next section we provide additional detail about 4 specific teaching methods: 1) concept mapping, 2) use of educational scaffolds, 3) actual or simulated case examples, and 4) evidence-based medicine as a teaching and learning method.

Concept Mapping

Concept mapping is a method of engaging learners to visually connect ideas (e.g., concepts) by diagramming explicit links between these ideas; this method is based on theoretical understandings of knowledge and its organization (see Chapter 10 for a more in-depth discussion). The technique allows learners to organize and represent knowledge as an interconnected network that might take the form of webs, decision trees, or Venn diagrams. Concept mapping can encourage learners to explore and make apparent connections that otherwise may go unseen; it allows learners to ask questions about relationships between concepts in ways that may not be represented in traditional texts or teaching materials. This teaching method may be used to reinforce causal reasoning.

Educational Scaffolds

Educational scaffolds are the cognitive equivalent of physical scaffolds, enabling one to reach a higher level of performance than possible without the aid. Educational scaffolds provide guidance to learners and clinicians in learning situations where they have limited experience. As learners progress, the scaffold is no longer needed (i.e., the scaffold fades). This concept was first described in child psychology, explaining development in the

Table 5-7. Practical Points: Applying Theory to Teach Clinical Reasoning

Teaching Tip	Theoretical Basis
Be explicit about building knowledge and knowledge organization • Store and retrieve facts about diseases as illness scripts • Connect and apply stored knowledge, including biomedical knowledge	Information processing
Identify and accurately represent problems • Use semantic qualifiers • Develop summary statements	
Develop both nonanalytic and analytic reasoning skills Think fast (nonanalytical) • Pattern recognition • Intuition and heuristics	
Think slow (analytical) • Hypothetico-deduction • Scheme-inductive thinking • Probabilistic reasoning (e.g., Bayesian)	
Foster motivation to monitor and improve reasoning • Commit to most likely diagnoses • Try to predict diagnostic test results	Deliberate practice self-regulated learning
Seek and provide timely feedback on reasoning • Use test results or clinical course as a source of feedback • Analyze and reflect on successes and failures in clinical reasoning	
Create opportunities for further practice and incremental improvement • Apply reasoning to new patients or problems • Practice harder: increase complexity; manage uncertainty/ambiguity; reason despite incomplete data	

"zone of proximal development," a zone just beyond the developmental zones already mastered (35).

>   ***Example:*** *A 12-month-old child is beginning to walk. He can pull up to a stand without assistance. He is able to walk but must hold*

on to a couch or hands of a parent to walk several steps. With this assistance he is able to walk several feet without difficulty.

A first-year medical student arrives at a clinical practice site to which he is assigned for the next 2 years. He has mastered skills in establishing rapport, professional behaviors with patients, and basic interview. He can gather the history of present illness, with some additional aids, specifically if he uses a disease or complaint-based template or a framework such as CODIERS that helps remind him about various cardinal features to gather.

Many educational scaffolds in common use in medical education support clinical reasoning, from simple mnemonics to more complex structures. In this section, we detail 6 scaffolds.

CODIERS
The mnemonic "CODIERS" is an example of a scaffold that enables learners to gather more thorough information from a patient's history. CODIERS provides the novice student with a guide to the details to be obtained during the interview: Character, Onset, Duration, Intensity, Exacerbating and Relieving factors, and other Symptoms. By recalling this scaffold, an early clinical student can gather much of the relevant history to assist with arriving at the diagnosis. With experience the scaffold becomes less important and the interview is guided by reasoning as information is gathered. The more advanced student may ask questions largely based on possible diagnoses considered (i.e., in a hypothesis-directed fashion) yet can still fall back on this scaffold as needed, ensuring that all of the important questions have been asked.

IDEA
Another example of a clinical reasoning scaffold is the mnemonic "IDEA," which reminds students to "tell me your IDEAs". IDEA stands for: 1) Interpretive summary, 2) Differential of diagnoses with commitment to which is most likely, 3) Explanation of rationale, and 4) Alternatives (36). This scaffold is useful in prompting learners to more explicitly articulate reasoning and can also be used to assess their reasoning.

Summary Statements With Illness Scripts
Instructing students to synthesize clinical information into a summary statement that uses the framework of an illness script (as described earlier in this chapter) is another way to provide a scaffold for learning. This scaffold prompts the student to seek out and identify the most pertinent information needed for clinical reasoning, even before sufficient experience and knowledge of diseases is available to guide this judgment.

Diagnostic Schema

Diagnostic schema (i.e., cognitive frameworks for approaching specific clinical problems) can aid students in the inductive reasoning process (37). Several textbooks incorporate the teaching of diagnostic algorithms, providing a scaffold for inexperienced clinical learners. Clinical guidelines often provide algorithms to aid their adoption as medical practice evolves. Schema serve as educational scaffolds.

> **Example:** *In acute kidney injury, diagnostic studies are interpreted to assess whether the injury is due to prerenal, intrarenal, or postrenal causes.*

Certain scaffolds are used to frame the teacher-learner dialogue around the reasoning process. These scaffolds aid in making reasoning explicit and provide a structure in which feedback can be given. The 2 most commonly used such scaffolds are SNAPPS and the microskills model.

Scaffolds That Frame the Teacher-Learner Dialogue

SNAPPS is an educational scaffold that is a 6-step, learner-centered technique for student case presentations (38). The steps are: Summarize the findings; Narrow the differential diagnosis; Analyze the differential diagnosis by comparing and contrasting alternatives; Probe the preceptor about uncertainties; Plan management; and, finally, Select an area for further learning related to the patient. This technique shifts the focus of the presentation from delivery of facts obtained from the patient to a discussion of the student's differential diagnosis, management plan, and areas of uncertainty related to the case (39). With this change in focus, the preceptor is better able to assess the student's clinical reasoning (38). Additionally, when students express their uncertainties, preceptors may respond by providing targeted teaching tailored to the student's uncertainties (40). SNAPPS, when combined with an educational prescription, also helps ensure that students research and read about their patient's problem (41). The Alberta Rural Physician Action Plan's Practical Doc site offers step-by-step instructions and videos about use of this scaffold in teaching students or residents (42). SNAPPS is a learner-centered technique, and implementation involves teaching learners to follow this model when presenting patients rather than intensive faculty development. This model integrates portions of tactics based on and drawn from information processing as well as self-regulated learning (Box 5-7).

The **One-Minute Preceptor** (or microskills model) is another teaching scaffold (43). In contrast to SNAPPS, which is a scaffold for learners to use, this is a model for teachers, specifically those who work with students

> **Box 5-7. SNAPPS Presentations**
>
> *S*ummarize briefly the history and findings
>
> *N*arrow the differential diagnosis to 2 or 3 relevant possibilities
>
> *A*nalyze the differential diagnosis by comparing and contrasting the possibilities
>
> *P*robe the preceptor by asking questions about uncertainties, difficulties, or alternatives
>
> *P*lan management of the patient's medical issues
>
> *S*elect a case-related issue for self-directed learning
>
> Data obtained from reference 38

and residents in the clinical setting. When clinical preceptors follow this model they generally feel they are able to glean more useful information from the learner's presentation. Teachers and learners spend the same amount of time on the learners' presentation as with unstructured teaching, but the teacher spends relatively more time listening and less time talking, increasing the opportunity for assessment of the learner (44, 45). Preceptors thus report more confidence assessing the learners' clinical reasoning abilities (44) and provide better feedback, particularly specific and higher-order feedback (45).

The model includes 5 steps. The first step is to **get a commitment** from the learner. After presenting the case, the learner may stop and wait for the teacher to supply the working diagnosis. Instead of giving the answer, the teacher asks, "So, what do you think is going on?" After the learner commits to an assessment, the learner may look to the teacher to confirm or refute the opinion. Before doing so, the teacher should **ask the learner for evidence** (second step) that he or she feels supports the assessment proposed (e.g., "I am interested in how you came to that diagnosis"). During the third step, the teacher **provides general rules;** these can be pearls or diagnostic schema, such as "Patients with cystitis usually present with pain on urination, frequency, urgency, and an abnormal urinalysis. Fever, flank pain, nausea and vomiting would be unusual, and this usually indicates the presence of pyelonephritis.").

In the fourth step, the teacher can **reinforce what was done correctly;** learners may or may not realize what aspects of their reasoning were accurate. The teacher provides feedback by focusing on the specific deed and the effect it had, such as "You considered the cost of the medication and the schedule of dosing in your selection of an antibiotic. This will increase

---

Box 5-8. Microskills Model

- Get a commitment
  - *What do you think is going on?*
- Probe for supporting evidence
  - *Why do you think this?*
- Provide general rules
  - *When this happens consider…*
- Reinforce what was done correctly
  - Tell them what they did right and the effect it had
- Correct mistakes
  - Tell them what they did right
  - Tell them what they did not do right
  - Tell them how to improve for the next time

Data obtained from reference 43

---

the likelihood that the patient will complete the course." In the case where the learner has demonstrated a misunderstanding, the teacher can **correct mistakes** (fifth step) (e.g., "You may be right to attribute this patient's altered mental status to the urinary tract infection. However, given the history of a recent fall in a patient on warfarin, an intracranial bleed should be considered as well.") (Box 5-8).

Actual or Simulated Patient Case Examples

To acquire expert clinical judgment, physicians-in-training need the opportunity for deliberate practice of reasoning, whether this practice is with actual or virtual (simulated) patients. Online simulations (virtual patients), while not as authentic as in-person simulations, can accomplish some clinical reasoning goals, such as ensuring exposure to key clinical experiences or undifferentiated patients and adding some of the nuance of a "real" clinical experience, such as the social environment (1). In other words, simulation can reduce the randomness of clinical experience by ensuring exposure of all students to important symptoms or diseases.

Simulations can be of low or high fidelity. In a study of early medical students, the level of fidelity did not clearly alter clinical reasoning performance (46). Higher-fidelity simulations, including role-play, dramatizations, or use of standardized patients that can be used to simulate human interactions and patient care in a more authentic way, may have greater value in scenarios associated with high stress or emotion or that are error intolerant (47). **High-fidelity simulations** may help provide safe environments for clinical students to advance skills with more complex cases, as in formative exercises with standardized patients, or to increase opportunities to demonstrate rapid application of knowledge and to interpret data, as in mock cardiopulmonary resuscitations. Simulations can be used to develop team skills or to practice skills needed for high-stakes, high-stress situations, such as end-of-life discussions or cardiopulmonary resuscitation, creating authentic opportunities to practice reasoning skills in more complex social environments.

Case-Based Discussions
We will now describe typical classroom and clinical approaches that use case examples in the teaching of clinical reasoning.

 Case-based instruction, as a term, applies to a collection of classroom-based techniques that allow for acquisition or retrieval of knowledge and its application in a context of how it might be used clinically (48). The complexity of the cases, the component of reasoning focus, and the level of guidance provided by the teacher or by scaffolds may be varied to suit the educational purpose.

> ***Example:*** *A small-group session during a pathophysiology course uses a series of cases to illustrate the mechanisms of anemia, providing students with opportunities to use a diagnostic algorithm.*
>
> *During a case conference (morning report), a senior resident presents a patient that she admitted to the hospital the night before. A faculty member guides the participants as they process and reason through the clinical information, first from the history, and then the examination and laboratory findings.*

When this instructional method is used, **case selection** is important, with particular attention to the educational purpose. Some cases may be better suited for teaching hypothesis generation; others, for Bayesian reasoning or causal reasoning. For the more novice learner, simple cases are more appropriate; with advanced learners, cases should be more complex and add authentic uncertainty, ambiguity, and errors. To best simulate clinical practice and develop reasoning skills in ways used with real patients, cases should be presented so that the patient's story and clinical information unfolds in a sequence similar to real patients and clinical situations.

 Coaching skills can be helpful to faculty teachers, who use case-based instruction to promote reasoning skills, whether the cases discussed are actual or simulated exemplars (13, 49). The teacher as clinical reasoning coach has multiple tasks to manage: 1) activating prior learner knowledge, 2) assessing learners' levels to individualize learning, 3) asking high-level questions, to promote thinking and active participation, and 4) role modeling lifelong learning skills. The case may be presented in chunks, allowing for individual processing, followed by group questions and comments. Learners can be encouraged to seek additional information about the case, and the coach may explore why the information was requested. Responses to questions provide opportunities for the coach to provide feedback on the answers. An initial differential can be developed and then refined as further information is obtained, with an ongoing give-and-take between the coach and the participants. The challenge for the coach is keeping everyone engaged while making the session challenging, yet not threatening. Coaches may elect to be blinded to the diagnosis so that learners can observe their think-aloud approach to the case.

Morning report conferences are a specific type of case-based instruction, commonly used in resident education. Morning reports typically occur in teaching hospitals 1 or more days a week for the purpose of presenting new admissions or recent cases for discussion. Cases are often presented as an unknown; the differential diagnosis, management, and potential medical errors are discussed. Educational programs have varied approaches to these conferences (50).

Morbidity and mortality (M&M) conferences use error as the stimulus for learning. An effective M&M conference has been described as one that identifies events that resulted in adverse patient outcomes, fosters discussion of adverse events, identifies and disseminates information and insights about patient care that are drawn from experience, reinforces accountability for providing high-quality care, and creates a forum in which physicians acknowledge and address reasons for mistakes (51). An M&M can explore reasoning errors. This is an excellent venue to discuss how heuristics and biases can lead to poor outcomes and to consider the strategies that might be designed to help avoid reasoning errors (52, 53).

Like case-based instruction, **problem-based learning** uses cases to provide learners with the opportunity to acquire and apply knowledge within clinically relevant contexts. What makes problem-based learning different, however, is that problem-based learning is a purely learner-centered approach in which the teacher delivers no content; instead, learners must identify and seek to fill knowledge gaps as a group. Problem-based learning was first developed in response to observations that students acquired knowledge and skills but struggled with applying knowledge to evaluate and manage patient problems (54). The stimulus for learning is a patient problem, a health delivery problem, or a research problem. Students interact with the problem by requesting actions, such as whether to receive more of the patient story, examine the patient, order tests, or offer treatment. In its original form, patients were represented as paper cases, with sequential revelation of information based on student actions. This pedagogical approach creates largely unstructured sessions that are guided by faculty through the careful production and assembly of problem materials prior to the sessions (54). Evidence to date has demonstrated no difference in physician competencies with this approach as compared with more traditional classroom-based approaches to medical education; documented benefits relate to improved coping with uncertainty, communication skills, and self-directed learning (55).

A capstone course in the final year of medical school is often created to advance clinical reasoning performance. This type of course allows focused time for learners to step back from their clinical work and develop specific components of reasoning. Capstone courses have focused on general concepts related to clinical reasoning or on specific tasks, such as physical diagnosis. Limited evidence exists regarding the effectiveness of this approach, but some evidence suggests that these types of courses can improve student confidence and skill (56).

Real Patient Cases
The clinical teacher can serve a unique role in modeling and guiding clinical reasoning. The clinical setting provides an unending source of patients and opportunities to practice clinical reasoning, but it is also an environment in which a teacher must be highly adaptable and draw on several different teaching tactics. It is important for clinical teachers to remember that learners are often in complex, unfamiliar environments and dealing with unfamiliar tasks. Teachers can best ensure that learners interact in a meaningful way by helping them to adapt (57). The clinical teacher should try to select appropriate patient encounters that continue to advance the learner's reasoning and ensure that students have sufficient opportunity to evaluate and independently reason through patient problems. Clinical teachers can simplify reasoning by focusing on one part and by making reasoning explicit, not just determining what to do but also explaining why. Clinical teachers who work with students and residents can support development of reasoning by focusing on 4 main teaching tasks: 1) teaching schema, general rules, or use of other educational scaffolds related to the problems and problem-solving as discussed previously; 2) giving attention to cognitive load and problem/case selection; 3) expecting explicit articulation of reasoning by the student and the teacher; and 4) promotion of self-regulated and lifelong learning, including evidence-based medicine.

Cognitive load can be a substantial problem in clinical settings. Without the presence of the expert diagnostician, the patient with septic shock may be seen simply as a patient with an unstructured set of symptoms (58). The expert diagnostician can chunk information (septic shock), while the less experienced learner is working with several disconnected pieces of information (headache, myalgia, lethargy, fever, low blood pressure, tachycardia, clammy extremities). When students are presented with too many pieces of information, it becomes more difficult for them to learn; they can experience cognitive overload. The clinical teacher can facilitate reasoning by trying to optimize cognitive load through techniques, such as breaking the encounter or reasoning into manageable steps (see Chapter 2).

The selection of cases with lower levels of complexity is another way to help reduce cognitive load. For beginners, focusing first on what is common and straightforward, allowing for early successes, and then increasing complexity over time can be beneficial. Consideration should be given to case complexity and learner's experience with the specific clinical problems being addressed. Cases can be varied to provide new opportunities to adapt and refine knowledge and promote use of different problem solving strategies, such as incorporating opportunities for scheme-induction, pattern recognition (or more deliberate illness scripts comparison), and hypothesis testing to confirm the diagnoses considered. To facilitate clinical learning, the teacher can have the learner focus on just one component of the encounter, such as performing a hypothesis-driven examination. Learners can benefit from direct observation to reinforce data-collecting skills, assessing hypothesis-driven history or examination skills. Early learners may not know what portions of the history and examination are most relevant, so preencounter direction may be critical for learning.

Despite attempts to select cases intended to reduce cognitive load, in some circumstances the learner will seem overwhelmed by the number of problems that a patient has. In this circumstance, the teacher can decrease cognitive load through use of the "goal-free principle" (58). Asking a learner to give a differential with commitment to the most likely diagnosis is a complex task. Instead, the clinical instructor can ask the learner to list as many diagnoses as possible that could be related to the symptoms given in the history or findings on examination. This goal-free task can then be followed up by discussion during which the instructor compares and contrasts the diagnoses, rather than having the learner attempt to do this. Another cognitive load reducing approach is the "worked example," where an approach to a clinical problem or presentation is given and the learner's task is to critique the proposed approach; this is a simpler task than justifying one's own approach to a problem (58). Both of these approaches are effective at reducing cognitive load and therefore providing the learner with sufficient working memory for the task at hand.

Example: A resident is overwhelmed by the complexity of the myriad symptoms with which a patient presents. The teacher decides to set a goal-free task, saying, "Let's start with just naming all of the different diseases that came to mind as you were gathering his symptoms." After soliciting the list of diagnoses, the teacher then quickly compares and contrasts the options.

A student gathers the history and performs the examination on a complex and ill patient. The teacher quickly offers a plan for what needs to happen next, ordering diagnostic tests and initiating treatment. The teacher engages the student: "I want you to take a moment to review my plan and see if you can explain the purpose and rationale behind the tests and treatments ordered."

Articulation of reasoning in the clinical setting is important from both the teacher, as a way to explicitly model reasoning, and the learner, to better assess strengths and opportunities for growth. Articulation of clinical reasoning can be assessed during oral case presentations (59) or upon review of written documentation. Work suggests that learners benefit when allowed time to slow down and reason more analytically before committing to an assessment or before writing notes; to allow for this time, learners should see fewer patients than an expert clinician, typically 1 to 2 for early learners and 3 to 4 for more advanced learners. Questions and prompts can be used to assess problem identification, request a summary, explore illness scripts, or request elaboration of causal networks. More advanced learners might be asked to highlight key defining and discriminating features of diseases, to form well-constructed summary statements, and to create prioritized and transformed problem lists. Incorporation of evidence-based medicine principles can aid in decision support and reinforce lifelong learning. Learners at all levels should be encouraged to combine both nonanalytical and analytic approaches in their diagnostic reasoning (8). A clinical teacher can assess the learner's level of reasoning, to "diagnose the learner." Feedback correcting factual and diagnostic errors helps learners advance in their skill (see Chapter 4).

Example: An early learner suggests a diagnosis. The teacher inquires, "Tell me what you know about this disease." Upon further discussion, the teacher prompts, "Let's review, who gets this disease? How does it typically present?" — use illness scripts.

A student presents a patient with shortness of breath. He considers both pulmonary embolism (PE) and heart failure to be possible diagnoses. The preceptor asks, "What features from the history or *exam would make heart failure more or less likely? What features support PE? What features do not support PE?" — reinforce key features and deductive reasoning.*

A resident presents a patient with type 1 diabetes, who now is experiencing fatigue and hypoglycemia. She considers adrenal insufficiency as a diagnosis. The supervising physician requests, "Tell me how you would summarize this patient's story." After hearing the summary, he further prompts, "What is the typical illness script for adrenal insufficiency?" — use tactics of summary statements and illness scripts.

Role model analytic reasoning. Residents will often independently and quickly arrive at a diagnosis or differential without effort by using nonanalytic reasoning. Clinical preceptors can aid in extending reasoning ability by asking questions that might foster learner reflection. Simply asking the questions, "What else could it be?" or "Is there anything that does not fit?" may help uncover an anchoring heuristic, availability heuristic, confirmation bias, and representativeness heuristic. These questions can be followed up by a quick discussion of these common heuristics and biases and how they can lead to missed diagnoses. A powerful way to drive this message home on rounds is for the clinical instructor to share with the team a personal experience with diagnostic error (32). The next question, "What are you most worried about?", can help to avoid missing the critical, "can't miss" diagnoses (60).

> ***Example:*** *A resident presents a young woman who has had 3 visits to emergency departments for episodes of chest pain, shortness of breath, and palpitations. He offers panic attack as the diagnosis. The teacher explores, "What else could it be? What diagnoses would you not want to miss?"*

Alternatively, one might be susceptible to an affective bias, one based on an emotional response or reaction; for example, when one does not want to consider a "bad diagnosis" in a likeable patient. A follow-up question of "How does this patient make you feel?" can help to illustrate that emotions that may alter reasoning. This question can also be very helpful in the patient that is not so likeable.

> ***Example:*** *A resident presents a new patient who comes in asking for alprazolam and oxycodone for persistent and worsening fibromyalgia. The patient is angry when the resident recommends aerobic exercise and treatment with low-dose tricyclic antidepressants,*

arguing that she is not depressed. The clinical preceptor notes that this can be a difficult situation, asking, "What was your initial gut reaction to her anger? Why do you think she was angry? How might your reaction affect how you interact with her?"

With the fast pace often seen in clinical settings and patients who have been evaluated by others, anchoring biases, premature closure, and other errors may emerge. To build reasoning ability, teachers can have learners critique these as "worked problems," as previously described. An anchoring bias may impair reasoning when a patient was assigned a diagnosis, as commonly occurs with hospital admissions. Initial work-ups may already be underway, with results coming to another physician for interpretation. In these circumstances, a discussion related to test characteristics and Bayesian probabilities can also provide an opportunity to analyze and explore reasoning. These types of discussion may help broaden the differential and avoid premature closure (61).

***Example:** A patient is admitted with shortness of breath and has underlying heart failure. The admitting resident attributed the dyspnea to heart failure exacerbation. The attending physician on rounds asks, "Is it possible that this patient may have another problem?" In exploring heart failure exacerbation as a cause, the attending asks, "Why now?"*

Evidence-based medicine (EBM) details a 6-step approach: 1) seeing a patient, 2) formulating a clinical question, 3) searching the literature, 4) critically appraising the literature, 5) applying evidence to the specific patient seen, and 6) reflecting on the process (24). The application of evidence to patients includes developing an understanding of Bayesian theory and allows for mathematical estimates to inform decisions regarding probability of a diagnosis or risks and benefits of treatment. Use of EBM as a teaching strategy for clinical reasoning can take a very teacher-directed approach (i.e., lecture or classroom) or can be integrated clinically and driven by the questions and answers generated by the learner. The original model for teaching and learning EBM was proposed as an approach to self-directed and practice-based learning (24). EBM can incorporated into clinical teaching by use of the SNAPPS-Plus presentation scaffold (41). Important concepts, such as pretest probability, number needed to treat, and LRs, can similarly be applied to solve patient problems, and EBM can encourage learners to give a pretest probability for each condition in a differential diagnosis. This estimate may often be a gestalt, but students should be encouraged to use prediction rules (e.g., Wells score) when available to calibrate or recalibrate their pretest probability estimation. Additionally, a discussion of LRs associated with tests ordered during the plan can support reasoning, allowing for estimation of post-test probability should a test result be positive or negative.

A discussion of teaching methods would be incomplete without discussion of the resources available to support independent learning or to augment the teaching methods above. Clinical image libraries or atlases can be used as a way of building pattern recognition for highly visual patterns, such as dermatologic findings, images, histopathology, or visible examination findings. Use of resources, such as *The New England Journal of Medicine*'s Images in Clinical Medicine, can augment case-based instruction. Practice with these sources can be an important supplement to personal clinical experience. Textbooks may list possible diagnoses for a given symptom that might support a novice in use of the hypothetico-deductive reasoning. Other textbooks compile various thinking schema that support inductive or scheme-inductive reasoning. Review of and practice with recognizing auditory patterns, such as heart murmurs, can also be incorporated into classroom activities and simulation and be used for independent practice and learning (62). It is yet unclear what threshold of exposure, or what repeated or spaced exposure is needed for long-term retention and mastery of clinical reasoning skills.

❖ Guide to Adapting Teaching

When planning one's approach to teaching clinical reasoning, it is important to consider many factors, but here we focus on the issues related to the level of the learner. It is important to point out that a given learner may appear to fall on a different part of the following spectrum, depending on familiarity with the patient's clinical problem. While these general categories are an oversimplification, we believe that they can assist the educator with their teaching approach.

Level of Learner

The reasoning skills of learners can range from novice to competent to expert. In general, the development of professional knowledge and competence involves initial adherence to taught rules and limited situational perception (i.e., ability to see contextual issues); this level correlates with the novice and advanced beginner. At intermediate levels, the increased knowledge and competence acquired by learners enables them to cope with multiple factors, to prioritize and to form, not just use, routines and maxims. This correlates with competent and proficient levels. The advanced learner acquires expertise, characterized by an intuitive grasp of situations and agility in applying analytical approaches to new situations (63).

Example: A first-year student will join our rheumatology practice weekly for the next 2 years. As he has not finished his preclinical work, what do I have him do when he does not have enough knowledge to evaluate my complex patients?

Novice and advanced beginners in clinical reasoning often have limited illness scripts and therefore rely more on educational scaffolds and analytical reasoning, particularly hypothesis testing (10, 64). Early learners typically start to build rich networks of knowledge, to connect past and current learning, and to organize knowledge in clinically applicable ways. In the clinical setting, information gathered from a patient's history or examination tends to be based on following a general template (scaffold) and is thus inefficient. With guidance, early learners typically start to identify what parts of the history and examination are most relevant and can purposefully seek findings, as one does in a hypothesis-driven interview or physical examination (65). Often, these learners can accurately document and present clinical information, and they start to use semantic qualifiers (i.e., adjectives that help to focus the differential diagnosis of a symptom, such as acute or chronic, dull or stabbing). With provision of enough time to process and with the use of educational scaffolds, these early learners can typically synthesize clinical information into a meaningful assessment that includes a one-line interpretive summary or patient illness script, and offer a differential diagnosis, although this is often not prioritized. Thus, the typical fundamental responsibility of a novice's teacher is to help students build illness scripts and to organize this knowledge effectively through specific symptom-based approaches/algorithms (Box 5-9).

Example: I have a clerkship student on my service early in her clinical years. Unlike the residents and fellows with whom I usually work, she becomes lost in patient details and has difficulty knowing what to do next. How do I help her?

Intermediate learners are those with emerging proficiency; these learners often have had some exposure to the clinical environment, yet not enough that much of what they do is automatic (66). Their reasoning tends to be more analytic, and they are often in the position of trying to take information learned in one context (a classroom or different clinical setting) and transfer it into a new environment. When interviewing a patient, they may proceed blindly through all components of the interview without forming a clear enough early impression (differential diagnosis) such that they can narrow the questions asked or focus the physical examination; they may struggle with the hypothesis-driven

---

Box 5-9. For the Novice and Advanced Beginner

- Novices benefit from scaffolds that help extend skills to the next level
  - For common diseases encountered in the practice, consider providing the student with a template that structures the history and examination to be gathered.
- Preclinical students can start to organize knowledge in ways that can be used to evaluate patients
  - Ask the student to outline the illness scripts for the common diseases seen in the practice. Have the student compare and contrast these diseases. Ask the student to identify basic science concepts that relate to patients seen; consider a concept map.
- Problem-solving skills can be practiced by breaking the process into component parts
  - Instead of asking for an assessment and plan, ask the student to identify the problems or key features with which a patient presents. Ask the student to "brainstorm" about what diseases that this patient might have, without asking for a critique of each.

---

history and examination (10). Case presentations of the intermediate student are often characterized by accurate reporting of the facts; however, when attempting to summarize, the intermediate learner is likely to include extraneous facts and is less likely to transform the patient's language using semantic qualifiers as compared with experts (22). When prompted to reason aloud, this learner is typically more likely to list potential causes of the key symptom, without attention to clinical priorities. Learners at this level may still struggle with the cognitive skills of comparing and contrasting between alternatives in the prioritized differential diagnosis. Inexperience also typically affects clinical decisions, which may be exhibited by the over-ordering of laboratory tests (67). Thus, the general goal for learners at this stage is to refine their analytic reasoning ability while they continue to develop their nonanalytic clinical reasoning. Supervised patient encounters are the key. By seeing more patients and patients with increasing complexity, students develop elaborated illness scripts. The teacher can take an active role in aiding this process by highlighting key features of illness scripts, especially epidemiology, and providing feedback on performance. With increased experience, these learners often

> ## Box 5-10. For the Intermediate Learner
>
> - Clinical students benefit when reasoning and knowledge organization can be made explicit.
>   - Make reasoning explicit by using scaffolds, such as problem lists and illness scripts. Ask her to "Tell me your IDEAs" as a way to make reasoning explicit.
> - Start with simple, typical cases or, with a complex patient, have the student focus on 1 step in reasoning
>   - Use classroom settings or simulation to practice skills. Focus the student on just 1 part of the reasoning process. Help the student reduce cognitive load by systematically listing problems and processing them. Help her explicitly prioritize and identify pertinence for each datum.
> - Share resources; foster motivation to learn reasoning.
>   - Create a safe environment in which she can list possible diagnoses and use hypothesis testing to reason through possibilities; provide resources to help generate possibilities. Share common published algorithms and pocket guides.

become more automatic in their thinking related to common conditions (Box 5-10).

> **Example:** *My senior resident is experienced with generally good judgment... At this point in training, he seems a bit bored with the routine and focuses on getting through patients as quickly as possible. He sometimes jumps to conclusions without obtaining a careful history or exam. I want to prepare him for independent practice when I will not be there to catch errors in judgment. What can I do to help him develop his clinical judgment further, balancing efficiency with avoidance of errors?*

Expert and nearly expert clinicians increasingly rely on nonanalytical reasoning, particularly for more common or straightforward problems, and refine the application of dual reasoning strategies (analytical and nonanalytical). Learners at this level will often form an early impression (problem representation) when interviewing a patient (10) that allows them to follow up the patient's initial history with focused questions and a focused physical examination that narrows the diagnostic possibilities. The initial list of possible diagnoses is often arrived at subconsciously

---

Box 5-11. For the Nearly Proficient and Proficient Diagnostician

- Foster reflection and self-regulation
  - Ask "what else could it be?" and "Is there anything else it could be?"
- Make it fun and nonthreatening; admit your own errors and uncertainty
  - Model self-monitoring. Share examples of your own reasoning errors and what contributed (emotions, pace)
- Commit to an assessment and seek feedback through subsequent test results or clinical course
  - Commit to a diagnoses based on examination or history before tests are obtained. Try to predict test results. Where prediction rules exist, reflect on "first impressions" and how this compared with the rule and outcome.

(nonanalytic). When presenting a patient, the learner at this stage typically can succinctly summarize the key findings, often using semantic qualifiers and transformative language (68), resulting in a brief but coherent picture of the patient's problem.

Continued development of clinical reasoning is tied to clinical practice and working alongside other professionals in the expert and nearly expert clinician. Advancement in clinical reasoning develops in clinical settings, in which the emotional factors, complexity of cases, and the need to adapt are authentic. A desire to deliver better patient care and improved outcomes is often a motivation to improve reasoning (69). It is, in part, the learner's recognition of his or her own increased accountability that helps the learner progress to becoming independently proficient (70). Opportunities for self-evaluation and reflection should be built in to experiences that deepen learning (69). As learners develop additional and more complex pictures of what different diseases "look" like, their illness scripts typically become more elaborated, as does the density of their knowledge structures (58). Moulton uses the term *judgment* to describe how expert diagnosticians react when confronted with uncertainties, or "indeterminant zones of practice," as she describes it. Experts typically self-monitor and slow down, to step back and take another look at a troubling case or situation. Helping our advanced learner and colleagues to reflect and recognize cues from the environment that should trigger a slower and more thoughtful approach is an important role for teachers (Box 5-11) (33).

❖ Conclusions

Nearly every approach to teaching clinical reasoning involves the use of patient cases, whether paper, virtual, or real. Learners need opportunities to actively engage with problems and apply knowledge and practice reasoning. Several techniques for classroom and clinical teaching strategies are described. These teaching tactics can be adapted and used with learners at all skill levels.

The majority of clinical reasoning curricula focus on the diagnosis of 1 or more symptoms, as have we in this book. Diagnosis of symptoms is only 1 of the 3 reasons why a patient seeks care. Patients typically come to see a health professional with 1 of 3 basic needs: 1) preventive health care advice, 2) chronic disease management, or 3) diagnosis and management of symptoms. Physicians engage in reasoning for all 3 encounter types. We believe the general teaching techniques that we have discussed are effective in diagnostic reasoning and can be applied to help learners develop the clinical reasoning needed to assess a patient's personal health risk or the status of a chronic disease.

REFERENCES

1. **Lang VJ, Kogan J Berman N, Torre D.** The evolving role of online virtual patients in internal medicine clerkship education nationally. Acad Med. 2013;88:1713-8.
2. **Nixon LJ, Aiyer, M, Durning S, Gouveia C, Kogan, JR, Lang, VJ, Hauer KE.** Educating clerkship students in the era of resident duty hour restrictions. Am J Med. 2011;124:671-6.
3. **Wilkerson L, Irby DM.** Strategies for improving teaching practices: a comprehensive approach to faculty development. Acad Med. 1998;73:387-96.
4. **Bargh JA, Chartrand TL.** The unbearable automaticity of being. Am Psychol. 1999; 54:462–79.
5. **Miller GA.** The magical number seven, plus or minus two: some limits on our capacity for processing information. Psych Rev. 1956;63:81-97.
6. **Schmidt HG, Rikers RM.** How expertise develops in medicine: knowledge encapsulation and illness script formation. Med Ed. 2007;41:1133-9.
7. **Kahneman D.** Thinking, Fast and Slow. New York: Farrar, Straus and Giroux; 2011.
8. **Eva KW, Hatala RM, LeBlanc VR, Brooks LR.** Teaching from the clinical reasoning literature: combined reasoning strategies help novice diagnosticians overcome misleading information. Med Educ. 2007;41:1152–8.
9. **Ark TK, Brooks LR, Eva KW.** The benefits of flexibility: the pedagogical value of instructions to adopt multifaceted diagnostic reasoning strategies. Med Ed. 2007;41:281-7.
10. **Bowen JL.** Educational strategies to promote clinical diagnostic reasoning. N Engl J Med. 2006;355:2217–25.
11. **Pelaccia T, Tardif J, Triby E, Charlin B.** An analysis of clinical reasoning through a recent and comprehensive approach: the dual-process theory. Med Educ Online. 2011;16. doi: 10.3402/mco.v16i0.5890.
12. **Woods NN.** Science is fundamental: the role of biomedical knowledge in clinical reasoning. Med Educ. 2007;41:1173-7.

13. **Kassirer JP.** Teaching clinical reasoning: case-based and coached. Acad Med. 2010; 85:1118–24.

14. **Kuipers B, Kassirer JP.** Causal reasoning in medicine: analysis of a protocol. Cogn Sci. 1984;8:363-85.

15. **Norman GR, Brooks LR.** The non-analytical basis of clinical reasoning. Adv Health Sci Educ Theory Pract. 1997;2:173-84.

16. **Patel VL, Evans DA, Groen GJ.** Reconciling basic science and clinical reasoning. Teach Learn Med. 1989;1:116-21.

17. **Boshuizen HPA, Schmidt HG.** On the role of biomedical knowledge in clinical reasoning by experts, intermediates and novices. Cogn Sci. 1992;16:153-84.

18. **Rikers RM, Loyens S, te Winkel W, Schmidt HG, Sins PH.** The role of biomedical knowledge in clinical reasoning: a lexical decision study. Acad Med. 2005;80:945-9.

19. **Weed LL.** Medical Records, Medical Education, and Patient Care: The Problem-Oriented Record as a Basic Tool. Cleveland: Press of Case Western Reserve University; 1970.

20. **Weed LL.** Knowledge Coupling: New Premises and New Tools for Medical Care and Education. New York: Springer-Verlag; 1991.

21. **Hartung DM, Hunt J, Siemienczuk J, Miller H, Touchette DR.** Clinical implications of an accurate problem list on heart failure treatment. J Gen Intern Med. 2005;20:143-7.

22. **Bordage G, Lemieux M.** Semantic structures and diagnostic thinking of experts and novices. Acad Med. 1991;66:S70-2.

23. **Kogan J, Nixon J, Lang V.** Beyond the virtual patient: new SIMPLE features to enhance your course or clerkship. Presented at Alliance for Academic Internal Medicine National Meeting. 10–14 October 2012, Phoenix, AZ.

24. **Sackett DL, Straus SE, Richardson WS, Rosenberg W, Haynes RB.** Evidence-Based Medicine: How to Practice and Teach EBM. 2nd ed. Edinburgh: Churchill Livingstone; 2000.

25. **McGee S.** Simplifying likelihood ratios. J Gen Intern Med. 2002;17:646-9.

26. **Goodman SN.** Toward evidence-based medical statistics. 2: The Bayes factor. Ann Intern Med. 1999;130:1005-13.

27. **Mamede S, Schmidt, HG, Rikers RM, Custers EJ, Splinter TA, van Saase JL.** Conscious thought beats deliberation without attention in diagnostic decision-making: at least when you are an expert. Psych Res. 2010;74:586-92.

28. **Medow MA, Lucey CR.** A qualitative approach to Bayes' theorem. Evid Based Med. 2011;16:163-7.

29. **Lucey CR.** From problem lists to illness scripts: teaching clinical problem solving in small groups" Association of Program Directors in Internal Medicine Fall Meeting. 17–20 October 2002. Washington, DC.

30. **Mamede S, Schmidt HG, Penaforte JC.** Effects of reflective practice on the accuracy of medical diagnoses. Med Educ. 2008;42:468-75.

31. **Groopman J.** How Doctors Think. Boston: Houghton Mifflin; 2007

32. **Trowbridge RL.** Twelve tips for teaching avoidance of diagnostic errors. Med Teach. 2008;30:496-500.

33. **Moulton CA, Regehr G, Mylopoulos M, MacRae HM.** Slowing down when you should: a new model of expert judgment. Acad Med. 2007;82:S109-16.

34. **Meyer AN, Payne VL, Meeks DW, Rao R, Singh H.** Physicians' diagnostic accuracy, confidence, and resource requests: a vignette study. JAMA Intern Med. 2013;173:1952-8.

35. **Griggs RA.** Psychology: A Concise Introduction. New York: Macmillan; 2010.

36. **Baker E, Ledford, C, Liston B.** Teaching, evaluating, and remediating clinical reasoning. Acad Med Insight. 2010;8:12-3, 7.

37. **Mandin H, Jones A, Woloschuk W, Harasym P.** Helping students learn to think like experts when solving clinical problems. Acad Med. 1997;*72:*173-9.
38. **Wolpaw TM, Wolpaw DR, Papp KK.** SNAPPS: A learner-centered model for outpatient education. Acad Med. 2003;78:893–8.
39. **Wolpaw, T, Papp KK, Bordage G.** Using SNAPPS to facilitate the expression of clinical reasoning and uncertainties: a randomized comparison group trial. Acad Med. 2009; 84:517-24.
40. **Wolpaw T, Côté L, Papp KK, Bordage G.** Student uncertainties drive teaching during case presentations: more so with SNAPPS. Acad Med. 2012;87:1210-7.
41. **Nixon J, Wolpaw T, Schwartz A, Duffy B, Menk J, Bordage G.** SNAPPS-plus: an educational prescription for students to facilitate formulating and answering clinical questions. Acad Med. 2013;89:1174-9.
42. **SNAPPS.** Alberta Rural Physician Action Plan. Practical Doc. Available at: http:// www. practicaldoc.ca/teaching/practical-prof/teaching-nuts-bolts/snapps. Retrieved August 24, 2014.
43. **Neher JO, Gordon KC, Meyer B, Stevens N.** A five-step "microskills" model of clinical teaching. J Am Board Fam Pract. 1992;5:419-24.
44. **Aagaard EA, Teherani A, Irby DM.** Effectiveness of the one-minute preceptor model for diagnosing the patient and the learner: proof of concept. Acad Med. 2004;79:42-9.
45. **Salerno SM, O'Malley PG, Pangaro LN, Wheeler GA, Moores LK, Jackson JL.** Faculty development seminars based on the one-minute preceptor improve feedback in the ambulatory setting. J Gen Intern Med. 2002;17:779-87.
46. **La Rochelle JS, Durning SJ, Pangaro LN, Artino AR, van der Vleuten CP, Schuwirth L.** Authenticity of instruction and student performance: a prospective randomised trial. Med Educ. 2011;45:807-17.
47. **Issenberg SB, McGaghie WC, Petrusa ER, Lee Gordon, D, Scalese RJ.** Features and uses of high-fidelity medical simulations that lead to effective learning: a BEME systematic review. Med Teach. 2005;27:10-28.
48. **Cameron T, Ferguson K, Hagemann H, McCoy L, Stoddard H, Smothers V, Ballard A.** Curriculum Inventory Standardized Instructional and Assessment Methods and Resources. MedEdPORTAL iCollaborative. August 2012. Available at: www.mededportal. org/icollaborative/resource/498. Accessed 16 February 2015.
49. **Gifford KA, Fall LH.** Doctor coach: a deliberate practice approach to teaching and learning clinical skills. Acad Med. 2014;89:272-6.
50. **Cooke M, Irby DM, O'Brien BC.** The resident's experience: graduate medical education. In: Cooke M, Irby DM, O'Brien BC. Curriculum Didactics: Meetings and Conferences. C San Francisco, CA: Jossey-Bass; 2010:121-4.
51. **Orlander JD, Fincke BG.** Morbidity and mortality conference: a survey of academic internal medicine departments. J Gen Intern Med. 2003;18:656-8.
52. **Norman GR, Eva KW.** Diagnostic error and clinical reasoning. Med Educ. 2010;44: 94-100.
53. **Graber ML, Kissam S, Payne VL, Meyer AN, Lenfestey, N, Tant E, et al.** Cognitive interventions to reduce diagnostic error: a narrative review. BMJ Qual Saf. 2012;21:535-57.
54. **Barrows HS, Tamblyn RM.** Problem-Based Learning: An Approach to Medical Education. New York: Springer; 1980.
55. **Neville A.** Problem based learning and medical education forty years on a review of its effects on knowledge and clinical performance. Med Princ Pract. 2009;18:1-9.
56. **Nixon J, Harris I.** A one-month course can improve students' confidence and skill at physical diagnosis [Abstract]. Presented at Master of Health Professions Education

Summer Conference. July 29-30, 2004; Chicago, Illinois. Available at: www.uic.edu/com/mcme/mhpeweb/2004-proceedings.pdf. Accessed 16 February 2015.

57. **Fraser S, Greenhalgh T.** Complexity science: coping with complexity, educating for capability. BMJ. 2001;323:299-303.

58. **van Merrienboer JJ, Sweller J.** Cognitive load theory in health professional education: design principles and strategies. Med Educ. 2010;44:1365-2923.

59. **Dell M, Lewin L, Gigante J.** What's the story? Expectations for oral case presentations. Pediatrics. 2012;130:1-4.

60. **Croskerry P.** The cognitive imperative: thinking about how we think. Acad Emerg Med. 2000;7:1223-31.

61. **Kurzenhauser S, Hoffrage U.** Teaching Bayesian reasoning: an evaluation of a classroom tutorial for medical students. Med Teach. 2002;24:516-21.

62. **Wayne D, Cohen E, Singer B, Moazed F, Barsuk J, Lyons E, Butter J, McGaghie W.** Progress toward improving medical school graduates' skills via a "boot camp" curriculum. Simul Healthc. 2014;9:33-9.

63. **Eraut M.** Developing Professional Knowledge and Competence. London: Falmer Press; 1994.

64. **Cuthbert L, B Du Boulay B, Teather D.** Expert/novice differences in diagnostic medical cognition: a review of the literature. Brighton, United Kingdom: Sussex University; 1999.

65. **Yudkowsky R, Otaki J, Lowenstein T, Riddle J, Nigori H, Bordage G.** A hypothesis-driven physical examination learning and assessment procedure for medical students: initial validity evidence. Med Educ. 2009;43:729-40.

66. **Croskerry P.** A universal model of diagnostic reasoning. Acad Med. 2009;84:1022-8.

67. **Iwashyna TJ, Fuld A, Asch DA, Bellini LM.** The impact of residents, interns, and attendings on inpatient laboratory ordering patterns: a report from one university's hospitalist service. Acad Med. 2011;86:139-45.

68. **Bordage G.** Why did I miss the diagnosis? Some cognitive explanations and educational implications. Acad Med. 1999;74(Suppl):S138-43.

69. **Ajjawi R, Higgs J.** Using hermeneutic phenomenology to investigate how experienced practitioners learn to communicate clinical reasoning. Qual Rep. 2007;12:612-38.

70. **Carracio C, Benson BJ, Nixon LJ, Derstine P.** From the educational bench to the clinical bedside: translating the Dreyfus developmental model to the learning of clinical skills. Acad Med. 2008;83:761-7.

BIBLIOGRAPHY

Dell M, Lewin L, Gigante J. What's the story? expectation for oral case presentations. Pediatrics. 2012;130:1-4.

Eva KW. What every teacher needs to know about clinical reasoning. Med Educ. 2005;39:98-106.

Irby DM. What clinical teachers in medicine need to know. Acad Med. 1994;69:333-42.

Major CH, Palmer B. Assessing the effectiveness of problem-based learning in higher education: lessons from the literature. Acad Exchange Q. 2001;5:4-9.

McGee S. Evidence-based Physical Diagnosis Elsevier Health Sciences; 2007

Rencic J. Twelve tips for teaching expertise in clinical reasoning. Med Teacher. 2011;33:887-92.

Weed LL. Medical records that guide and teach. N Engl J Med. 1968;278:593-599, 652-657.

6

Assessment of Clinical Reasoning

Valerie J. Lang, MD, FACP

Lambert Schuwirth, MD, PhD

Steven J. Durning, MD, PhD, FACP

Joseph J. Rencic, MD, FACP

C linical reasoning is arguably the core professional competency of the practicing clinician—an ability absolutely necessary (although not sufficient) to be a competent physician. Many clinician educators believe that they can accurately recognize strong and weak clinical reasoning, although many struggle if asked to deconstruct the basis for this belief. However, individual faculty and educational institutions need to justify their appraisals and assessments. In one sense we live in a golden era where reliable standardized tests can help us provide these justifications. Standardized examinations (e.g., licensing examinations) can aid in this justification and do prognosticate future practice performance to a certain extent (1–3). However, they are not sufficient to assess clinical reasoning in its entirety because they assess it only in the comfortable environs of a test-taking center. To complete the assessment picture, faculty in the authentic settings of hospital wards and offices must vouch for learners' clinical reasoning, although they may spend as little as 2 weeks with learners and may rarely directly observe them. In this challenging setting, an evidence-based, systematic approach to clinical reasoning assessment is needed. This chapter highlights key principles to consider in assessing clinical reasoning gleaned from educational research and describes tools that can be used to achieve the goals of assessing, as well as improving, our learners' clinical

KEY POINTS
- Clinical reasoning is not an isolated skill but depends on the content of the problem and the context in which the problem is addressed.
- Clinical reasoning should be assessed with a broad sample of content domains and within a variety of contexts.
- There is no single "gold standard" for assessing clinical reasoning.
- There are a variety of tools for assessing clinical reasoning, including diverse standardized testing formats and workplace-based assessment tools.
- The purpose of the assessment, as well as the resources available to develop, administer, and score an assessment, should be considered when selecting a tool.
- A program of assessment using a variety of tools over multiple episodes should be used to determine competence in clinical reasoning.
- Assessment drives learning and is an essential component of teaching clinical reasoning.

reasoning. Finally, it describes future directions in clinical reasoning assessment.

❖ Goals of Assessment

Assessment clearly drives learning (4). Learners study the content that will help them "ace" the test. Learners also look to experts for clues to what is most important to learn. Assessments provide those clues to the novice. If the test calls for memorization, they will memorize; if problem solving, they will learn to solve problems. Educators recognize that assessments (e.g., tests) not only measure performance but also enhance learning (5). This concept has transformed the modern assessment paradigm. "Assessment *for* learning" is beginning to complement "assessment *of* learning" as the clarion call of medical educators. Within this modern paradigm, maximizing learning clearly becomes a fundamental goal of assessment.

Naturally, the question arises, "How does one create an assessment system that maximizes learning?" The answer in the traditional assessment of learning paradigm was to create a robust structure and process for formative assessment. Formative assessment refers to assessments that focus primarily on learner improvement by being specific, timely, regular, low-stakes, and bidirectional (i.e., learner and assessor contribute), as opposed to focusing on a final grade (i.e., summative assessment) (5). Formative assessment contrasts with summative assessment, which stratifies and promotes learners with "final examination"–type unidirectional assessment instruments selected for their discriminating, rather than teaching, properties (5). This traditional dichotomy has been recognized as artificial by the assessment for learning paradigm. Therefore, any instrument or strategy used in an assessment system should pass a simple litmus test: "Will this assessment maximize our learners' ability to become better doctors?" The application of this litmus test can be profoundly transformative.

As an example, consider the assessment strategy of secure test bank questions. While studying for a test enhances learners' knowledge, imagine the additional knowledge gained by allowing students to review and understand their mistakes. If an institution applied this litmus test to their clinical reasoning assessment strategy, it would certainly reflect on and potentially modify their approach. This approach may have disadvantages (e.g., loss of exam security); however, we believe that a focus on assessment for learning, tempered by practical considerations, maximizes the potential educational gains for learners.

Beyond this primary goal of assessment, a secondary goal is determining competency for progression to the next level of education or for unsupervised practice. Undergraduate and graduate medical education institutions rely on multiple strategies, including scalable, psychometrically sound assessment measures (e.g., standardized multiple-choice question tests), multisource global performance summaries of clinical rotations, objective structured clinical examinations (OSCEs), and direct observation of real patient encounters with a structured scoring form (e.g., the American Board of Internal Medicine's Mini-Clinical Evaluation Exercise [Mini-CEX]), to determine competence (6). Assessing clinical reasoning is a key aspect of competency determination but poses significant challenges (7). These challenges will be highlighted in subsequent sections.

❖ History of Assessment of Clinical Reasoning

Although the role of rote knowledge and its relevance for medical competence may have been the subject of debate at times in the past decades, the centrality of clinical reasoning has never been contested. It is seen as the holy grail of medical competence and performance. It is therefore not surprising that many methods and instruments to assess clinical reasoning have been developed in the past.

The traditional method used to assess clinical reasoning was the bedside oral examination, in which the patient case was used to examine the learner's ability to understand and explain the key findings (e.g., symptoms, physical examination, laboratory results, and other features needed to diagnose a patient) and provide a rationale for a differential diagnosis and management plan. Although perceived as valid (i.e., measuring what you hope or want to measure), the oral examination was also considered subjective and unreliable (i.e., results were inconsistent or not reproducible across different raters and learners), and therefore more structured and standardized assessment methods were sought (8).

An intuitive approach to assessing reasoning was to simulate real patient encounters using structured oral examinations, paper-and-pencil–based tests, and, later on, computer-based simulations. Typically the candidate was provided with the initial complaint and then had to ask the relevant history questions, "perform" the relevant physical examinations, and order additional diagnostic tests. The candidate would receive only the information she or he asked for in this process. All relevant information elicited by the candidate plus the correct diagnosis and therapy were scored. It was thought that by mimicking the patient encounter as carefully as possible, the clinical reasoning process would be assessed most validly. The most well-known examples of this approach were the Patient Management Problems (9) and the computer-based exam project, but there were many others to follow. Patient Management Problems have been used in various forms throughout the world. One form was the problem box, which was really a box with a patient scenario on paper, and audio (tape cassette) and visual (slide carousel) information. On the paper containing the scenario, history-taking questions could be asked, physical examinations could be "performed," and additional diagnostics could be "ordered" by rubbing the appropriate box with a felt-tip pen to elicit the information, written with latent ink. Alternative forms included the P4 (Portable Patient Problem Pack) deck, which was a deck of cards with the questions, physical examination procedures, and other information on the front and the answer on the back (to be conducted with an examiner), and the structured oral examinations. The computer-based exam involved the same approach but responses were provided by the computer.

Although these long (e.g., multiple questions on the same case) simulations appeared valid, serious issues with this approach developed. Experts, who were asked to provide scores for each decision a candidate could make, disagreed not only on the specific scores for each decision but also on what would be the optimal pathway through the simulation. This is often called the idiosyncrasy of the problem-solving process. There was more agreement, however, on the outcome of the process (the diagnosis and treatment) and some clearly essential decisions (10).

In addition, performance on one case did not predict performance on any other case; a candidate could perform very well on one case and very poorly on another. This so-called context specificity (see Chapter 3) is a serious threat to reliability because it makes large samples of cases necessary for the test to become reliable enough for high-stakes decisions. Because each case took considerable time to complete, total testing time had to be extremely long (10–12). A third problem arose upon discovery that the performance of experts on these tests was lower than that of intermediates (e.g., recently graduated doctors). This was unexpected—experts can be assumed to outperform intermediates instead of the other way around—and it cast serious doubts on the validity of the long scenario approach to assessing clinical reasoning (13, 14).

Based on these major concerns two main streams in assessment followed. The first focused on assessing the final decision step, and the other focused on capturing the most relevant parts of the reasoning process. Examples of the former are key features exam (KFE) cases (15, 16) and extended matching items (EMIs) (17), and the typical approach for the latter is the script-concordance test (18). Both KFEs and EMIs use short descriptions of a clinical problem—or vignettes—associated with questions that ask for essential decisions only. In KFE cases the type of decision can vary with the case (most often diagnosis and treatment). EMIs start with a panel of possible answers/options and followed by the vignettes. The candidate is asked to select the most appropriate option for each of the vignettes, where options can be selected more than once and some may not be applicable in any of the vignettes. These methods aimed to mitigate the effects of idiosyncrasy and content specificity by focusing more on the outcome or essential decisions (experts agree more on those decisions). By using short cases a broader sampling could be achieved, which had a positive effect on reliability.

In conceptualizing assessment programs, Miller's triangle has become very popular (19). This model suggests that a complete assessment program should include 4 aspects of a competence: "knows," "knows how," "shows how," and "does." Knowing and being able to apply knowledge to solve problems in unauthentic test situations are represented by the bottom 2 layers. Demonstration of skills in a test situation (as in an OSCE) is the third layer. The developments in assessing clinical reasoning in simulated patient-based examinations and OSCEs were felt to sufficiently address the first 3 levels of Miller's triangle, but there was still a need to include the authentic assessments of what learners do in actual practice at the "does" level.

Therefore, current approaches, which are still in development, tend to return to less structured assessment and increasingly involve on-the-spot human judgment more, especially in workplace-based assessment.

This may come across as having gone full circle; however, it is not merely a return to unreliable and arbitrary assessment but rather the result of a better understanding of the relationships between subjectivity and reliability (20), construct validity (21), and the nature of clinical reasoning (22).

❖ Principles of Assessing Clinical Reasoning

The most important finding with respect to clinical reasoning is that it is not a generic skill (22). It is highly associated with a good working knowledge about the problem at hand as well as prior experience. The chances of successful management of a clinical case drop dramatically if the problem-solver does not have sufficient, well-organized, relevant knowledge or experience. This in itself explains context specificity; because optimal care provided to a patient is situation specific (e.g., knowledge and experience), so are clinical reasoning and problem-solving.

Successful clinical reasoning is also associated with understanding the so-called deep structure of the problem (e.g., understanding Kussmaul breathing from a viewpoint of the acid-base balance disturbance rather than merely as a set of symptoms) (23). Understanding this deep structure is important because it facilitates "transfer" or the ability to see similarities and differences between 2 seemingly unrelated cases, for example, hyperventilation in an anxiety attack and Kussmaul breathing in diabetic ketoacidosis.

Finally, the role of clinical reasoning has to be understood in terms of "chunking." Chunking is the process by which humans can store and process larger bits of information (chunks) in their working memory and use them to solve a problem (24). In mathematics, for example, the problem "$12 \times 12 = x$" can be stored as one chunk and the solution is an automated "144." With "$17 \times 18 = x$" the problem is normally represented by 3 chunks—"17," "×," and "18"—and the solution requires analyses. With the problem "$3867 \times 2492 = x$" the number of chunks is considerably higher. One of the dominant theories about the development of clinical expertise therefore states that development starts with the connection of isolated facts into so-called semantic networks, which aggregate into illness scripts (one-chunk representations of a certain disease, like pneumococcal pneumonia) and finally include contextual factors (e.g., typical appearance of a patient) to aggregate into instance scripts (25). Various other theories portray slightly different views, but they seem to converge on the notion that clinical problem-solving expertise is associated with efficiency of the process and reliance on recognition of the problem (or large chunks of the problem). The more popularized version of chunking (and connectionism) is the system 1/system 2 reasoning (nonanalytical/analytical reasoning) model (26).

❖ Validity Considerations

The principles and theories described above as well as in Chapter 3 are important in determining the validity of instruments for assessing clinical reasoning. The validity of an assessment pertains to the extent to which the instrument measures what it is meant to assess. Determining the validity of clinical reasoning instruments is not easy because the process of clinical reasoning cannot be observed directly (i.e., it is a "latent" construct). It has to be inferred from the choices people make in clinical cases (their clinical decision-making) or from people's verbalizations of their own thinking processes (e.g., in think-aloud procedures). Both at best approximate clinical reasoning, and therefore the validity of any assessment instrument will have to be established by arguments, judgments, and research outcomes. Throughout the 20th and 21st centuries, different views on validity have been developed, but they mostly agree that no assessment can be valid in itself; rather, each assessment is always valid only for a certain purpose (and often only in a certain context) (20). Therefore, validity of an assessment of clinical reasoning can be established only when a clear conception of what clinical reasoning is has been formed.

It may be clear that in the case of clinical reasoning a predictive validity approach ("Does my 'new' test predict the outcome on a gold standard well?") does not work. Because there is no gold standard, there is nothing to validate assessment methods against. Since the seminal work of Cronbach and Meehl (27), validity has been approached by critically investigating the relationship between test scores and expectations about them given the purpose of the assessment. A simple example is: Do experts, who are reasonably expected to be good clinical-reasoners, perform better on the test than non-experts (or intermediates)? From this it is clear that the intermediate effect was a major argument against the validity of the long-branched simulations.

The most current approach to validity is the one formulated by Kane (Table 6-1) (21). He sees validity as a chain of arguments. The first link in the chain is from observation to score, the second from observed score to universe score, the third from universe score to target domain, and the final one from target domain to construct. When we apply this to taking a blood pressure to establish a patient's health, then the first inference is from observing the sphygmomanometer and listening to the Korotkoff tones to a numerical value (120/80 mmHg). The second is by repeating the measurement several times to ensure that any conclusion is not drawn on only one measurement and to improve generalizability or reliability. The third is from the generalizable blood pressure to cardiovascular status (triangulating it, for example, with heart auscultation and pulse). Finally, there is an inference from cardiovascular status to health (e.g., incorporating lungs, kidneys, liver).

Table 6-1. Kane's Validity Argument

Link	Observation	Observed Score	Universe Score	Target Domain	Construct
Example	Observing the sphygmomanometer and listening to Korotkoff tones	Numeric value for blood pressure (e.g., 120/80)	Repeat measurement multiple times to improve reliability or generalizability	Cardiovascular status (e.g., triangulated with cardiac auscultation and pulse)	General health (e.g., incorporating lungs, kidney, liver)

Information obtained from reference 21.

The same approach can be taken with any test that tries to capture clinical reasoning. There is the decision on how to score the answers to the questions, the generalizability of the scores, the combination of various test results to assess clinical decision-making, and finally combining these results with others to make the inference from clinical decision-making to clinical reasoning. By now it may be clear that validating any new approach to assessment of clinical reasoning will require much more than a single study; it will require a carefully planned program of research.

In ensuring the validity of an individual test without trying to validate a whole new approach, several steps need to be taken. The most important steps include those listed in Box 6-1, organized by Messick's framework for validity evidence (28).

Box 6-1. Steps to Ensure the Validity of an Individual Test

▶ Content
- The blueprint (a table detailing how many questions should deal with each of the topics of the test) needs to be constructed.
- The items need to be written such that they are an optimal predictor for problem-solving ability. False-positive responses (a student answering an item correctly despite insufficient ability) and false-negative responses (a student answering an item incorrectly despite sufficient ability) must be avoided.
- The scoring system needs to be considered carefully. Typical considerations include whether to assign

continued

Box 6-1. Steps to Ensure the Validity of an Individual Test (continued)

weights to certain questions (the standard suggestion is not to do this) (4, 20).

▶ Internal structure
  • The number of items or assessment episodes (e.g., direct observations) needs to be high enough to increase reliability or generalizability. Insufficient sampling results in *construct underrepresentation*.
  • The difficulty of the assessment and ability of the assessment to discriminate between high and low performers need to be determined.

▶ Response process
  • Any source of error must be excluded as much as possible (e.g., poor item formulation, distractions during the assessment) to avoid error influencing the score, a concept known as *construct-irrelevant variance*.

▶ Consequences
  • The principle of proportionality is applied: that is, the consequences of the test result are in proportion with the validity of the assessment process. Low-stakes consequences may be based on simple observations or simple tests, but high-stakes decisions always require ample assessment and the generation of rich data. A high-stakes decision on the basis of a single test— and certainly on a single case—is not defensible.

▶ Relationship to other variables
  • Performance should be compared with that of other assessments; if the new assessment correlates perfectly, then it may not add new information, although it might have value if it's more resource-efficient to administer. In general, performance should improve with increasing expertise.

❖ Challenges of Clinical Reasoning Assessment

Clinical Reasoning Assessment as an Inference

The previous "principles" section pointed out that clinical reasoning ability is inferred from learners' diagnostic accuracy and clinical decision-making. If learners make the correct diagnosis in multiple contexts, then assessors assume that they reason well and adequate learning has occurred. However, what if learners regularly miss the correct diagnosis? Then educators typically will attempt to understand and correct the learner's reasoning process to improve the outcome (i.e., diagnostic accuracy). Herein lies the dilemma. Because it's likely that some elements of every reasoning process are subconscious, learners will inaccurately rationalize why certain decisions were made when probed by an assessor. Imagine a learner who fails to clearly describe the patient's presenting symptoms and signs. The assumption is that the learner has an issue with problem representation, but it could be that the learner lacked adequate illness scripts to collect the appropriate data and recognize which data to prioritize. Practically speaking, the best assessors can do in most cases is to identify and provide feedback on learners' errors based on probing questions that attempt to uncover the flaws in their clinical reasoning process. This feedback approach still likely has some educational value, despite the limitations described.

No Gold Standard for the Clinical Reasoning Process

As previously mentioned, the clinical reasoning process is idiosyncratic, determined by the interaction of clinician knowledge and experience, patient factors, and the context of the encounter—in other words, it is situation specific. The bottom line for measuring "success" is making the correct diagnosis and choosing the correct management plan. This approach is problematic because learners can make the correct diagnosis with flawed intermediate steps that could lead to diagnostic failure with the next similar case. Furthermore, there are many acceptable solution paths to the correct answer, and experts may therefore vary in their strategies and approaches. In other words, clinical reasoning is not a linear phenomenon. Although it is unlikely that this challenge will be overcome completely, novel approaches, such as microanalytic techniques or concept mapping (see Chapter 11), might provide further insights into factors that prognosticate success (e.g., meta-cognitive awareness).

Clinical Uncertainty

Even if we assume that we could determine a "gold standard" clinical reasoning process, clinical uncertainty provides another challenge to its assessment. In cases with clear diagnoses and uncomplicated management, assessment is relatively straightforward (e.g., a patient with chest pain and acute ST-segment elevation in the anterior leads has a myocardial infarction and needs reperfusion). However, the range of reasonable diagnostic and therapeutic approaches expands in complicated or complex cases due to uncertainty and contextual factors, including patient preferences. A potential solution is to think of clinical reasoning and clinical decision-making under uncertainty using the analogy of a strike zone. A range of reasonable diagnoses and actions (like the boundaries of a strike zone) exist that qualify as competent clinical reasoning. Although this analogy fits, it prompts the question, "How do we standardize the strike zone?" Just as umpires have different levels of ability in calling strikes as well as differing opinions about the exact location of the strike zone, clinicians have varying levels of clinical reasoning ability as well as differing opinions about what constitutes "good" clinical reasoning within a specific clinical context (i.e., a "strike zone" of reasonable clinical decisions). Who should arbitrate what constitutes a diagnostic reasoning "strike zone" under conditions of uncertainty? Should it be a panel of generalists, subspecialists, or a mix of both? On which criteria should they be selected (e.g., experience, reputation)? One might argue that clinically uncertain and/or ambiguous scenarios should be excluded from high-stakes assessment given these and other challenges. In fact, as described previously, this argument has led to our current assessment strategies of standardized tests and OSCEs. However, this approach assumes that learners and physicians who do well in conditions of certainty will perform equally well under conditions of uncertainty. Such a hypothesis/assumption certainly deserves further study.

Clinical Reasoning as a Context-Specific Phenomenon

As previously described in this chapter and Chapter 2, clinical reasoning performance is also highly dependent on context, or the specifics of an individual situation or encounter. Given 5 different presentations of chest pain, an individual clinician's diagnostic performance from one case to the next will vary, even if the final diagnoses and treatments are the same. That is, there is a poor correlation of clinician diagnostic performance within the same diagnoses (poor intraclinician reliability). The different factors within the clinical situation (e.g., patient gender, health care setting, doctor affect) can have powerful effects on clinical reasoning outcomes. To account for context specificity in assessing reasoning, an even larger sampling of clinical reasoning performance is essential.

Clinical Reasoning as a Construct

Clinical reasoning is a construct that consists of a combination of multiple interacting elements (e.g., medical knowledge, communication skills, physical examination skills). When different tools (post-encounter form versus checklist versus oral presentation) have been used together to assess clinical reasoning, a low level of correlation between their data has been observed (29), suggesting that each instrument may measure different aspects of clinical reasoning. Therefore, one might think that global summary ratings by faculty best measure the "whole" construct of clinical reasoning. However, the previously described challenges, inter-rater "unreliability," lack of direct observation, and context specificity cast some doubt on their ability to serve as the gold standard of clinical reasoning assessment. Given the reality that no magic-bullet instrument that assesses all aspects of clinical reasoning exists, we recommend using multiple tools that evaluate different aspects of clinical reasoning (e.g., medical knowledge tests, direct observations, global summary, think-aloud, chart stimulated recall). The ideal number and proportion of different tools to maximize clinical reasoning assessment accuracy have not been determined, but we believe that too many instruments (more than 5) may overwhelm faculty and reduce their ability to use each individual tool effectively.

Considerations for Teachers

Key Practical Questions

The principles and considerations described in the previous sections should inform any clinical reasoning assessment strategy. To incorporate these assessments into a comprehensive program, the following questions should be answered:

1. What instruments will you use for clinical reasoning assessment?
2. In what settings will you assess clinical reasoning?
3. Will the assessment be standardized or unstandardized?
4. Are there adequate resources for the development, administration, and scoring of the assessment?
5. Will faculty and/or administrators have time to develop and/or administer the assessment?
6. Do faculty and/or administrators have the expertise to develop and/or rate performance accurately (i.e., is faculty development needed)?
7. Are other resources available (e.g., standardized patients, protected time for the learner, chart notes)?

Institutions face at least 2 important challenges in terms of developing a program of clinical reasoning assessment: 1) obtaining meaningful data and 2) using those data to improve learner, faculty, and institutional performance. The second challenge is beyond the scope of this chapter but has been recently discussed elsewhere (30). We will defer discussion of written examinations until the next section and focus comments on global summaries and direct observation of clinical reasoning.

Several insights have emerged from the literature regarding assessment instruments. First, several studies suggest that only 2 constructs, patient care/clinical ability and professionalism/interpersonal and communication skills, account for most of the variance in global assessments of clinical performance (31, 32). Clinical reasoning likely falls within both, but more the first category; it is worth recognizing that global assessments will not provide a pure assessment of clinical reasoning (even if the question is directly asked). For those using the Accreditation Council for Graduate Medical Education (ACGME) Milestones structure, these may provide greater discriminatory capability for clinical reasoning, but that hypothesis remains unproven. Within the milestones framework, one could imagine constructing enstrustable professional activities around clinical reasoning, but these have not been described in the literature to this point.

The role of workplace-based (i.e., direct observation) assessment instruments deserves comment. It is natural to focus emphasis on the choice of instrument; however, at least 1 study suggests that an instrument may account for less than 10% of the variance in assessment (33). Nevertheless, certain characteristics of instruments and implementation strategies improve their likelihood of measuring the ability of interest (Box 6-2). The caveat to using the pearls listed in Box 6-2 is that they have not been directly shown to be useful for assessing clinical reasoning; however, it seems reasonable to assume that they would be of some benefit in improving clinical-reasoning assessment as well. The form should be relatively self-explanatory, easy to use, not too long, and narrative rather

---

Box 6-2. Pearls for Assessing Clinical Performance in the Workplace Setting

1. Acquire 7–11 assessments by different raters to obtain reliable (>0.7–0.8) global summaries of clinical performance (34).
2. To obtain results that correlate with typical performance, do not inform learners that they are being assessed (e.g., unannounced standardized patients) (35).
3. Keep ratings forms short; most variance in clinical performance assessment derives from patient care and professionalism (36).
4. Use forms that include narratives for anchors because they can enhance the effects of feedback.
5. Train raters to improve comfort with instruments and provide feedback on their stringency or leniency, recognizing that evidence that training improves ratings' accuracy is limited (37).

than numeric. Recent literature suggests that instruments should align with the expertise of the assessor (38). More structured forms help novice and intermediate assessors. Practically speaking, creating tiered versions of assessment instruments based on assessor expertise is not realistic, but allowing adequate space for narrative comments will allow expert assessors to add their judgments to a structured form. However, even when these prerequisites are met, we must recognize that the "perfect" form does not exist (39).

If the tool alone is not sufficient to obtain useful data, then faculty development would seem to be the critical factor in improving assessment (see Chapter 8). Unfortunately, faculty development training exercises for improving clinical skills rating have demonstrated improvement in stringency but no significant improvement in inter-rater reliability (37). Despite this, faculty development interventions, especially a structured means of providing feedback on stringency or leniency, seem vital to standardizing performance scoring between "hawks" and "doves." Further study is needed to elucidate the best means of developing faculty to increase the likelihood of obtaining meaningful observations of learner performance.

Given these global considerations, what practical tips regarding clinical reasoning assessment specifically can be provided?

1. Combine standardized assessment instruments (e.g., written tests or OSCEs) with authentic workplace-based assessment instruments (e.g., global assessments, Mini-CEX).

This approach is a standard of practice given that no single assessment instrument can capture the entire construct of clinical reasoning. Clinical reasoning clearly consists of more than medical knowledge. Therefore, it is essential to include instruments that assess learners in clinical settings to obtain a more comprehensive understanding of their clinical reasoning.

2. Use a valid and reliable instrument for workplace-based clinical reasoning assessment.

The Mini-CEX has the most robust reliability evidence, although it assesses clinical reasoning only by having faculty assess learners' judgment on a 1–9 scale with optional comments. Its validity is difficult to impeach. However, without anchors describing the specific behaviors that should be assessed, it is likely that different raters may focus on different aspects of clinical reasoning. Its specificity and utility for learning clearly depend upon meaningful comments. Many other tools, which include behavioral anchors, have been studied. Kogan and colleagues have created a comprehensive review on the topic (40).

3. Faculty development is important to improve comfort with assessment and to increase stringency.

Training faculty is an essential component of developing a strong clinical reasoning assessment program (37). Dhaliwal has published a successful workshop structure for faculty development in clinical reasoning, although the evidence for its utility is limited to self-reported satisfaction (41) and a systematic review by Steinert and colleagues suggest that longer-term initiatives are more likely to be successful (42).

4. Developing a system of clinical reasoning assessment that is both horizontal (i.e., within rotations and throughout a given year) and vertical (i.e., between years) is essential.

Horizontal clinical reasoning assessment has been the standard approach for years, with most of the focus on the clinical years. The entrustable professional activities (43) and recent ACGME Milestone initiatives (44) have focused attention on learner development over years of training. Milestones for clinical reasoning development have not been specifically defined, although many of the milestones ask evaluators to assess components of clinical reasoning.

❖ Assessment Methods

The following section briefly describes a variety of tools for both standardized and workplace-based assessment of clinical reasoning. While not exhaustive, this section highlights some of the major pros and cons of each tool (Table 6-2).

Because clinical reasoning is context-specific, assessment tools should be chosen accordingly. Standardized exams (e.g., written exams or OSCEs) enable the assessment of all learners across the same predetermined set of problems and can sample a broad set of content domains within limited testing time. However, standardized assessments place learners in artificial contexts (e.g., a computer-testing center) and therefore don't assess all aspects of clinical reasoning. Workplace-based assessments take place in more authentic contexts, where physicians or future physicians actually practice. However, they are performed with a more idiosyncratic group of patient cases. The content and complexity of each case may vary among different learners in the same group. It is not necessary that all workplace-based assessment occurs with the same content, as long as the quality of the assessments is similar (45). A balance of standardized and workplace-based assessments is important as part of a program of assessment.

Assessment tools consist of a stimulus and a response. For assessing clinical reasoning, the stimulus is typically a written or computer-based patient case, an actor or simulator portraying a patient, or a real patient with a real chief complaint. The response is the procedure for ascertaining the learner's ability. In a standardized exam, this often consists of a question

Table 6-2. Standardized Methods for Assessing Clinical Skills of Medical Trainees

Assessment Method	Stimulus Format	Response Format	Reliability*	Resource Inten-sity† (Develop/Administer)	Advantages	Disadvantages	Examples	Recommended Assessment Uses‡
Standardized assessment methods								
Multiple-choice questions	Case vignette	Single best answer from a short list of options	High	High/low	Familiar to learners; predicts performance on future multiple-choice exams	Mixed effects of cueing; limited ability to predict clinical performance	USMLE	Knowledge and clinical reasoning; common and rare problems
Key-features exam	Case vignette	Multiple selections from short or long list; free text; partial credit and "poison responses"	Moderate-high	High/low	Predictive of performance in clinical practice	Significant training required to develop exam	Medical Council of Canada Qualifying Exam, Australian GP Fellowship Exam, medical student progress exams	Application of knowledge to make key decisions to solve common clinical problems
Extended-matching items	Case vignette	Single best answer from a shared long list of options for multiple vignettes about a common topic	High	High/low	Tests pattern recognition		USMLE	Diagnostic reasoning
Script concord-ance tests	Case vignette	Weighting of how new data affect the likelihood of a hypothesis on 5-point Likert scale	High	High/low	Allows partial credit for choices where experts reasonably disagree	Require a panel of experts to establish an answer key; optimal scoring method is unclear	Preclinical and clinical students, residents, fellows, faculty	Ability to interpret new information in situations of uncertainty; illness scripts

Method	Description	Format			Strengths	Limitations	Setting	Assesses
Short-answer	Case vignette or question about comparing/contrasting diagnostic or therapeutic approaches	Free text	Low-moderate	Moderate/high	Avoids cueing; allows learners to explain their underlying reasoning	Limited breadth of content can be tested; faculty time to score the essays	Undergraduate medical courses	Formative feedback; progress testing
Clinical reasoning problems	Case vignette	Free text development of hypotheses; weighting of how each key finding affects each hypothesis on Likert scale	Unknown	High/low-moderate	Identifies accuracy of illness scripts; avoids cueing of differential diagnosis	Limited to diagnostic reasoning, not management; cueing of key findings	Medical students	Diagnostic knowledge/illness scripts
Concept maps	Broad clinical topic	Diagram depicting relationship between features of the topic	Unknown	Moderate/high	Identifies accuracy of illness scripts; avoids cueing	Requires training of learners; limited breadth of material can be tested	Undergraduate medical courses	Structure and depth of knowledge on a single topic
Oral exams	Case vignette, standardized patient, or real patient encounter	Verbal questions and answers; structured or unstructured	Low-moderate with structured interview and training	Moderate/high	Avoids cueing; allows examiners to probe learners' underlying reasoning and ability to think on their feet	Biases of examiners (e.g., examinee attire or projected confidence)	Specialty board certification	Ability to synthesize complex data and articulate thought process; formative feedback
OSCEs	Trained actor portraying a patient using standard script	Checklist by observer or SP assessing history, physical, communication skills; post-encounter note or form	Low-moderate	High/high	Assessment of application of knowledge and reasoning in standardized clinical scenarios	Requires training of standardized patient; scoring tool may overly reward thoroughness	USMLE Step 2 Clinical Skills	Ability to select relevant data to gather while conducting a history and physical examination; involvement of patient in shared decision-making

continued

Table 6-2. Standardized Methods for Assessing Clinical Skills of Medical Trainees (continued)

Assessment Method	Stimulus Format	Response Format	Reliability*	Resource Intensity† (Develop/Administer)	Advantages	Disadvantages	Examples	Recommended Assessment Uses‡
High-fidelity simulations (with technology assistance)	Mannequin or task trainer, with or without confederates	Observation of trainee performing history, physical, or procedures; managing illness in real time; checklist or global assessment form	Low-moderate	High/high	Assessment of clinical decision-making in rare but important scenarios	Requires trained staff to operate equipment and act as confederates	Cardiac/respiratory arrest simulations	Ability to make decisions in real time, especially in critical situations; communication with interdisciplinary team in decision-making
Workplace–based assessment methods								
Chart-stimulated recall/review	Documentation of encounter with a real patient	Verbal questions and answers; unstructured	Unknown	Low/moderate	Allows examiners to probe learners' underlying reasoning	Medical decision-making may reflect other physicians' decisions	Residency milestone assessment	Formative feedback to learners with high level of independence
Oral case presentations	Oral presentation of a real patient encounter	Unstructured or structured (One-Minute Preceptor model or SNAPPS framework)	Unknown	Low/moderate	Triggers readily available; woven into patient care and instruction	Breadth of topics limited by available patients; influence of other providers' assessments of patient	Inpatient rounds; clinic sessions; morning report conferences	Formative feedback

| Direct observation of clinical or procedural skills | Real task with real patient (e.g., data-gathering, counseling) | Scoring form (e.g., Mini-CEX) with Likert scale and verbal feedback | Low-moderate | Low/high | Triggers readily available; woven into patient care and instruction | Coordination of encounter with learner, patient, and observer availability; observer training improves observation skills | Internal medicine residency milestones | Ability to select correct data to gather while conducting a history and physical examination; involvement of patient in shared decision-making; formative feedback |
| Global assessments | Interactions over the course of a clinical rotation | Scoring form, typically with Likert scale and narrative comments | Low- moderate | Low/moderate | Triggers readily available; woven into patient care and instruction | Reliability low and affected by factors unrelated to the learner | End-of-rotation assessment of medical students, residents, fellows, and faculty | Summative assessment for clinical rotations |

Mini-CEX = Mini-Clinical Evaluation Exercise; OSCE = objective structured clinical examination; SP = standardized patient; USMLE = United States Medical Licensing Examination.

*In general, reliability increases with increased number of items, and therefore longer assessment time. For the purposes of this table, reliability was estimated according to reports within a typical amount of assessment time. For learners on longer clinical rotations, a sufficient number of workplace-based assessments may be gathered to increase reliability.

†For resource intensity description, see Box 3.

‡General recommendations; specific tools may be useful for additional purposes.

Box 6-3. Resource Intensity for the Standardized Methods for Assessing Clinical Skills of Medical Trainees*

Development
- ► Low: No prior preparation required to develop the stimulus/response options (it is already available)
- ► Moderate: Some preparation required to develop the stimulus/response options
- ► High: Significant preparation required to develop the stimulus/response options

Administration
- ► Low:
  - No or little time required to administer and/or score the response (e.g., automatically scored)
  - May require proctoring, but not necessarily by faculty
- ► Moderate:
  - Some faculty time required to administer the assessment tool and/or score the response OR
  - Some resources not routinely available during patient care required to administer the assessment tool and/or score the response
- ► High:
  - Significant faculty time required to administer the assessment tool and/or score the response OR
  - Significant resources not routinely available during patient care required to administer the assessment tool and/or score the response

*See Table 2.

---

stem with predetermined options ("selected response") or free text ("constructed response"). In assessing a learner with a standardized or real patient, the response may be direct observation of the learner's bedside assessment, an oral presentation, or a written note.

Standardized Examinations

Multiple-Choice Questions

Multiple-choice questions are perhaps the most widely known standardized testing format and are frequently used in high-stakes testing in the United States, as well as in lower-stakes, locally developed exams. To assess clinical reasoning, the stimulus is typically a clinical vignette, followed by a question and a short list of answer options, usually 3 to 5. The response is a single best answer.

Because multiple content areas can be tested in a short period, multiple-choice exams can have high reliability. Performance on multiple-choice examinations in medical training predicts performance on future multiple-choice examinations (46, 47), and limited data show a positive correlation with practice performance (48). In comparison to questions with free text responses, multiple-choice questions can cue learners (49). However, the cuing effect depends on the difficulty of the question; on difficult questions, learners are more likely to be cued to the correct response, while on easy questions, learners are more likely to be cued to an incorrect response (49). The single-best-answer response format limits the types of questions that can be written, and many locally developed exams have item-writing flaws and/or few validity data (50, 51). However, an excellent resource for writing high-quality multiple-choice questions is available from the National Board of Medical Examiners (52). Another resource provides guidance on the creative process of developing material for test questions (53).

Key Features Exams
The key features approach was originally designed to replace longer cases known as Patient Management Problems, which are now obsolete as a form of standardized testing (16). Key features are defined as the critical steps in identifying or resolving a clinical problem (54). Long cases are distilled down to the key branch points in clinical decision-making, where identifying a critical piece of information would lead to a correct diagnosis or a crucial step in the management would determine the patient's outcome (16). The stimulus is a case vignette, and the learner may be asked 1 or multiple questions (usually 2 to 3) about the case (55). The responses may be free text or selected from a predetermined list.

The scoring of key features exams is different from scoring of multiple-choice exams. Multiple correct responses may be allowed if selecting multiple options would be expected in an authentic scenario, although only the key features earn points. Partial credit is provided for each key feature, although each full case counts equally within the exam. Decisions that might harm the patient ("poison responses") can cause loss of all points for a key feature, but not the full case (56). Computer formats, where answers cannot be changed after they are submitted, allow the case to unfold with new information. Computer-based exams with predetermined lists of options can be scored automatically (57, 58), but free text responses must be scored manually.

Key features exams are used for the high-stakes Canadian Qualifying Exam at the end of medical school (16) and in other high- (59) and moderate-stakes (58, 60, 61) settings but are seldom used in the United States (62). Performance on key features cases is significantly associated with performance in clinical practice, including likelihood of a retained complaint against a practitioner, and likelihood of patient adherence to antihypertensive regimens (1, 63).

Disadvantages of key features exams include the extensive training required to develop the cases and the complexity of the scoring system. There are several excellent guidelines for designing and writing key features cases (56, 59, 64).

Extended-Matching Items

EMIs are similar to multiple-choice items in that each question has a single best answer (65). A set of 2 or more clinical vignettes is used as the stimulus. All the vignettes in a group are arranged to assess content in a similar subject area (e.g., pneumonia). All vignettes in a group share a single, longer set of answer options; 8 options provide optimal discrimination among learners within a limited testing time (66).

Advantages of the EMI format include the ability to test diagnostic reasoning for a variety of clinical presentations in a short period and the high reliability (67). In addition, the lists of answer options do not cause a cuing effect (67). The National Board of Medical Examiners provides an excellent resource on writing high-quality EMIs (52).

Script Concordance Tests

Script concordance tests assess the ability to interpret new data in a constructed scenario (68). The script concordance test evolved from illness script theory (69). Illness scripts are ways of organizing information about an illness, such as the clinical features, epidemiology, management, and underlying pathophysiology (70). Illness scripts become richer with increased experience, and performance on script concordance tests tends to improve with experience (71). However, illness scripts are idiosyncratic; one expert's path to a correct answer may differ from another's; therefore, the exam is scored based on responses by a panel of multiple experts (72).

The stimulus is a brief case vignette followed a hypothesis (e.g., a potential diagnosis or management plan) (73). Then the examinee is given an additional piece of data (e.g., a physical finding or laboratory result) and asked in which direction (negative or positive) and to what degree the new data affect the likelihood of the hypothesis (73). The response is in the form of a Likert scale, usually with 5 points, including a neutral response (from −2 to +2) (73). Each vignette may be followed by multiple questions. Multiple guidelines on constructing script concordance tests are available (74, 75).

There are many different approaches to scoring script concordance tests. The most common is to give the test to a panel of 10 to 15 experts, then use their responses to weigh each response (72). For example, if 60% of experts choose one option and 40% choose another option, then examinees who choose the first option receive full credit for the item and examinees who choose the latter option receive partial credit.

An advantage of script concordance tests is that they enable the assessment of clinical reasoning in scenarios where experts may reasonably disagree on the correct answer. Multiple content areas can be tested in a short period, increasing the reliability of the exam (68). However, there are several areas of controversy. Many sources of error may not be reflected in reliability estimates, including interpanel, interpanelist, and test–retest measurement error (76). Examinees may improve their scores simply by avoiding the extreme ends of the Likert scales (76). Reference panelists may answer questions differently because of deficits in factual knowledge (76), and the composition of the panel (direct supervisors versus other in the community) can affect scores (77). The optimal approach to scoring is disputed (78, 79), as is the assumption that script concordance tests assess only clinical reasoning and not other dimensions (80).

Short-Answer Essays

A short-answer essay may have a variety of stimuli, such as a clinical vignette, a question about an individual's own experience with a case, or a question asking the learner to compare different management approaches to a clinical problem (81). The response is free text.

An advantage of the short-answer essay is that it allows the learner to articulate his or her thinking process and provide more complex explanations than formats with predetermined lists of answer options. This is especially important for assessing reasoning with complex clinical scenarios that do not have a clear, correct answer (82). Learners tend to use scheme-inductive reasoning, as opposed to hypothetico-deductive reasoning, to answer essay questions (83). A disadvantage is that each essay must be scored manually. A scoring rubric or guidelines about content, format, and clarity are typically developed as a guide (81), but the consistency of scoring has been questioned for decades (82, 84). Because of the time necessary to complete each essay, the breadth of content domains that can be tested in a given amount of time is limited. In general, essay questions are best suited for assessing depth, rather than breadth, of reasoning.

Clinical Reasoning Problems
With a clinical reasoning problem, a brief clinical vignette is provided as the stimulus, and learners are then asked to provide their leading differential diagnosis (85). In some forms, the learner is asked to list the key findings, and in some forms the key findings are provided. The examinee is asked to estimate in which direction and to what degree each key finding affects the likelihood of each diagnosis, typically using a 5-point Likert scale from −2 to 2+. The exam is scored similarly to a script concordance test.

An advantage of clinical reasoning problems is that they avoid cuing by asking the examinee to develop a differential diagnosis. They may be useful for understanding examinees' illness scripts. A scoring rubric must be developed to accommodate variations in how the diagnoses are described (e.g., "CHF" versus "acute systolic congestive heart failure"). Scoring must be done manually or with sophisticated computer programming. Studies of clinical reasoning problems have shown improvement in performance with progression through medical school, but no validity data are available outside of medical student education (85, 86).

Concept Maps
Concept maps are designed to assess the structure and depth of knowledge about a clinical topic (87). The stimulus is simple; learners are asked to map their knowledge of a topic, using nodes and arrows with propositions to illustrate how different concepts interact with each other. They may show hierarchies, crosslinks, and examples. For example, if asked about deep venous thrombosis, a learner may map out predisposing factors; rank the importance of inciting factors; and show the clotting cascade, diagnostic tools, and treatment regimens. Scoring can be performed in different ways (87–90), but combining the number of propositions with the quality or importance of propositions gives the highest reliability (89). Concept maps have been used with medical students for assessment (90) and to enhance critical thinking in problem-based learning (91) and with residents (87, 89).

An advantage of concept maps is that, rather than simply assessing whether a learner has the right answer to a question, it assesses the correctness, richness, and organization of knowledge about a more general topic. Disadvantages are that each question takes time to answer, limiting the amount of content that can be assessed; approximately 4 to 5 sessions were needed to achieve adequate reliability (89). Learners must be trained in the mapping approach (88, 89). Faculty must be trained in the scoring approach, and it takes time for faculty to score the results. In 1 study, rater variation was low (89), and in another, inter-rater reliability improved with improvement in the quality of the maps (87).

Oral Exams

In an oral exam, the examinee must respond verbally to a series of questions presented by the examiners. The stimulus may be a predetermined set of questions about clinical scenarios, simulated clinical encounters, or a review of the learner's records of patient care (92, 93).

An advantage of oral exams is that, like short essays, they allow the learner to articulate his or her underlying thinking processes. Oral exams also enable assessment of the learners' ability to communicate and "think on their feet." A disadvantage is that they introduce unique biases unrelated to clinical-reasoning ability. Learners' attire (94) and projected confidence (94, 95) can affect the examiners' interpretation of performance. Conducting an oral exam is also resource intense; examiners must be trained, and significant time is required for each examination (96). The breadth of content that can be tested in a given amount of time is also limited. Despite these limitations, oral exams are still used for high-stakes testing (92, 93, 97).

Objective Structured Clinical Examinations

OSCEs have some overlap with other high-fidelity simulations. In an OSCE, the learner moves through a series of stations designed to assess various clinical skills. The stimulus is typically a trained actor portraying a standardized patient (SP). The SP has a script and in some cases can mimic abnormal physical findings. Depending on the scenario, the learner may interview, examine, and/or counsel the SP. The learner is typically assessed by the SP, who can document which history questions were asked and which physical exam maneuvers were performed, and rate the learner's communication skills. Faculty examiners may score the encounter, either synchronously (with the faculty in the exam room) or asynchronously (with the faculty member observing a recording of the SP encounter). The scoring tool is often a checklist and/or a global rating scale. For additional assessment of the learner's clinical reasoning, a post-encounter form (29, 98), a note (e.g., SOAP [subjective, objective, assessment, and plan] note), or an oral exam may be included. These typically ask the learner to synthesize the case, identify the key findings, develop a prioritized differential diagnosis, and describe a plan (29).

The United States Medical Licensing Examination (USMLE) uses an OSCE for the Step 2 Clinical Skills Exam, and Canada uses an OSCE for the Qualifying Exam at the end of medical school (99, 100). Many medical schools have incorporated OSCEs into their locally developed exams (101).

Multiple studies have shown weak correlations between OSCE performance and performance on multiple-choice exams, suggesting that OSCEs assess a different construct (102–104).

An advantage of the OSCE is that it places learners in more authentic situations than does a written exam, and it requires learners to demonstrate how they would use their clinical reasoning to gather information from a patient. A disadvantage of OSCEs is that they are resource-intense to develop and administer (105, 106). SPs must be trained and are usually paid a fee for their time. Checklists or postencounter forms must be developed to score the encounter. If the stations are observed, then examiners must commit time to observing the SP encounters or grading the notes, post-encounter forms, or oral exams after the SP encounter. Raters are subject to a contrast effect bias, when the performance of previous examinees affects ratings of subsequent examinees (107). Women tend to perform better on data gathering and written communication skills (108). Some evidence also suggests a sequence effect, where actual performance changes through the course of the testing day (109). Reliability can vary but improves with increasing the number of stations (110, 111), increasing the number of examiners per station (110), and narrowing the scoring checklist to focus on actions that are most important for establishing a diagnosis, rather than rewarding thoroughness (112). Variable weighting of scores for each checklist item does not improve reliability (113).

High-Fidelity Simulations (Other Than Standardized Patients)
High-fidelity simulations can take a variety of forms. OSCEs with SPs are high-fidelity simulations; however, mannequins, parts of mannequins, or other equipment can also be used to simulate a clinical encounter or procedure. For assessment of clinical reasoning, the stimulus is often an urgent or emergent clinical scenario (114, 115). Typically a mannequin is used to simulate a patient, and other actors (known as "confederates") may portray family members or other members of the health care team. Technically sophisticated mannequins can be programmed to simulate cardiovascular and/or respiratory instability. The simulation may be followed by a debriefing, in which a trained facilitator probes the reasoning underlying decisions that were made during the scenario (116). In a 2012 survey of 90 U.S. and Canadian medical schools, 72 (80%) used simulation to assess critical thinking or decision-making (117).

Advantages of high-fidelity simulations include the capacity to assess learners' ability to "think on their feet." Because real emergencies may be infrequent, simulations provide a window into the learners' performance in seldom-observed but important scenarios (118). Because multiple learners and/or confederates may be involved in the simulation, they provide an opportunity to assess clinical decision-making within a team structure. The major disadvantage is the resources needed to develop, administer, and score the simulations (117). Technically sophisticated mannequins are expensive; administering the assessment requires trained programmers to operate the mannequin, actors, or actual health care providers (such as pharmacists or nurses) to portray members of the team, as well as faculty time to observe the simulation and debrief the examinee afterward. The advantage of high-fidelity simulation over less expensive, low-fidelity simulations for instructional purposes is heavily disputed (119, 120); however, there is little research on high-fidelity simulation for assessment purposes, and even less research on simulation for assessment of clinical reasoning. One study revealed that, unlike self-assessment of technical skills during a simulation, self-assessment of nontechnical skills (including cognitive and communication skills) correlated poorly with expert assessment (121). Another study showed poor inter-rater reliability in the assessment of nontechnical skills (122). One study showed that a weighted instrument discriminated between novice and expert learners (123). There is some evidence that, as with SP cases, a global assessment scale has higher reliability than checklists (124).

Workplace-Based Assessments

Chart-Stimulated Recall

The stimulus for chart-stimulated recall is the leaner's own records of patient care, such as an admission note. Similar to an oral exam, the examiner probes the learner's reasoning underlying the decisions documented in the patient record (125). A worksheet may be used to guide the review (125, 126).

An advantage of chart-stimulated recall is that it requires little preparation, and the content is grounded in authentic clinical cases for which the learner had responsibility. It also enables learners to articulate their underlying thought processes, which may not be as well represented in the chart (125). A disadvantage is that it requires synchronization of the examiner's and learner's schedules to implement.

Oral Case Presentations

Actual patient cases are often presented orally for instructional purposes, as in a morning report conference, or for patient care purposes, during rounds or a clinic session. There is little validity evidence for oral presentations as an assessment tool; however, 2 frameworks have been studied for presenting cases in a manner that elicits the learner's clinical reasoning. The One-Minute Preceptor (OMP) model (also known as the 5-step microskills model) is more instructor-driven, while the SNAPPs model is more learner-driven. In the OMP model, the following framework is used by the instructor when the learner presents a case (127):

- Get a commitment (e.g., differential diagnosis)
- Probe for supporting evidence (e.g., how the key findings of the case support or refute each diagnosis)
- Teach general rules
- Reinforce what was done right
- Correct mistakes

With the SNAPPs framework the learner must be oriented to presenting the case using a 6-part mnemonic (128):

- Summarize briefly the history and findings
- Narrow the differential diagnosis to 2 or 3 possibilities
- Analyze the differential diagnosis by comparing/contrasting the possibilities
- Probe the preceptor by asking questions
- Plan management for the patient's medical issues
- Select a case-related issue for self-directed learning

Neither framework has a specific scoring tool for evaluating the learners' clinical reasoning, but OMP and SNAPPS increase learners' articulation of a differential diagnosis and underlying clinical reasoning and increase faculty's confidence in being able to assess them (128, 129).

Advantages of using the oral case presentation, with or without the OMP or SNAPPS framework, are the ready availability of cases and the opportunity to weave assessment within the context of actual patient care without significantly affecting efficiency (129). A disadvantage of the oral case presentation is that patients may have been evaluated by other physicians and "handed off" to the learner (130); the oral presentation may reflect other physicians' input rather than the learner's own clinical reasoning (37).

Direct Observation of Clinical Skills and Direct Observation of Procedural Skills

The stimulus for direct observation of clinical skills or direct observation of procedural skills is an encounter with or a procedure on a real patient. An examiner observes the learner performing bedside clinical skills, such as interviewing, physical examination, counseling, or procedures. Scoring is typically done using a tool with a Likert scale and/or behavioral anchors or a checklist. The Mini-CEX tool has the most validity evidence for use in direct observation of clinical skills, although many other tools are available;

a 2009 systematic review found descriptions of 55 different tools (40). The clinical encounter is followed by a feedback session with the observer and the examinee. Direct observation may be used to determine which data the learner chooses to gather during the history and physical examination, which should be driven by their diagnostic hypotheses, or what decisions the learner makes during a procedure. The feedback session may be used to probe the learner's underlying reasoning.

An advantage of direct observation is that it can be used opportunistically in the workplace, and it may be woven into the care of a patient for whom the learner and evaluator have shared responsibility. However, direct observation requires the observers to coordinate their availability with the learner's and patient's availability. The ability to correctly identify aspects of a learner's performance with direct observation can improve with training (131).

Global Assessments
After a clinical rotation, fellows, residents, and students are typically evaluated by their faculty, residents, and/or peers. The rating form often contains a Likert scale or behavioral checklists and spaces for providing narrative comments.

An advantage of global assessments is that they are based on authentic day-to-day performance in the workplace. Many factors can affect the accuracy of global assessments, including the likability of the learner, gender discordance with the assessor, the leniency or stringency of the assessor, and the delay in time between assessment and completion of the form (37). However, the reliability of global assessments can be improved using guidelines outlined in Table 6-2.

❖ Future Directions in Assessment

Several potential future directions in the assessment of clinical reasoning are worth mentioning here. Some of these are discussed in other chapters and therefore are only briefly mentioned below. As discussed earlier in this chapter, assessing clinical reasoning is challenging because of the nature of our current approaches, which are based on inferences about what the individual decision-maker is thinking. With this in mind we propose that future efforts need to be better informed by theory, incorporate intermediate steps, be more situated in the workplace, and more closely align with biology. The experience with the Patient Management Problem format, in which widespread implementation preceded fundamental research, shows that developing theoretical foundations for assessment tools may reduce waste of money, time, and resources.

Advancing the theory of clinical reasoning offers assessment opportunities, as theory can serve as a "lens" or perspective for our assessment approaches with predictions that can be tested. As per the theoretical concepts in Chapter 3, clinical reasoning theory is broad in its origins and development; however, much remains to be learned for the teaching of clinical reasoning. Examples include the need for additional theory to help assess how learners develop clinical reasoning, as well as what happens to clinical reasoning ability as physicians age. Our theories are also limited by the focus on the individual decision-maker as opposed to the system, culture, and teams (see Chapter 3). Theory can and should drive the development as well as the evaluation of the tools that we construct to assess clinical reasoning. Some of the theories that offer promise to the future assessment of clinical reasoning include self-regulated learning, situativity, cognitive load, and dual process (described in more detail in Chapter 3).

Another future direction is incorporating the intermediate steps in the process. We are learning that clinical reasoning is not a singular process (an individual can use multiple paths and strategies to arrive at the "answers") and thus assessing intermediate steps (optimally theoretically driven) could lead to important advances in our assessment of clinical reasoning. This becomes even more important, we believe, with moving from diagnostic reasoning (where there are a limited number of answers or a single potential answer for a patient's presentation that may be arrived at through a variety of paths) to therapeutic reasoning, which must also account for the patient's circumstances and preferences. Therapeutic reasoning, by its nature, is more "value driven" or "ethics driven" than arriving at the diagnostic label and also varies more in what might constitute acceptable practice. Examples of work in this area of intermediate steps include milestones and entrustable professional activities. These approaches may help because they represent "sign posts" or intermediate steps for developing expertise in clinical reasoning (milestones) and the needed performance domains to meet these intermediate steps (entrustable professional activities). Concept maps and script-concordance tests, as well as more open-ended response queries (versus multiple-choice questions, which also have an important role), can help in this manner. Furthermore, cases that "evolve" and incorporate feedback to the leaner offer promise in this regard. Advances have been made in the topics of learning analytics and virtual patients, such as MedU and i-Human, that offer means of better understanding (and assessing) the intermediate steps and trajectories of clinical reasoning performance.

We are also learning that clinical reasoning in vitro (in a research "laboratory") can differ from clinical reasoning in vivo (in practice settings).

Theories such as situativity, which are more inclusive than standard theoretical approaches of today, offer a means to better understand what is happening in the workplace. Furthermore, studying clinical reasoning in the workplace allows us to unravel vexing phenomena, such as context specificity.

Aligning with biology also offers an important means of advancing the assessment of reasoning. After all, this is our Achilles heel—we do not directly "observe" the reasoning of the participant; we infer it from behaviors. Potential means of exploration in this regard include more directly measuring the thought processes of physicians, such as through functional magnetic resonance imaging or positron emission tomography, as well as physiologic measures of cognitive effort, such as pupil size, heart-rate variability, and galvanic skin response. While these physiologic measures may not be easily incorporated into regular practice (with the exception, perhaps, of heart-rate variability, which is becoming more feasible with mobile technology) such measurements can provide the needed reliability and validity data of assessments that could be more easily incorporated into our usual assessment practices.

REFERENCES

1. **Tamblyn R, Abrahamowicz M, Dauphinee D, et al.** Physician scores on a national clinical skills examination as predictors of complaints to medical regulatory authorities. JAMA. 2007;298:993-1001.
2. **Wenghofer E, Klass D, Abrahamowicz M, et al.** Doctor scores on national qualifying examinations predict quality of care in future practice. Med Educ. 2009;43:1166-73.
3. **Ramsey PG, Carline JD, Inui TS, Larson EB, LoGerfo JP, Wenrich MD.** Predictive validity of certification by the American Board of Internal Medicine. Ann Intern Med. 1989;110:719-26.
4. **Schuwirth LW, Van der Vleuten CP.** Programmatic assessment: from assessment of learning to assessment for learning. Med Teacher. 2011;33:478-85.
5. **Larsen DP, Butler AC, Roediger HL 3rd.** Test-enhanced learning in medical education. Med Educ. 2008;42:959-66.
6. **Harlen W, James M.** Assessment and learning: differences and relationships between formative and summative assessment. Assess Educ 1997;4:365-79.
7. **Schuwirth L.** Is assessment of clinical reasoning still the Holy Grail? Med Educ. 2009;43:298-300.
8. **Harden RM, Gleeson FA.** Assessment of clinical competence using an objective structured clinical examination (OSCE). Med Educ. 1979;13:41-54.
9. **Berner ES, Hamilton LA Jr, Best WR.** A new approach to evaluating-problem-solving in medical students. J Med Educ. 1974;49:666-72.
10. **Swanson DB, Norcini JJ, Grosso LJ.** Assessment of clinical competence: written and computer-based simulations. Assess Eval Higher Educ. 1987;12:220-46.
11. **Norman GR, Smith EK, Powles AC, Rooney PJ, Henry NL, Dodd PE.** Factors underlying performance on written tests of knowledge. Med Educ. 1987;21:297-304.

12. **Eva KW, Neville AJ, Norman GR.** Exploring the etiology of content specificity: Factors influenceing analogic transfer and problem solving. Acad Med. 1998;73:s1-5.
13. **Schmidt HG, Boshuizen HP.** On the origin of intermediate effects in clinical case recall. Memory Cogn. 1993;21:338-51.
14. **Schmidt HG, Boshuizen HP, Hobus PP.** Transitory stages in the development of medical expertise: the "intermediate effect" in clinical case representation studies. Proceedings of the 10th Annual Conference of the Cognitive Science Society. Montreal, Canada: Lawrence Erlbaum Associates; 1988:139-45.
15. **Bordage G.** An alternative approach to PMP's: the "key-features" concept. In: Hart IR, Harden R, eds. Further Developments in Assessing Clinical Competence, Proceedings of the Second Ottawa Conference. Montreal: Can-Heal Publications Inc; 1987:59-75.
16. **Page G, Bordage G.** The Medical Council of Canada's key features project: a more valid written examination of clinical decision-making skills. Acad Med. 1995;70:104-10.
17. **Case SM, Swanson DB.** Extended-matching items: a practical alternative to free response questions. Teach Learn Med. 1993;5:107-15.
18. **Charlin B, Brailovsky C, Leduc C, Blouin D.** The Diagnostic Script Questionnaire: a new tool to assess a specific dimension of clinical competence. Advanc Health Sci Educ. 1998;3:51-8.
19. **Miller GE.** The assessment of clinical skills/competence/performance. Acad Med. 1990;65:S63-7.
20. **Van der Vleuten CP, Norman GR, De Graaf E.** Pitfalls in the pursuit of objectivity: issues of reliability. Med Educ. 1991;25:110-8.
21. **Kane M.** Validation. In: Brennan RL, ed. Educational Measurement. Westport: ACE/Praeger; 2006:17-64.
22. **Elstein AS, Shulmann LS, Sprafka SA.** Medical Problem-Solving: An Analysis of Clinical Reasoning. Cambridge, MA: Harvard Univ Pr; 1978.
23. **Chi MTH, Glaser R, Rees E.** Expertise in problem solving. In: Sternberg RJ, ed. Advances in the Psychology of Human Intelligence. Hillsdale, NJ: Lawrence Erlbaum Associates; 1982:7-76.
24. **Chase W, Simon H.** Perception in chess. Cogn Psychol 1973;4:55-81.
25. **Schmidt HG, Boshuizen HP.** On acquiring expertise in medicine. Special Issue: European educational psychology. Educa Psychol Rev. 1993;5:205-21.
26. **Kahneman D.** Thinking, Fast and Slow. New York: Farrar, Strauss, and Giroux; 2011.
27. **Cronbach L, Meehl P.** Construct validity in psychological tests. Psychol Bull. 1955;52:281-302.
28. **Downing SM.** Validity: on meaningful interpretation of assessment data. Med Educ. 2003;37:830-7.
29. **Durning SJ, Artino A, Boulet J, et al.** The feasibility, reliability, and validity of a post-encounter form for evaluating clinical reasoning. Med Teach. 2012;34:30-7.
30. **Donato AA.** Direct observation of residents: a model for an assessment system. Am J Med. 2014;127:455-60.
31. **Verhulst SJ, Colliver JA, Paiva RE, Williams RG.** A factor analysis study of performance of first-year residents. J Med Educ. 1986;61:132-4.
32. **Ramsey PG, Wenrich MD, Carline JD, Inui TS, Larson EB, LoGerfo JP.** Use of peer ratings to evaluate physician performance. JAMA. 1993;269:1655-60.
33. Landy **FJ, Farr JL.** Performance rating. Psychol Bull. 1980;87:72-107.
34. **Williams RG, Klamen DA, McGaghie WC.** Cognitive, social and environmental sources of bias in clinical performance ratings. Teach Learn Med. 2003;15:270-92.

35. **Kopelow ML, Schnabl GK, Hassard TH, et al.** Assessing practicing physicians in two settings using standardized patients. Acad Med. 1992;67:S19-21.
36. **Ramsey PG, Carline JD, Blank LL, Wenrich MD.** Feasibility of hospital-based use of peer ratings to evaluate the performances of practicing physicians. Acad Med. 1996;71:364-70.
37. **Holmboe ES, Hawkins RE, Huot SJ.** Effects of training in direct observation of medical residents' clinical competence: a randomized trial. Ann Intern Med. 2004;140:874-81.
38. **Govaerts MJ, Schuwirth LW, Van der Vleuten CP, Muijtjens AM.** Workplace-based assessment: effects of rater expertise. Adv Health Sci Educ. 2011;16:151-65.
39. **Noel GL, Herbers JE Jr, Caplow MP, Cooper GS, Pangaro LN, Harvey J.** How well do internal medicine faculty members evaluate the clinical skills of residents? Ann Intern Med. 1992;117:757-65.
40. **Kogan JR, Holmboe ES, Hauer KE.** Tools for direct observation and assessment of clinical skills of medical trainees: a systematic review. JAMA. 2009;302:1316-26.
41. **Dhaliwal G.** Developing teachers of clinical reasoning. Clin Teach. 2013;10:313-7.
42. **Steinert Y, Mann K, Centeno A, et al.** A systematic review of faculty development initiatives designed to improve teaching effectiveness in medical education: BEME Guide No. 8. Med Teach. 2006;28:497-526.
43. **ten Cate O.** Nuts and bolts of entrustable professional activities. J Grad Med Educ. 2013;5:157-8.
44. **Iobst W, Aagaard E, Bazari H, et al.** Internal medicine milestones. J Grad Med Educ. 2013;5:14-23.
45. **Schuwirth L, Swanson D.** Standardised versus individualised assessment: related problems divided by a common language. Med Educ. 2013;47:627-31.
46. **Zahn CM, Saguil A, Artino AR Jr, et al.** Correlation of National Board of Medical Examiners scores with United States Medical Licensing Examination Step 1 and Step 2 scores. Acad Med. 2012;87:1348-54.
47. **Dong T, Swygert KA, Durning SJ, et al.** Is poor performance on NBME clinical subject examinations associated with a failing score on the USMLE step 3 examination? Acad Med. 2014;89:762-6.
48. **Norcini JJ, Boulet JR, Opalek A, Dauphinee WD.** The relationship between licensing examination performance and the outcomes of care by international medical school graduates. Acad Med. 2014;89:1157-62.
49. **Schuwirth LW, van der Vleuten CP, Donkers HH.** A closer look at cueing effects in multiple-choice questions. Med Educ. 1996;30:44-9.
50. **Jozefowicz RF, Koeppen BM, Case S, Galbraith R, Swanson D, Glew RH.** The quality of in-house medical school examinations. Acad Med. 2002;77:156-61.
51. **Kelly WF, Papp KK, Torre D, Hemmer PA.** How and why internal medicine clerkship directors use locally developed, faculty-written examinations: results of a national survey. Acad Med. 2012;87:924-30.
52. **National Board of Medical Examiners.** Item Writing Manual. Available at www.nbme.org/publications/item-writing-manual-download.html. Accessed March 16, 2014.
53. **Draaijer S, Hartog R, Hofstee J.** Guidelines for the design of digital closed questions for assessment and learning in higher education. e-JIST. 2007;10:1-29.
54. **Bordage G, Brailovsky C, Carretier H, Page G.** Content validation of key features on a national examination of clinical decision-making skills. Acad Med. 1995;70:276.

55. **Norman G, Bordage G, Page G, Keane D.** How specific is case specificity? Med Educ. 2006;40:618-23.

56. **Medical Council of Canada.** Guidelines for the development of key feature problems and test cases, version 3. Ottawa, Ontario: Medical Council of Canada; August 2012.

57. **Schuwirth LW, van der Vleuten CP, Stoffers HE, Peperkamp AG.** Computerized long-menu questions as an alternative to open-ended questions in computerized assessment. Med Educ. 1996;30:50-5.

58. **Fischer MR, Kopp V, Holzer M, Ruderich F, Jünger J.** A modified electronic key feature examination for undergraduate medical students: validation threats and opportunities. Med Teach. 2005;27:450-5.

59. **Farmer EA, Hinchy J.** Assessing general practice clinical decision making skills: the key features approach. Austral Fam Phys. 2005;34:1059-61.

60. **Rademakers J, Ten Cate TJ, Bar PR.** Progress testing with short answer questions. Med Teach. 2005;27:578-82.

61. **Hatala R, Norman GR.** Adapting the key features examination for a clinical clerkship. Med Educ. 2002;36:160-5.

62. **Trudel JL, Bordage G, Downing SM.** Reliability and validity of key feature cases for the self-assessment of colon and rectal surgeons. Ann Surg. 2008;248:252-8.

63. **Tamblyn R, Abrahamowicz M, Dauphinee D, et al.** Influence of physicians' management and communication ability on patients' persistence with antihypertensive medication. Arch Intern Med. 2010;170:1064-72.

64. **Page G, Bordage G, Allen T.** Developing key-feature problems and examinations to assess clinical decision-making skills. Acad Med. 1995;70:194-201.

65. **Case SM, Swanson DB.** Extended-matching items: a practical alternative to free-response questions. Teach Learn Med. 1993;5:107-15.

66. **Swanson DB, Holtzman KZ, Allbee K.** Measurement characteristics of content-parallel single-best-answer and extended-matching questions in relation to number and source of options. Acad Med. 2008;83:S21-4.

67. **Fenderson BA, Damjanov I, Robeson MR, Veloski JJ, Rubin E.** The virtues of extended matching and uncued tests as alternatives to multiple choice questions. Human Pathol. 1997;28:526-32.

68. **Lubarsky S, Charlin B, Cook DA, Chalk C, van der Vleuten CP.** Script concordance testing: a review of published validity evidence. Med Educ. 2011;45:329-38.

69. **Brailovsky C, Charlin B, Beausoleil S, Cote S, Van der Vleuten C.** Measurement of clinical reflective capacity early in training as a predictor of clinical reasoning performance at the end of residency: an experimental study on the script concordance test. Med Educ. 2001;35:430-6.

70. **Charlin B, Boshuizen HP, Custers EJ, Feltovich PJ.** Scripts and clinical reasoning. Med Educ. 2007;41:1178-84.

71. **Humbert AJ, Miech EJ.** Measuring gains in the clinical reasoning of medical students: longitudinal results from a school-wide script concordance test. Acad Med. 2014;89:1046-50.

72. **Gagnon R, Charlin B, Coletti M, Sauve E, van der Vleuten C.** Assessment in the context of uncertainty: how many members are needed on the panel of reference of a script concordance test? Med Educ. 2005;39:284-91.

73. **Lubarsky S, Dory V, Duggan P, Gagnon R, Charlin B.** Script concordance testing: from theory to practice: AMEE Guide No. 75. Med Teach. 2013;35:184-93.

74. **Fournier JP, Demeester A, Charlin B.** Script concordance tests: guidelines for construction. BMC Med Inform Decis Mak 2008;8:18.
75. **Dory V, Gagnon R, Vanpee D, Charlin B.** How to construct and implement script concordance tests: insights from a systematic review. Med Educ. 2012;46:552-63.
76. **Lineberry M, Kreiter CD, Bordage G.** Threats to validity in the use and interpretation of script concordance test scores. Med Educ. 2013;47:1175-83.
77. **Charlin B, Gagnon R, Sauve E, Coletti M.** Composition of the panel of reference for concordance tests: do teaching functions have an impact on examinees' ranks and absolute scores? Med Teach. 2007;29:49-53.
78. **Wilson AB, Pike GR, Humbert AJ.** Analyzing script concordance test scoring methods and items by difficulty and type. Teach Learn Med. 2014;26:135-45.
79. **Lubarsky S, Gagnon R, Charlin B.** Scoring the script concordance test: not a black and white issue. Med Educ. 2013;47:1159-61.
80. **Wilson A, Pike G, Humbert A.** Preliminary factor analyses raise concerns about script concordance test utility. Med Sci Educ. 2014;24:51-8.
81. **Oermann M.** Developing and scoring essay tests. Nurse Educator. 1999;24:29-32.
82. **Elstein AS.** Beyond multiple-choice questions and essays: the need for a new way to assess clinical competence. Acad Med. 1993;68:244-9.
83. **Heemskerk L, Norman G, Chou S, Mintz M, Mandin H, McLaughlin K.** The effect of question format and task difficulty on reasoning strategies and diagnostic performance in internal medicine residents. Advanc Health Sci Educ. 2008;13:453-62.
84. **Abrahamson S.** A Study of the objectivity of the essay examination. Acad Med. 1964;39:65-8.
85. **Groves M, Scott I, Alexander H.** Assessing clinical reasoning: a method to monitor its development in a PBL curriculum. Med Teach. 2002;24:507-15.
86. **Lee A, Joynt GM, Lee AK, et al.** Using illness scripts to teach clinical reasoning skills to medical students. Fam Med. 2010;42:255-61.
87. **West DC, Pomeroy JR, Park JK, Gerstenberger EA, Sandoval J.** Critical thinking in graduate medical education: a role for concept mapping assessment? JAMA. 2000;284:1105-10.
88. **West DC, Park JK, Pomeroy JR, Sandoval J.** Concept mapping assessment in medical education: a comparison of two scoring systems. Med Educ. 2002;36:820-6.
89. **Srinivasan M, McElvany M, Shay JM, Shavelson RJ, West DC.** Measuring knowledge structure: reliability of concept mapping assessment in medical education. Acad Med. 2008;83:1196-203.
90. **Azarpira N, Amini M, Kojuri J, et al.** Assessment of scientific thinking in basic science in the Iranian second national Olympiad. BMC Res Notes. 2012;5:61.
91. **Veronese C, Richards JB, Pernar L, Sullivan AM, Schwartzstein RM.** A randomized pilot study of the use of concept maps to enhance problem-based learning among first-year medical students. Med Teach. 2013;35:e1478-84.
92. **American Board of Obstetrics and Gynecology.** 2014 Bulletin for the Oral Examination for Basic Certification in Obstetrics and Gynecology. Available at www.abog.org/bulletins/current/basic.oral.bulletin.pdf. Accessed March 16, 2014.
93. **American Board of Emergency Medicine.** Oral examination description and content specifications. Available at https://www.abem.org/public/emergency-medicine-(em)-initial-certification/oral-examination/oral-examination-description-and-content-specifications. Accessed March 16, 2014.

94. **Burchard KW, Rowland-Morin PA, Coe NP, Garb JL.** A surgery oral examination: interrater agreement and the influence of rater characteristics. Acad Med. 1995;70:1044-6.

95. **Rowland-Morin PA, Burchard KW, Garb JL, Coe NP.** Influence of effective communication by surgery students on their oral examination scores. Acad Med. 1991;66:169-71.

96. **Mount CA, Short PA, Mount GR, Schofield CM.** An end-of-year oral examination for internal medicine residents: an assessment tool for the clinical competency committee. J Grad Med Educ. 2014;6:551-4.

97. **de Virgilio C, Yaghoubian A, Kaji A, et al.** Predicting performance on the American Board of Surgery qualifying and certifying examinations: a multi-institutional study. Arch Surg. 2010;145:852-6.

98. **Williams RG, Klamen DL, Markwell SJ, Cianciolo AT, Colliver JA, Verhulst SJ.** Variations in senior medical student diagnostic justification ability. Acad Med. 2014;89:790-8.

99. **Brailovsky CA, Grand'Maison P.** Using evidence to improve evaluation: a comprehensive psychometric assessment of a SP-based OSCE licensing examination. Advance Health Sci Educ. 2000;5:207-19.

100. **Tamblyn R, Abrahamowicz M, Brailovsky C, et al.** Association between licensing examination scores and resource use and quality of care in primary care practice. JAMA. 1998;280:989-96.

101. **Simon SR, Volkan K, Hamann C, Duffey C, Fletcher SW.** The relationship between second-year medical students' OSCE scores and USMLE Step 1 scores. Med Teach. 2002;24:535-9.

102. **Rifkin WD, Rifkin A.** Correlation between housestaff performance on the United States Medical Licensing Examination and standardized patient encounters. Mt Sinai J Med. 2005;72:47-9.

103. **Harik P, Cuddy MM, O'Donovan S, Murray CT, Swanson DB, Clauser BE.** Assessing potentially dangerous medical actions with the computer-based case simulation portion of the USMLE step 3 examination. Acad Med. 2009;84:S79-82.

104. **Saber Tehrani AS, Lee H, Mathews SC, et al.** 25-year summary of US malpractice claims for diagnostic errors 1986–2010: an analysis from the National Practitioner Data Bank. BMJ Qual Safe. 2013;22:672-80.

105. **Petrusa ER, Blackwell TA, Rogers LP, Saydjari C, Parcel S, Guckian JC.** An objective measure of clinical performance. Am J Med. 1987;83:34-42.

106. **Grand'Maison P, Lescop J, Rainsberry P, Brailovsky CA.** Large-scale use of an objective, structured clinical examination for licensing family physicians. CMAJ. 1992;146:1735-40.

107. **Ramineni C, Clauser BE, Harik P, Swanson DB.** Contrast effects in the USMLE step 2 clinical skills examination. Acad Med. 2008;83:S45-8.

108. **Swygert KA, Cuddy MM, van Zanten M, Haist SA, Jobe AC.** Gender differences in examinee performance on the step 2 clinical skills data gathering (DG) and patient note (PN) components. Advance Health Sci Educ. 2012;17:557-71.

109. **Ramineni C, Harik P, Margolis MJ, Clauser BE, Swanson DB, Dillon GF.** Sequence effects in the United States Medical Licensing Examination (USMLE) step 2 clinical skills (CS) examination. Acad Med. 2007;82:S101-4.

110. **Brannick MT, Erol-Korkmaz HT, Prewett M.** A systematic review of the reliability of objective structured clinical examination scores. Medical education 2011;45:1181-9.

111. **Carraccio C, Englander R.** The objective structured clinical examination: a step in the direction of competency-based evaluation. Arch Pediatr Adolesc Med. 2000;154:736-41.

112. **Yudkowsky R, Park YS, Riddle J, Palladino C, Bordage G.** Clinically discriminating checklists versus thoroughness checklists: improving the validity of performance test scores. Acad Med. 2014;89:1057-62.

113. **Sandilands DD, Gotzmann A, Roy M, Zumbo BD, De Champlain A.** Weighting checklist items and station components on a large-scale OSCE: is it worth the effort? Med Teach. 2014;36:585-90.

114. **Aylward M, Nixon J, Gladding S.** An entrustable professional activity (EPA) for hand-offs as a model for EPA assessment development. Acad Med. 2014;89:1335-40.

115. **Mudumbai SC, Gaba DM, Boulet JR, Howard SK, Davies MF.** External validation of simulation-based assessments with other performance measures of third-year anesthesiology residents. Sim Healthc. 2012;7:73-80.

116. **Arora S, Ahmed M, Paige J, et al.** Objective structured assessment of debriefing: bringing science to the art of debriefing in surgery. Ann Surg. 2012;256:982-8.

117. **Passiment M, Sacks H, Huang G.** Medical simulation in medical education: results of an AAMC survey. Washington, DC: Association of American Medical Colleges; 2012.

118. **Spillane L, Hayden E, Fernandez R, et al.** The assessment of individual cognitive expertise and clinical competency: a research agenda. Acad Emerg Med. 2008;15:1071-8.

119. **Norman G, Dore K, Grierson L.** The minimal relationship between simulation fidelity and transfer of learning. Med Educ. 2012;46:636-47.

120. **Issenberg SB, McGaghie WC, Petrusa ER, Lee Gordon D, Scalese RJ.** Features and uses of high-fidelity medical simulations that lead to effective learning: a BEME systematic review. Med Teach. 2005;27:10-28.

121. **Arora S, Miskovic D, Hull L, et al.** Self vs expert assessment of technical and non-technical skills in high fidelity simulation. Am J Surg. 2011;202:500-6.

122. **Morgan PJ, Kurrek MM, Bertram S, LeBlanc V, Przybyszewski T.** Nontechnical skills assessment after simulation-based continuing medical education. Sim Healthc. 2011;6:255-9.

123. **Lipner RS, Messenger JC, Kangilaski R, et al.** A technical and cognitive skills evaluation of performance in interventional cardiology procedures using medical simulation. Sim Healtc. 2010;5:65-74.

124. **Hall AK, Pickett W, Dagnone JD.** Development and evaluation of a simulation-based resuscitation scenario assessment tool for emergency medicine residents. CJEM. 2012;14:139-46.

125. **Goulet F, Jacques A, Gagnon R, Racette P, Sieber W.** Assessment of family physicians' performance using patient charts: interrater reliability and concordance with chart-stimulated recall interview. Eval Health Prof. 2007;30:376-92.

126. **Schipper S, Ross S.** Structured teaching and assessment: a new chart-stimulated recall worksheet for family medicine residents. Can Fam Phys. 2010;56:958-9, e352-4.

127. **Aagaard E, Teherani A, Irby DM.** Effectiveness of the one-minute preceptor model for diagnosing the patient and the learner: proof of concept. Acad Med. 2004;79:42-9.

128. **Wolpaw T, Papp KK, Bordage G.** Using SNAPPS to facilitate the expression of clinical reasoning and uncertainties: a randomized comparison group trial. Acad Med. 2009;84:517-24.

129. **Salerno SM, O'Malley PG, Pangaro LN, Wheeler GA, Moores LK, Jackson JL.** Faculty development seminars based on the one-minute preceptor improve feedback in the ambulatory setting. J Gen Intern Med. 2002;17:779-87.

130. **Lang VJ, Mooney CJ, O'Connor AB, Bordley DR, Lurie SJ.** Association between hand-off patients and subject exam performance in medicine clerkship students. J Gen Intern Med. 2009;24:1018-22.

131. **Holmboe ES.** Faculty and the observation of trainees' clinical skills: problems and opportunities. Acad Med. 2004;79:16-22.

7

Faculty Development and Dissemination

Jennifer R. Kogan, MD
Eric S. Holmboe, MD, FACP

❖ Introduction

To help ensure effective teaching, it is important that faculty are prepared to teach. This preparation is particularly relevant in the context of a changing landscape of medical education and health care delivery that requires teachers to have new competencies and to model and teach skills that they themselves might not have learned explicitly during their own training. To meet these evolving needs, faculty must acquire new knowledge and skills (1–3).

Given the centrality of effective clinical reasoning to high-quality patient care and the importance of being knowledgeable about diagnostic errors, it is incumbent upon training programs to ensure its graduates are competent at clinical reasoning (see Chapter 1 for a discussion about differentiating clinical reasoning and diagnostic errors). Therefore, educators must effectively teach clinical reasoning, provide learners with feedback, make summative assessments of competence, and remediate learners when appropriate. Educators who oversee the implementation of educational initiatives to improve trainee clinical reasoning must optimize the contributions of the teachers who are involved as educators (4). Even if there is an innovative educational program about clinical reasoning with an outstanding syllabus, clear learning objectives, exciting and novel instructional strategies, and

KEY POINTS

- Extrapolate from more general faculty development practices when creating a faculty development program about clinical reasoning because the literature on faculty development initiatives specifically focused on clinical reasoning is sparse.
- Follow the general steps recommended for curriculum development (e.g., Kern's 6-step approach) when creating a faculty development program about clinical reasoning.
- Use educational strategies in faculty development programs that have been shown to improve teaching effectiveness, such as experiential learning, opportunities for practice and feedback, peer role-modeling, and mixing instructional methods (didactic and interactive).
- Consider longitudinal faculty development programs and programs that are designed to develop and or enhance social networks and communities of practice.

well-thought-out assessment tools, efforts will be compromised if faculty are not prepared for their teaching and assessment roles (4).

While most medical educators learned history-taking, physical examination, and differential diagnosis as a part of clinical problem-solving during their own medical training, fewer have learned specific techniques related to clinical reasoning (5). Realistically, an even smaller number have been trained to teach and assess clinical reasoning or remediate learners who struggle (5). In fact, faculty's level of knowledge and skills related to addressing learners' clinical reasoning difficulties is heterogeneous (5). For example, a principal method faculty use to assess their trainees is questioning to probe clinical reasoning. These questions also are crucial for helping trainees learn clinical reasoning (6). However, faculty often fail to explore the logic and rationale behind their trainees' decisions (7). Teaching clinical reasoning is particularly challenging because educators often need to be able to deconstruct their own diagnostic thinking and explain their metacognitive processes (the awareness or analysis of one's own thinking process) in order to articulate their own clinical reasoning to their students (8). This can be very difficult to do, even when faculty have a strong grounding in clinical reasoning theory.

Therefore, to assure the effective teaching, assessment, and remediation of clinical reasoning, it is necessary to assist faculty in acquiring the requisite knowledge and skills. Faculty need to develop the teaching skills that will enable them to ask questions that emphasize components of the reasoning process, such as clinical key features and findings, and incorporate lessons from research on cognition (6). To achieve this goal, faculty development is essential because teaching clinical reasoning requires the use of a range of strategies to accommodate diverse student learners (i.e., students, residents, fellows) in a variety of teaching contexts (e.g., one-on-one versus group teaching; lecturing versus teaching in the clinical training environment) (8).

The goal of this chapter is to provide readers with suggestions for how to develop and implement a faculty development program to improve the effectiveness of their faculty's teaching, assessing, and remediating of clinical reasoning. We acknowledge, up front, the paucity of published research or commentary on faculty development focused on clinical reasoning. In fact, to our knowledge, almost no published studies describe faculty development initiatives showing that a faculty development program improves teachers' understanding of clinical reasoning teaching methods or enhances the intent or ability to use these methods (9). Additionally, there is no clear consensus on how clinical reasoning might best be taught or how it should be assessed (10). In light of these limitations, we have approached this chapter by describing what is known, more generally, about best practices in faculty development and applying that to faculty development focused on clinical reasoning. While it is an assumption, our belief is that what has been shown to work in other types of faculty development contexts can be useful for clinical reasoning. Throughout this chapter, we use the word *faculty*, which typically connotes the physicians responsible for educating medical students, residents, and fellows. However, "faculty" development programs also advance training programs, institutions, and nonphysician health care professionals.

We first provide a broad overview and rationale for why it is important to have faculty development to help prepare faculty to teach, assess, and remediate clinical reasoning. We then describe a framework, or steps, for developing, implementing, and evaluating a faculty development program related to clinical reasoning. Many of the steps required for creating a faculty development program are similar to the 6 steps advocated by Kern and colleagues for curriculum development (11, 12). When we describe instructional strategies, we highlight faculty development approaches shown to improve teaching effectiveness in general (because there is little information, as already mentioned, on faculty development specific to clinical reasoning). In doing so, we share faculty development practices that are effective in other contexts. Finally, we highlight the need for ongoing research that can inform best practices for faculty development in the future.

❖ Rationale for Faculty Development

Faculty development is defined as a broad array of activities that institutions use to renew, assist, or prepare faculty in their existing or evolving roles as teachers, researchers, and administrators (13, 14). Although faculty development often requires resources and time, precious commodities in our current training and health care delivery environment, many factors justify faculty development. First, it can enhance faculty members' abilities to teach more efficiently and effectively. Additionally, faculty development is justified because it 1) provides for the continuing professional growth of the institution's teachers, 2) is an essential component of ongoing program quality improvement, 3) advances the scholarship of teaching, and 4) is required by accreditation bodies (i.e., Liaison Committee on Medical Education and Accreditation Council for Graduate Medical Education) (4).

Faculty development specifically focused on clinical reasoning also may improve the clinical reasoning of the teachers themselves. This would further justify faculty development because it improves not only teaching skills but faculty's care of their own patients. Our preliminary research shows that when faculty are trained in the assessment of trainees' clinical skills (i.e., history-taking, physical examination, and counseling), they perceive that this training improves not just their skills as educators but also their skills providing care to their own patients (15). The same may be true of faculty development about clinical reasoning. Learning to teach clinical reasoning likely improves or enforces internal abilities that are then translated to patient care. This highlights the potential "dual benefit" of faculty development.

An important goal of faculty development is that it stimulates faculty to reflect on what they want to accomplish in their teaching and what they and their learners must do to achieve these goals. Without faculty development, faculty may view teaching and its associated responsibilities as an expectation of others, rather than a privileged responsibility (4). Faculty development can professionalize the educational activities of teachers, enhance educational infrastructure, and increase accountability (16, 17). In addition to helping faculty understand that developing a more nuanced understanding of teaching improves their continuing professional development, it also can create opportunities for participants to explore teaching and learning as an evidence-based practice (18). Individuals who voluntarily and regularly participate in faculty development 1) perceive that it fosters personal and professional growth, 2) value learning and self-improvement, 3) believe topics are relevant to their needs, and 4) appreciate the opportunity to network with colleagues (19).

Successful faculty development should ideally lead to improved teaching performance, such as acquisition of novel teaching skills, assessment abilities, and enhanced curricular planning and implementation (20). Successful faculty development also should ideally lead to improved learning outcomes for learners (20). In a Best Evidence in Medical Education (BEME) systematic review of faculty development initiatives designed to improve teaching effectiveness, Steinert and colleagues showed that faculty development has been associated with participants' increased motivation and enthusiasm for teaching and an increased self-awareness of teaching abilities (both strengths and limitations) (20). This synthesis of the evidence also demonstrated a relation between faculty development and educators' enhanced understanding of, and willingness to try, learner-centered techniques and skills that increase student participation (20). Faculty participating in faculty development to improve teaching effectiveness report increased abilities to assess learners' needs, promote learner reflection, and provide feedback (20).

❖ Steps for Developing a Faculty Development Program for Clinical Reasoning

This section describes the important steps for developing a faculty development program in clinical reasoning, including planning, implementation, and evaluation. These steps highlight how important it is that faculty development programs be systematically planned and implemented. Table 7-1 provides an overview of principles of good practice in faculty development, using Kern's framework for curriculum development and as described by McLean and colleagues (11). Because no studies have described program development specifically related to clinical reasoning, we again remind readers that the steps outlined below are presumed best practices for curriculum development and for creating, implementing, and evaluating faculty development programs to improve teaching effectiveness in general.

Step 1: Problem Identification

The first step in planning a faculty development program is to determine the purpose of the proposed faculty development. What is the problem you are trying to solve? What is the broad aim? Broadly speaking, faculty development as it relates to clinical reasoning involves 3 areas: teaching clinical reasoning, assessing clinical reasoning, and remediating clinical reasoning. Which of these areas will be important for you to cover in your faculty development program will depend on the expected roles and responsibilities of the teachers. For example, are you interested in improving the

Table 7-1. Overview of Steps for Developing a Faculty Development Program in Clinical Reasoning

Step 1	Identify the problem • Teaching, assessing, and/or remediating clinical reasoning
Step 2	Conduct a needs assessment • Faculty's own clinical reasoning skills • Faculty's skills teaching, assessing, remediating clinical reasoning
Step 3	Define goals and specific, measurable objectives • Knowledge, comprehension, application, analysis, synthesis, evaluation
Step 4	Select content of faculty development program and effective educational strategies • Include experiential learning • Present new knowledge/skills in the context of applying them to real-life situations • Allow opportunities for practice and feedback • Create informal, comfortable, flexible, nonthreatening settings • Use peers as role models • Use a variety of instructional methods (both didactic and interactive) • Consider longitudinal programs • Capitalize on pre-existing materials
Step 5	Implement the program • Consider resources • Determine timing • Identify participants • Incorporate concepts of workplace-based learning and communities of practice
Step 6	Evaluate program effectiveness • Assess outcomes (reaction, learning, behavior change, organizational/culture change) • Analyze and share findings with participants and key stakeholders

teaching of clinical reasoning? Or do you want to improve the ability of faculty to remediate learners who struggle with clinical reasoning? Are you interested in focusing on teaching clinical reasoning in the classroom or in the clinical workspace? Assessment and learning are intimately linked, as the adage "assessment drives learning" suggests. As you explore the questions regarding the focus of faculty development, be sure to also reflect on key links and areas of integration in the educational program. One strategy to help identify the purpose of the faculty development is to ask the following questions: 1) What is the current state of teaching, assessing, or remediating clinical reasoning? 2) What is the desired state? The purpose of faculty development is to bridge the gap between the current state and the desired state (11).

Step 2: Needs Assessment

Early on, when creating a faculty development program, it is important to perform a needs assessment of both faculty teachers and institutional needs to ensure that the faculty development program addresses faculty and institutional goals. This step is often missing from many faculty development programs designed to improve teaching effectiveness (20). Similar to quality improvement in clinical medicine, a needs assessment allows participants to identify a performance gap before the onset of the faculty development program. It helps ensure that faculty development content aligns with needs. A needs assessment also is important to ensure that faculty are on-board with the initiative and see the need for the development. If they do not see the need, it is unlikely they will attend a faculty development program. Engaging potential participants is valuable, particularly for faculty who are busy with multiple competing clinical, research, and academic demands. Finally, a needs assessment allows faculty to leave the faculty development program with a plan for what they will do and how they will measure the effectiveness of their newly acquired knowledge and skills (21). Table 7-2 summarizes sources of information for the needs assessment.

Faculty's Own Clinical Reasoning Abilities

For faculty to effectively teach, assess, and remediate learners, faculty themselves should possess good, if not excellent, clinical skills (22–25). That is, for their role as teachers, facultys' own clinical skills matter. Therefore, part of an initial needs assessment should be helping faculty members recognize their own approaches to clinical reasoning and what strengths and potential weaknesses they possess. This is important because some faculty might find themselves in the awkward position of having to teach content (i.e., Bayesian reasoning, taxonomy of diagnostic errors) that they themselves have not yet mastered.

There are several approaches for performing a needs assessment of faculty's own clinical reasoning abilities. Simply, one could ask faculty to complete a brief survey or self-assessment of their understanding of clinical reasoning concepts. Alternatively, one could review the growing literature to identify the common diagnostic errors that occur in clinical care (26).

Table 7-2. Sources of Information for Needs Assessment

Faculty's own clinical reasoning abilities

Literature describing common diagnostic errors in clinical care

Institutional morbidity and mortality conferences

Medical records review for undesirable outcomes (i.e., readmissions, emergency room visits)

Faculty's skills in teaching, assessing and remediating clinical reasoning

Faculty self-assessment

Educational leaders (core faculty, program directors, clerkship directors, deans, chairs)

Institution quality and safety officers

Learners (subjective needs, objective review of assessments of their clinical reasoning)

Anticipated curriculum

Potential objectives of clinical reasoning curriculum

Roles/responsibilities of teachers to meet curricular objectives

These areas could be the focus of faculty development content. Another approach would be to review past morbidity and mortality conferences at one's own institution to see how often and what types of diagnostic errors were committed in each situation. These could then be target areas for faculty development. A recent study by Singh and colleagues suggested a relatively straightforward approach to examining the potential prevalence of diagnostic errors in the local environment (27). The investigators used a systematic rubric of known factors in diagnostic errors to review the medical records of patients seen unexpectedly in the emergency department or clinic within 14 days of an index visit to the clinic. Their study found that diagnostic error at the index visit was a common cause for unanticipated returns for medical care (27). This technique can simultaneously inform a needs assessment of the nature of the diagnostic errors that can subsequently be used as part of the faculty development while providing rich data for quality improvement. However, this needs assessment approach (assessing diagnostic reliability rates) is relatively new and can be difficult to do in practice. While it may yield highly valuable information, it can be a significant undertaking requiring substantial institutional buy-in and resources. As such, most needs assessments will not use this approach; this may change, however, as the measurement field matures.

In addition to providing content for faculty development, each of these approaches could simultaneously promote faculty buy-in of the need for faculty development about their own clinical reasoning. Sharing these findings with faculty may help them to appreciate the scope of the problem and emphasize that diagnostic error is not just a trainee issue. In turn, faculty might then be more willing to reflect upon and identify their own learning needs.

Faculty's Skills as Teachers

Another important step in performing a needs assessment is to gather information on the faculty's teaching role. The faculty development agenda can be shaped by 1) reviewing the learning objectives of the clinical reasoning curriculum, 2) determining the roles and responsibilities of your teachers to meet those learning objectives, and 3) considering the topics most appropriate to cover (i.e., teaching in the clinical setting, small group facilitation, large group lecturing, providing feedback). Another strategy for performing a needs assessment is identifying the obstacles to teaching clinical reasoning. Identifying obstacles and then selecting a faculty development strategy to explicitly address these obstacles can help you get started in increasing interest for potential participants (4).

Written questionnaires/surveys, interviews, and or focus groups can be used to collect information for the needs assessment. There are at least five potential sources of information. First, prospective faculty participants could be asked to self-assess their confidence or competence teaching, assessing, or remediating learner's clinical reasoning. They could be asked broader questions, such as, "What is working well?" "What is not working well?" "What could be improved in our teaching of clinical reasoning?" Second, information could be obtained from other educational leaders within the institution (i.e., core faculty, program directors, department chairs, deans/associate deans, curriculum committees, medical education interest groups).

Third, discussions with the quality improvement and safety office may be particularly useful to see whether any patterns around diagnostic errors of trainees are common at the local institution. Fourth, learners (current or former) can serve as key informants. It can be useful to ascertain what learners perceive to be the strengths or weaknesses of their training/assessment in clinical reasoning. Learners can be asked what would be needed to improve their clinical reasoning. Eliciting learner perceptions is valuable because faculty development needs identified by the teachers may not be completely congruent with those identified by their learners. Objective measures of learner skills in clinical reasoning can also serve as a source of information that can guide faculty development content. Using formative or summative assessments of learners' clinical reasoning, such as performance on standardized tests, in-training exams, certification exams, and patient notes associated with standardized patient exams, can provide information about what is needed in faculty development. Fifth, the needs assessment could be guided by opinions or reports of national leaders in clinical reasoning. Regardless, when performing a needs assessment, it is helpful to remember that the more sources of information you acquire, the better you will be able to paint an accurate picture of actual needs.

Once you have collected all of the information from your needs assessment, you will need to synthesize the information that you have collected. It can be helpful to meet with other individuals who may be planning or participating in the faculty development to discuss the findings of the needs assessment. The goal is to identify key areas of need, keeping in mind that you will want to select areas that will be feasible to accomplish through your faculty development program. Finally, it is important to remember that in addition to performing an initial needs assessment up front, assessing faculty development needs iteratively helps address emerging needs (28).

Step 3: Define Goals and Specific Measurable Outcomes
After you have performed the needs assessment and analyzed your findings, you can identify what knowledge, skills, and attitudes will need to be acquired through the faculty development. A goal is a broad educational directive that communicates the overall purpose of the curriculum (e.g., improve the teaching of clinical reasoning in the clinical setting). Objectives are more specific educational directives (e.g., improve faculty's ability to use chart stimulated recall as a method to teach clinical reasoning).

When writing the learning objectives for your faculty development program, you should create learning objectives that will describe exactly what you want your faculty learners to be able to demonstrate after successful completion of the faculty development program. You can write objectives that describe 1) *knowledge/remembering* (ability to recognize/recall previously learned information), 2) *comprehension/understanding* (ability to grasp meaning, restate or interpret information in their own words), 3) *application* (ability to use information in new situations), 4) *analysis* (critical examination of the information, ability to separate material into component parts and show relationships between parts), 5) *synthesis* (ability to put together separate ideas to create new models), or 6) *evaluation* (ability to assess or judge value of learned information) (29, 30). As you write your objectives you should try to ensure that they are "SMART" objectives (specific, measurable, attainable, relevant, and time framed). Your objectives should be able to answer the following question: "*Who will do* (performance/behavior) *how much* (how well) of *what by when* and *where*." For example: "By the end of the clinical reasoning faculty development session [*by when and where*], each participant [*who*] will create [*will do*] one [*how much*] vignette to illustrate premature closure [*of what*]." It is helpful to refer to a list of performance verbs when writing objectives (29, 30). Many objective writing guidelines are readily available online (31).

Step 4: Curricular Content and Educational Strategies
The next step in creating a faculty development program is to choose the content of the faculty development program and the strategies that will be used to teach that content. Each of these substeps is described below.

Content of Faculty Development Programs for Clinical Reasoning
Decisions regarding the content of the faculty development program will be informed by the needs assessment that was conducted and the goals and specific measurable outcomes you identified. As mentioned previously, part of faculty development may be instructional content that helps faculty to improve their own clinical reasoning skills.

Teaching Clinical Reasoning　Given the variability in faculty's knowledge about clinical reasoning principles, it is important to make certain that faculty are knowledgeable about the components of the clinical reasoning process. For example, faculty development content might include instruction about the vocabulary of clinical reasoning, such as hypothesis generation and refinement, test interpretation, Bayesian reasoning, probabilistic reasoning, cognitive errors, treatment in uncertainty, tradeoffs between risk/benefits, treatment thresholds, analytic and nonanalytic processes in clinical reasoning, and dual processing theory (32, 33). Content could include approaches to teaching clinical reasoning (7), including how to select and use cases for teaching. The reader can use the information in Chapter 5 for additional suggestions on content related to teaching clinical reasoning. Faculty development might also review strategies to enhance clinician educators' ability to teach clinical reasoning (Table 7-3) (34).

Assessing Clinical Reasoning　Faculty development may focus on the assessment of clinical reasoning. When it comes to faculty development about assessment, one of the most important principles is to recognize the importance of training evaluators to use assessment tools. Often with new assessments, there is a tendency to focus the most time and energy on developing the assessment tool rather than training faculty to use it (35). The key to effective assessment is faculty development in assessment (36). However, little empiric research has addressed what constitutes effective faculty development to improve faculty's assessment of clinical reasoning. As such, what we describe here are steps identified as important for improving assessment in general.

Table 7-3. Areas of Focus for Faculty Development Workshops Teaching Clinical Reasoning as Based on 12 Tips for Teaching Clinical Reasoning

Tip	Relevant Content to Teach Faculty
1. Maximize learning from each patient encounter	• How to prepare learners for an encounter • How to give learners time to perform the evaluation and read/reflect on data • How to select patients on the basis of learner level
2. Minimize omission errors through active information-seeking	• How to encourage learners to do early hypothesis generation followed by confirmation and rejection • How to teach learners to avoid errors of omission
3. Capitalize on pathophysiologic knowledge to make diagnoses	• How to use pathophysiology concepts to help learners dissect complex or unfamiliar clinical problems
4. Use epidemiology	• How to highlight relevant epidemiology and disease prevalence
5. Explicitly compare diagnostic possibilities	• How to help learners build illness scripts by asking them to compare and contrast the most likely diagnostic possibilities • Teaching SNAPPS oral presentation model (45)
6. Be flexible when reasoning diagnostically	• How to teach learners to use an analytic approach to "cross-check" diagnoses identified through pattern recognition
7. Encourage learners to make commitments	• How to ask questions that encourage learners to commit to a diagnosis and develop an evaluation/treatment plan including pros/cons through stepwise questioning
8. Practice deliberately	• How to provide formative feedback to learners about clinical reasoning • How to identify additional learning opportunities that will help trainees expand their skills
9. Bring Bayesian reasoning to life	• Identify resources to help faculty calculate pretest probability

continued

Table 7-3. Areas of Focus for Faculty Development Workshops Teaching Clinical Reasoning as Based on 12 Tips for Teaching Clinical Reasoning (continued)

Tip	Relevant Content to Teach Faculty
10. Emphasize evidence-based decision-making	• How to role model evidence-based decision-making, such as doing high-quality evidence-based literature searches in the context of patient care
11. Diagnose the learners, not just the patients	• How to probe the learner to determine source of clinical reasoning difficulties
12. Be a coach	• How to role model, motivate, and provide feedback

Adapted from reference 34.

An essential step in assessment is ensuring the direct observation of the abilities that are going to be evaluated. Therefore, a potentially important content area for faculty development is elucidating the opportunities that faculty have to observe their trainees' clinical reasoning. This should also include a discussion about the barriers and constraints to the direct observation of clinical reasoning in the current system of education and patient care. This can be followed by a discussion of potential strategies to overcome these barriers. More explicitly, it may be helpful to identify how faculty can observe clinical reasoning during their direct supervision of trainees, during their indirect supervision (i.e., during case discussions), or during a review of their medical records (e.g., patient notes). Because the perspectives of assessors will always differ, decisions about how a trainee is doing require robust sampling and group decision-making. Robust sampling of tasks by a robust sample of assessors can improve the reliability, validity, quality, and defensibility of assessment decisions. However, despite the many "paths" to arriving at a diagnosis (different questions, exam sequence, selection of diagnostic tests), high-quality health care is "bounded": There are not limitless ways for trainees to have sound clinical reasoning.

An important focus of faculty development is to ensure that the teachers of clinical reasoning have a shared mental model of what effective clinical reasoning looks like. Typically, developing this shared mental model requires conversations that break down what is being assessed into its component parts. Many of the key components of effective clinical reasoning have been described and could be used as a platform for the shared mental model (see Chapter 6) (7, 37). One approach to faculty development would be to provide faculty with a pre-existing framework that articulates the various components of clinical reasoning. Alternatively, faculty could develop their own assessment framework through group discussions. This latter approach may take more time but often results in enhanced buy-in for the assessment tool.

The third step in assessment is synthesizing one's observations to make a judgment about how the trainee is doing relative to some standard. Faculty development can focus on developing consensus about how *satisfactory* is defined, preferably in descriptive terms and not the usual Likert-type scales (38). This will require covering such topics as normative assessment (judging how well an individual performed by comparing them to other individuals) versus criterion referenced assessment (judging how well an individual performed by comparing them to a set standard). Given the expanding role of competency-based medical education, there is an increased role for grounding assessment in the concepts of criterion referenced assessment based on concepts of entrustment (i.e., can the trainee be trusted to perform the skill unsupervised?) (39–41). These may be new and unfamiliar terms for many faculty. To help define *satisfactory* or *competent*, faculty development can include frame-of-reference training. Such training defines and applies the standard by which to judge performance. Some of the steps involved in frame-of-reference training include 1) reviewing examples of different performance levels of clinical reasoning, 2) judging these examples by using behaviorally based frameworks, 3) getting feedback on the accuracy of one's assessments, and 4) discussing discrepancies between scripted examples (strengths/errors) and participants' assessments (42). Faculty should receive feedback on their range of scores compared with those of their coevaluators. Training faculty to assess clinical reasoning should include assessment in straightforward cases as well as more complicated cases that involve diagnostic uncertainty and a range of reasonable diagnostic and management strategies.

Faculty development about assessment of clinical reasoning should be informed by the instruments or methods that are being used to assess learners' clinical reasoning. For example, will learners' clinical reasoning be assessed by their clinical interactions with patients, through their patient presentations, or through written notes? Will assessors be completing the Mini-Clinical Evaluation Exercise (35) or doing chart stimulated recall (43, 44)? Will they be assessing students using SNAPPS (45)? These are just a few examples to demonstrate that the strategies used to assess clinical reasoning in a training program will inform the content of the faculty development program. See Chapter 6 to learn more about approaches to assessing clinical reasoning. Content of the faculty development may also be influenced by whether assessment focuses on feedback or evaluation. Although there are recommendations for best practices in delivering feedback (46), to our knowledge no studies specifically describe how to give feedback about clinical reasoning. By breaking down the process of clinical reasoning into discrete steps with questions, however, self-regulated learning offers one potential way to do so (see Chapter 10).

Remediating Clinical Reasoning Faculty development may focus on faculty's skills in remediating learners with clinical reasoning difficulties. Some faculty may be knowledgeable about key concepts pertinent to clinical reasoning and remediation methods; however, few faculty deeply understand underlying principles (5). Given the challenges that many faculty have in remediating clinical reasoning, an important content area of faculty development may be to teach strategies that help faculty to diagnose and remediate clinical reasoning difficulties. See Chapter 9 to review practices for remediating learners in clinical reasoning that could then be taught to faculty as part of a faculty development program.

Educational Strategies

In this section we provide an overview of educational strategies that improve teaching effectiveness. We then describe how to select instructional methods and capitalize on predeveloped materials.

Overview of Effective Educational Strategies A systematic review has delineated some key features of faculty development programs associated with improved teaching effectiveness (20). Table 7-1 summarizes these features. First, experiential learning, defined as applying what has been learned during and after faculty development, practicing skills, and receiving feedback on skills, is important. Faculty need to have the opportunity to practice what they learn (20). Second, participants should receive systematic, constructive feedback (20). Third, using peers as role models and allowing participants to exchange information and ideas are valuable. Colleagues participating in faculty development together can help to promote and maintain change (20). Fourth, it is beneficial to use a variety of instructional methods to meet learning objectives, such as combining small group discussions, interactive exercises, and role plays. In continuing medical education, sessions that include both an interactive and a didactic component have the best outcomes; interactive sessions alone or lectures alone are less effective (47, 48). Fifth, longer faculty development programs that extend over time may lead to better outcomes than one-time interventions, such as short courses or workshops (20). In part, this may be related to the fact that when a group meets over time, the members can create communities of learning and networks.

In addition to these best practices, effective faculty development programs also should adhere to the principles of learning theory. It is beneficial for faculty participants to negotiate their learning objectives and drive their own educational process, techniques that have promoted learner-centeredness (49, 50). Faculty will learn knowledge and skills most effectively when they are presented in the context of applying new knowledge to real-life situations (51). Learning should not be separated from the context in which it is used (52). Indeed, the best time to learn anything is when the material is immediately useful. In addition, faculty should be motivated to learn (53). A sense of relatedness (feeling like a part or member of a community), having a sense of autonomy, and a sense of competence help drive motivation for learning (53). Because learning builds from and is linked to the environment, the situations, and the culture in which learners find themselves, it is important ensure that the learning environment aligns explicit and implicit curricula (54). Having hands-on practical experience is beneficial (55). A core method of education should be the analysis of experience (51). Faculty should have the opportunity to solve problems and transfer this experience to other situations and to practice (56). In addition, the educational setting should be informal, comfortable, flexible, and nonthreatening (51). The cognitive load (the mental energy required to think about something) should be considered so that learners have an optimal amount of developmentally appropriate work that challenges them as learners but does not exceed their capacity (57).

Selecting Instructional Methods   Given the abundance of available instructional methods that can be used in a faculty development program (Table 7-4), it is important to carefully consider which of these methods you will choose to use on the basis of your goals and objectives. Instructional methods include lectures (in-person or online), small group discussions, interactive exercises, role plays, and simulations and videotape reviews of performance. Faculty can watch DVDs or complete online training programs. Computer-based learning opportunities may be useful when faculty are distributed across sites. Through the creation of various web-based learning programs, faculty development can be customized according to the individualized needs of a given participant (58). Web-based modules can be stand-alone activities, can be combined with other learning activities, or can serve as a platform for discussion groups (59). Massive online open courses (MOOCs) may be another vehicle for faculty development (60). Recently, Coursera launched a MOOC in clinical problem-solving that contains information and instruction in teaching (61). While ultimate completion rates of MOOCs tend to be low, Lucey presented early results of the clinical problem-solving MOOC at the 2014 MedBiquitous Annual Conference (62). While Lucey reported high levels satisfaction for those who completed this MOOC, peer review of these

Table 7-4. Instructional Methods for Faculty Development

Internal faculty development programs
Disseminate journal articles or newsletters
Grand rounds
Seminars (1 h–90 min)
Standardized patients and/or standardized students
Workshops (>2 h)
External faculty development programs
Education tracks at national meetings (e.g., American College of Physicians, specialty society meetings, Alliance of Academic Internal Medicine, Association of American Medical Colleges)
Longitudinal train-the-trainer programs

Adapted from reference 7.

results and validation of this approach for its ability to improve clinical reasoning and teaching are needed.

Instruction that includes experiential learning provides opportunities for guided practice and feedback (micro-teaching). Micro-teaching and working on specific skills with the opportunity to practice are particularly well-received instructional strategies (58). Micro-teaching can occur in the clinical environment or can be simulated through the use of role plays and or objective structured teaching encounters (OSTEs). OSTEs consist of a simulated teaching scenario involving a standardized learner in which the "teacher" is given feedback, often guided by a predetermined behaviorally based scale or checklist to assess teaching performance. Frameworks to guide the use of OSTEs for faculty development have been published (63). Faculty participating in OSTEs (not necessarily about teaching clinical reasoning) have found them to be a rewarding experience and have perceived that they lead to improved teaching abilities; however, there are fewer data that OSTEs actually improve teaching evaluations or teaching performance (64, 65).

Peer coaching is a work-based faculty development method in which teachers help each other to reflect on and improve their teaching (66). One component of peer coaching is peer observation of teaching, in which a peer observes and gives feedback and support to a faculty member; the goal is for collaboration between the two individuals (66). Receiving feedback and reflection are important components of deliberate practice (see Chapter 2) (67, 68). Although peer observation of teaching clinical reasoning has not been specifically described, a study has demonstrated how peer observation of teaching problem-based learning, small group teaching, case-based teaching, and ward-based teaching was considered useful and relevant to faculty's teaching practice. In this study, peer observation of teaching was viewed as nonthreatening, and participants felt it enhanced the quality of their teaching and promoted professional development (69).

Given the abundance of available teaching strategies, it is most important to select instructional methods that are best suited to achieve the goals and objectives you have identified for your faculty development program. For example, increasing faculty's knowledge of the vocabulary of clinical reasoning might be effectively covered through independent reading or a brief lecture, either in person or through a web-based module. In contrast, increasing ability in teaching clinical reasoning during case-based discussion may be more effectively taught through experiential exercises, role-playing, or peer observation of teaching. Second, faculty development programs should use a variety of educational methods that promote experiential learning, reflection, feedback, and immediacy of application. Activities that help participants to transfer their new skills back into the workplace are important (20). As described previously, a mixed-strategy approach is beneficial (i.e., mini-lectures, group discussion, role-playing, feedback) (70, 71). It is sometimes helpful to think about instructional methods by categorizing them according to the context of learning (individual versus group) and formality (informal or formal) (72).

Capitalize on Pre-existing Materials   Given the emerging importance of faculty development, many individuals and institutions are starting to create faculty development programs focused on clinical reasoning. There is no need to "reinvent the wheel" and create a program from scratch when existing programs or resources may be available. You can find existing faculty development programs through several avenues, including searches of MedEdPORTAL (an educational repository for peer-reviewed educational tools and programs) (73), web-based searches (e.g., using key word searches, such as "faculty development" and "clinical reasoning"), or PubMed searches (4). Many medical education societies and professional societies have listservers through which to ask colleagues about their experience running faculty development focused on clinical reasoning. Finally, the Society to Improve Diagnosis in Medicine is a relatively new group that is developing and posting educational resources on their website to help faculty in teaching clinical reasoning (74). Not uncommonly, many will be eager and willing to share their educational programs, as well as their successes and challenges.

Below we provide 2 examples from the literature that describe the structure of faculty development programs specifically focused on clinical reasoning. A Google search ("faculty development" and "clinical reasoning") also yielded several faculty development workshops. Table 7-5

Table 7-5. Faculty Development Workshops for Clinical Reasoning

Workshop Title	Institution/ Facilitators	Description
Problems of clinical reasoning: diagnosis and treatment http://www.mcgill. ca/familymed/ node/1978	McGill University Dr. Daniel Ince-Cushman	The workshop will begin with a plenary session whereby participants will learn of the different types of situations in clinical reasoning that are encountered with learners in medical education; followed by in case discussions in a practical session to learn how to help learners overcome these problems. Learning objectives: At the end of the workshop, participants will be able to: 1. Name 5 types of clinical reasoning problems in medical education and for each type 2. Give examples of representative behaviors 3. Phrase questions that confirm or refute your hypothesis 4. Be able to propose remediation strategies
Teaching Clinical Reasoning Skills http://education. med.ufl. edu/faculty-development/ faculty-affairs/ faculty-development-skills-in-education/ miscellaneous-other-teaching-clinical-reasoning-skills/	University of Florida College of Medicine Jay Lynch, MD	Description: This presentation explores the notion of clinical reasoning and how to teach and evaluate such skills. The content will include attempts to define clinical reasoning, review literature regarding pedagogy in this area, and describe a specific small group strategy used during the Medicine Clerkship to develop clinical reasoning skills in 3rd year medical students. Format: This is a 30-40 minute didactic presentation which can be modified as needed for a specific audience

continued

Table 7-5. Faculty Development Workshops for Clinical Reasoning (continued)

Workshop Title	Institution/ Facilitators	Description
How to assess clinical reasoning in your learners www.med.ualberta. ca/about/faculty/ development/ teachingmastery/ clinicalreasoning	University of Alberta	Clinical diagnostic reasoning is a key component to clinical competence. However, observation and assessment of clinical diagnostic reasoning skills in medical trainees is a complex task. The learning objectives of this 90 minute interactive workshop are to provide you with a simple schematic tool to help you systematically observe, assess, and provide quality feedback on your learners' clinical diagnostic reasoning performance. An introductory inter-active presentation will outline existing evidence and conceptual frameworks regarding observation and assessment of clinical diagnostic reasoning, and demonstrate a simple schematic tool to aid in this observation, assessment, and feedback. The schematic tool will be demonstrated in several simulations of learner-preceptor clinical diagnostic reasoning scenarios, followed by a group discussion

summarizes the programs, their formats, and their objectives. One caveat with use of pre-existing materials is that not all have been peer reviewed. Therefore, careful review of materials is important before they are adopted. In addition, it is important to seek permission for materials you might choose to adopt.

Example 1: Faculty Development Workshop to Teach Clinical Reasoning
Dhaliwal described a 2-hour workshop in which the goal was "to distill

the clinical reasoning literature and use technology based analogies in an interactive format to make the [clinical reasoning] lexicon familiar for front-line teachers who promote and remediate clinical reasoning on a daily basis" (9). This faculty development workshop, which was highly rated by faculty participants and was associated with an intent to change teaching practice, has been delivered at least 19 times over 6 years to both core faculty and community faculty (9). Table 7-6 summarizes the structure of the workshop.

In the first hour of the workshop, the clinical reasoning process was simplified into 4 components that teachers could evaluate and intervene on during daily patient care discussions: data collection, problem representation, illness script contents, and illness script comparison and selection. These components were discussed through didactic and interactive exercises. In the second hour, workshop participant were divided into groups to analyze examples of 3 trainee patient presentations, each with a different clinical reasoning challenge. The cases used were 1) a trainee with excellent reasoning but a missing illness script, 2) a book-smart resident who cannot represent problems when he takes on a leadership role as a second-year resident, and 3) a student with uncertain knowledge and a disorganized differential diagnosis. Participants were asked to assess each of the 4 steps in the reasoning model and propose an educational plan for the most significant deficit.

Example 2: SNAPPS Model for Patient Presentations   Another example of faculty development to improve effectiveness in teaching clinical reasoning is teaching faculty to use the SNAPPS model for patient presentations. The SNAPPS model provides a structure for students' patient presentations. This structure can help faculty elucidate students' diagnostic reasoning and uncertainties (45). The study describing the implementation of SNAPPS suggests that faculty could learn this technique during a 20-minute, one-on-one orientation with a study investigator. This training occurred within 2 weeks of working with a student. Training included viewing an 11-minute instructional DVD explaining and demonstrating the SNAPPS technique. The faculty member had an opportunity to ask questions about the technique. Faculty also received a 3×5-inch laminated card highlighting the 6 steps of the SNAPPS technique. On the day before working with the student, the preceptor received a phone call reminding him or her that the student would be using the SNAPPS technique for patient presentations (45). Of note, students in this study were also trained to use the SNAPPS technique, so it is unclear to what extent faculty training was responsible for the effectiveness of the SNAPPS presentations. Subsequent publications demonstrated that students using the SNAPPS technique expressed twice

Table 7-6. Example of a Faculty Development Workshop Agenda for Teaching Clinical Reasoning: Content and Methods

Time	Content focus	Method/Task
15 min	Introduction • Practice describing clinical reasoning phenomena using domain-specific vocabulary	Small group discussions: 1. Describe "black box" of reasoning 2. Explain inverse association between data gathered and diagnostic accuracy
10 min	Clinical reasoning introduction • Summary of relevant literature • Clinical reasoning 4-step model	Didactic presentation
15 min	Illness script • Explore illness script structure and development • Develop analogy between illness script and computer file • Develop analogy between illness script and Wikipedia page	Dyads compare and contrast personal illness scripts for pneumonia; group discussion
15 min	Problem representation • Explore problem representation as a teaching tool • Develop analogy between problem representation and Google search terms	Dyads create and compare problem representation for a written case; group discussion
5 min	Script selection • Outline cognitive challenges that arise in script comparisons and selections • Develop analogy between Google search and results • Introduce prioritized differential diagnosis	Didactic presentation
55 min	Application of clinical reasoning model • Three case studies of learners with clinical reasoning issues • Participants diagnose clinical reasoning issue and propose educational plan to improve or remediate	Small group discussions followed by facilitated large group discussion
5 min	Summary and evaluation • Matrix of steps and teaching methods • Session evaluation	Facilitated large group discussion

From reference 9.

as many diagnoses in their presentations, justified their diagnosis more, and were more likely to contrast 2 diagnostic possibilities (75).

Step 5: Program Implementation
In this section we discuss how to implement a program. We describe how to identify necessary resources, how to make decisions about timing, and how to determine the setting and participants. We specifically emphasize the importance of incorporating concepts of workplace-based learning and communities of practice.

Resources
The type of faculty development program to be implemented will be influenced by the available resources: money, space, technology, human resources, print materials, and time. Given the benefit of experiential learning in faculty development programs to improve teaching effectiveness, resources may include standardized students, standardized patients, or video-recording technology.

Administrative support is an invaluable resource. Administrative tasks include coordinating speakers, notifying participants about the session, reserving a room, coordinating refreshments, sending out reminders (to speakers and participants), tracking attendance, making handouts, and ensuring session evaluation (or helping to obtain continuing medical education accreditation for the session). Administrative support is particularly important for sustaining longitudinal programs (4).

Resources also include faculty development speakers. Experts in clinical reasoning within the institution may be able to present at the faculty development session. However, sometimes external experts can lend credibility to a program. The value of an external speaker and enhanced credibility and validation of the topic must be weighed against the additional cost inherent in securing an external speaker (4). As resources are identified, identifying potential funding sources is necessary. Funding sources might include schools of medicine (the dean's office), offices of graduate medical education, the hospital (as part of patient quality and safety initiatives), and other departmental leadership.

Timing
In planning a faculty development workshop, it is important to decide on the timing. This is a particularly important consideration in light of faculty members' other clinical, research, and administrative responsibilities. The faculty development must be timed in such a way that individuals can actually attend.

Faculty development can occur as a 1-time seminar or workshop or as a longitudinal series delivered over time. A single workshop may be more feasible and can replace an existing conference or meeting that faculty already attend (i.e., department or division grand rounds). Alternatively, a workshop can occur at a time distinct from existing conferences and meetings. The duration of a workshop could range from an hour to a half-day or full day. Longitudinal seminars, which occur over days, weeks, or months, have the additional benefit of producing communities of learners. They also allow participants to apply new knowledge and skills and then return to the group to share experiences, challenges, and successes. This process facilitates peer learning. In addition, longitudinal programs provide opportunities for practice and reflection, essential elements of deliberate practice and the development of expertise (67).

Setting

Faculty can improve their understanding of clinical reasoning by participating in local faculty development programs that occur within the medical school, residency program, or hospital. Programs may be offered by teaching academies in their institutions. They can attend faculty development programs at regional or national meetings as well. Increasingly, social media are being used as a way to overcome the barrier of faculty being able to attend "in-person" faculty development. Social media can help to disseminate content asynchronously, and some platforms (e.g., Facebook, Twitter, blogs) can help to create communities of learning (76).

Participants

In general, faculty development programs will have groups of learners. Some faculty development programs are conducted on a one-on-one basis, rather than in a group setting (45). However, these can be time and resource intensive.

It is necessary to decide whether your faculty development program will include participants from a single discipline, specialty, or department (e.g., internal medicine) or from multiple specialties (e.g., internal medicine, pediatrics, and family medicine). Faculty development participants could include teachers of medical students, residents, and/or fellows. Including faculty from multiple specialties who teach across the medical education continuum can provide economies of scale and minimize resource utilization because multiple faculty can participate simultaneously and similar programs are not run many times in different disciplines. It is relatively easy to imagine how teaching central concepts in clinical reasoning (e.g., dual processing theory, diagnostic errors) is not necessarily specialty or trainee level specific. However, the more practical aspects of application may require groups who teach in similar contexts or have similar learners. Including members of the interprofessional care team may be helpful because clinical reasoning often occurs in teams (77).

A second consideration is thinking about whether participants are individual faculty members who may not necessarily work together or groups/teams of faculty who typically work together (e.g., a clinical practice or the general medicine hospitalist group). The creation of social networks and communities of learners is important for encouraging the adoption of the curricular innovation and sustaining it. For example, you might focus your faculty development efforts on the core faculty, who are likely to be faculty who are enthusiastic about clinical teaching, or the hospitalist group or core outpatient preceptors, who have high exposure to trainees.

Finally, it is important to decide whether participation is voluntary or mandatory. Common barriers to participating in faculty development include volume of clinical work and lack of protected time, logistic factors (such as timing and location), and a perceived lack of financial reward and recognition for teaching (19, 78). If faculty development is mandatory, it will be necessary to ensure that the program is feasible to attend and that accommodations are made to ensure attendance (e.g., relief from clinical responsibilities). A method for tracking attendance is also necessary. Regardless of whether participation is voluntary or mandatory, it is worthwhile to try to have incentives to attend (e.g., continuing medical education credit).

Incorporating Concepts of Work-based Learning and Communities of Practice Into Faculty Development
While most of the literature has described faculty development as formal, structured activities such as workshops and seminars, fellowships, or other longitudinal programs, there is an increasing focus on the role of informal learning and the value of faculty development in building communities of practice (16, 19). Because many faculty "learn on the job," work-based learning, defined as learning for, at, and from work (17), is central to the development of teaching skills. Faculty development can help faculty see their everyday teaching experiences as learning experiences and help them to reflect on these experiences with other colleagues (16). This essentially brings faculty development to the workplace itself (16).

The concept of a community of practice is also becoming increasingly important in the faculty development literature (16). A community of practice has been defined as a "persistent, sustaining social network of individuals who share and develop an overlapping knowledge base, set of beliefs, values, history and experiences focused on a common practice and/or mutual enterprise" (79). Faculty development in medical education can help educators feel they are part of a community; can help build networks among faculty members; and provide opportunities for faculty to exchange ideas, support each other; and sustain relationships (16).

Increasingly, it has been recognized that the degree to which an individual in a social network is connected to other individuals in that network significantly influences that individual's adoption of an educational innovation or new pedagogical methods (80). In fact, being connected to a community of educators may be more effective and predictive of adopting new educational innovations than participating in an educational workshop (80). Therefore, when thinking about offering faculty development programs, it is important to consider faculty members' social networks and capitalize on them to improve the implementation of medical education innovations (79). This network approach to faculty development programs seems to be important to the success of the program (81). Social networks can be created by including medical faculty with high centrality (connections to other faculty) and viewing faculty development initiatives as a way to build and maintain communities of practice (80). This approach to faculty development can be contrasted with a more traditional, linear model of faculty development, which focuses on a single teacher.

Factors That Support the Formation of Successful Faculty Development Programs in Medical Education
In implementing a faculty development program, it is important to consider factors that are important to supporting the formation of a successful faculty development program in medical education. Again, few examples of faculty development programs have specifically focused on clinical reasoning, so we extrapolate from the experiences of faculty development programs in medical education in general.

One model that supports the formation of a successful faculty development program is the fishhook model of faculty development (81). The model is based on 7 key factors: 1) environmental readiness, 2) commitment and vision of a mobilizer, 3) recruitment of key stakeholders and leaders to committees, 4) formation of a collaborative network structure, 5) accumulation of networking capital, 6) legitimacy, and 7) flexibility (81).

The success of a new faculty development program, in part, is associated with the presence of an environment that supports the educational initiative and the program (81): that is, do your institutional or program leadership and/or faculty believe that enhancing the teaching, assessment, or remediation of clinical reasoning important? Second, the program must have the commitment and vision of a mobilizer. Mobilizers actively orchestrate the initiation and formation of the faculty development program. With respect to clinical reasoning, mobilizers might be individuals who are passionate about and invested in improving the clinical reasoning of fellow faculty members and learners. Potential mobilizers might be educational leadership (clerkship, residency, or fellowship program directors or core faculty) or "master" clinicians who have reputations for being outstanding "clinical reasoners." They would likely understand clinical reasoning concepts (i.e., Bayesian reasoning). Although evidence is lacking, mobilizers may be highly respected, easily approachable, and trusted teachers who also remain active in the clinical care of patients.

A key role for a mobilizer is to identify and recruit the key stakeholders and leaders. These individuals are also interested in clinical reasoning. The mobilizers, key stakeholders, and leaders need to form a collective identity by identifying common objectives and aligning their interests (clinical reasoning) into a shared vision. Through this desired shared vision, prospective participants become motivated and are willing to invest their time, energy, and knowledge into the faculty development program. Involving key stakeholders and leaders early can enhance visibility and increase legitimacy and knowledge of local needs and access to local champions and future collaborators. This, in turn, leads to the growth of a collaborative network structure in which more faculty, divisions, or departments become involved. By making connections with others in the network, individuals can achieve more than if they had acted alone (81). Legitimacy or credibility of the program is enhanced with institutional support from key stakeholders and leaders (i.e., medical school, residency, fellowship, or hospital leadership). Finally, faculty development programs must be flexible by responding to the evolving needs of teachers and changing external conditions.

Step 6: Evaluating the Effectiveness of Your Faculty Development Program

As with any medical education program, it is important to evaluate the faculty development program. Part of evaluation includes assessing the quality of the program and its teachers. More important, and whenever possible, evaluation of program effectiveness should assess the degree to which participants acquired the knowledge and skills as set forth by the goals and objectives of the faculty development program: that is, how well have participants acquired the desired predefined knowledge, skills and attitudes? Have participants met the goals and objectives of the faculty development program (the goals and objectives articulated in step 3 above)?

As with any type of program evaluation, evaluation systems should be feasible. Feasibility benchmarks include 1) effectiveness (90% of possible evaluations are captured), 2) consistency (data are recorded and stored without degradation, 3) efficiency (no more than 10% of program director's time or administrator's time needed), and 4) cost-effectiveness (evaluation should not be more than 5% of the operating budget) (82).

There are many ways to measure the effectiveness of a faculty development program. Kirkpatrick's hierarchy (Figure 7-1) can be used to define how to measure the effectiveness of the faculty development program (83). At the base of Kirkpatrick's hierarchy is *reaction:* measuring participants' satisfaction with the faculty development program or its teachers. This tends to be the most common way to assess faculty development programs (1, 20). Program evaluation would include evaluating participants' satisfaction with the program and its teachers, perceptions of program usefulness and acceptability, and value of the activity (1).

You will need to decide how to collect these evaluations. Choices include paper or web-based evaluations. Increasingly, evaluations can be completed on smartphones or other mobile devices. You will need to decide whether to collect faculty evaluations "just in time," immediately after the faculty development program concludes, or wait until some distal point in time. Identifying which approach results in a higher response rate may help inform how to collect evaluations because a high response rate is essential to make reproducible and valid assertions about the program. Evaluation forms can be designed to collect quantitative data (numbers) or qualitative data (words, narrative).

The next level of assessment in Kirkpatrick's hierarchy is *learning:* measuring participants' change in attitudes, knowledge, or skills. In research describing the effectiveness of faculty development programs, learning is often assessed via participants' self-assessed acquisition of knowledge, skills, and attitudes (1, 20). Examples of attitudes that can be measured include changes in motivation, self-confidence, and enthusiasm

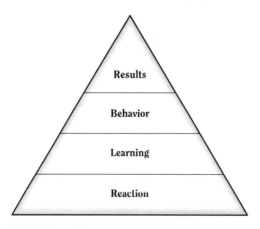

Figure 7-1 Kirkpatrick's hierarchy.

for teaching (1). Changes in participants' attitudes, knowledge, or skills can be measured through pre-post program evaluation using validated scales (11). Although common, this approach, when used alone, is not fully adequate because self-assessment is often inaccurate (84, 85).

The next level of Kirkpatrick's hierarchy is *behavior:* measuring participants' change in behavior. Behavior change can be measured in several ways. First, faculty's commitment to change forms can be reviewed. After faculty development, participants can be asked to list changes they plan to make as a result of the faculty development and rate their level of commitment (low to high) to making the change. At a predetermined point in time (e.g., 3 months later), participants can be asked whether their intended changes were complete, still in progress, incomplete, or not undertaken (86). Another way to measure behavior change is by observing and assessing participants' actual teaching, either in real time or through video review of a teaching encounter. Alternatively, faculty's skills could be measured though OSTEs. "Standardized students" have been used as a more objective evaluative measure of teaching effectiveness (87, 88). As described earlier, OSTEs are modeled on the concepts and principles used for objective structured clinical examinations (89). Although OSTEs are used in faculty development courses focused on assessing and improving faculty and residents' clinical teaching skills, they can also serve as a way to measure teaching effectiveness (90). Standardized students are trained to simulate clinical teaching challenges related to clinical reasoning. The standardized student then completes rating scales on the participants' use of effective and ineffective teaching strategies related to clinical reasoning. If desired, the standardized student, with or without a facilitator present, can provide feedback to the participant at the end of the simulated encounter. The resources needed for training standardized students and reimbursement for training and testing time are similar to those for standardized patients. Therefore, assessment of faculty development using OSTEs requires time and money.

The highest level of Kirkpatrick's hierarchy (and most difficult to measure) is *results:* measuring whether the system/organizational practice has changed. Change in the organization has 3 components. First is change in organizational culture or practices. Second is measuring whether there is a benefit to students. For example, does the faculty development improve students' ability to engage in effective clinical reasoning with fewer diagnostic errors? This could be measured by looking at how students perform on clinical reasoning exercises. Third is patient benefit. For example, do patient outcomes improve as a result of the faculty development (e.g., is there improved clinical reasoning that leads to more effective use of diagnostic testing or fewer diagnostic errors)? The approach of Singh and colleagues, which was previously highlighted, could be a potential mechanism to study change in diagnostic errors (27). However, assessing results is notoriously difficult. As such, despite the importance of measuring "results," how the organization is changed by the faculty development is rarely measured given the lack of feasibility of collecting such data.

The final step in creating a faculty development program is to report the results of the evaluation to participants and to stakeholders. This is important because it helps to identify future needs of the faculty development program. Reviewing the results of the evaluation can also identify any unintended outcomes (11). This information can subsequently be used to modify the existing faculty development program.

❖ Need for Additional Research

Given the paucity of studies on faculty development programs to improve faculty's ability to teach, assess, and remediate clinical reasoning, the medical education community must study and publish their faculty development efforts. Studies that use rigorous research methods and that are designed in the context of a theoretical or conceptual framework are needed (1, 58). When possible, these studies should not only assess satisfaction of learners and teachers but also evaluate changes in attitudes and teaching behaviors (83). Multiple sources of data should be collected with validated instruments to evaluate the effect of the faculty development program (1, 58). Understanding the effect of faculty development on the behavior of organizations (organizational culture, patient care) are lofty but important goals (1, 58).

❖ Summary

To maximize the effectiveness of faculty responsible for teaching, assessing, and remediating clinical reasoning, it is imperative to prepare faculty for their roles. It is incumbent, therefore, to have effective faculty development programs. The steps required to create a faculty development program are similar to the steps required to develop a curriculum: problem identification, needs assessment, goals and objectives, curricular content and educational strategies, implementation, and evaluation. Faculty development programs will probably need to address faculty's own clinical reasoning as well as their teaching abilities. Although evidence on the most effective strategies to use in a faculty development program about clinical reasoning is limited, evidence-based best practices are believed to enhance teaching effectiveness. These practices include experiential learning, opportunities for practice and feedback, peer role-modeling, and mixing instructional methods (didactic and interactive). There may be particular benefit in creating longitudinal faculty development programs and programs designed to develop and/or enhance social networks and communities of practice. As with any curriculum, it is very important to evaluate the faculty development program as a means of continuing quality improvement as well as to identify evolving faculty needs. Given the few existing faculty development programs specifically focused on clinical reasoning, there is great need for the medical education community to study, publish, and disseminate their faculty development efforts.

REFERENCES

1. **Leslie K, Baker L, Egan-Lee E, Esdaile M, Reeves S.** Advancing faculty development in medical education: a systematic review. Acad Med. 2013;88:1038-45.
2. **Ullian JA, Stritter FT.** Faculty development in medical education, with implications for continuing medical education. J Contin Educ Health Prof. 1996;16:181-90.
3. **Wilkerson L, Irby DM.** Strategies for improving teaching practices: a comprehensive approach to faculty development. Acad Med. 1998;73:387-96.
4. **DaRosa DA, Simpson D, Roberts N, Lund M, Marcdante KW.** 2012. Faculty Development. In: Morgenstern BZ, ed. Clerkship Directors Guidebook. 4th ed. New York: Gegensatz Press:531-66.
5. **Audétat MC, Dory V, Nendaz M, Vanpee D, Pestiaux D, Perron N, et al.** What is so difficult about managing clinical reasoning difficulties? Med Educ. 2012;46:216-27.
6. **Holmboe ES, Ward DS, Reznick RK, Katsufrakis PJ, Leslie KM, Patel VL, et al.** Faculty development in assessment: the missing link in competency-based medical education. Acad Med. 2011;86:460-7.
7. **Bowen JL.** Educational strategies to promote clinical diagnostic reasoning. N Engl J Med. 2006;355:2217-25.
8. **Groves M.** Understanding clinical reasoning: the next step in working out how it really works. Med Educ. 2012;46: 444-6.
9. **Dhaliwal G.** Developing teachers of clinical reasoning. Clin Teach. 2013;10:313-17.
10. **Durning SJ, Artino AR, Schuwirth L, van der Vleuten C.** Clarifying assumptions to enhance our understanding of clinical reasoning. Acad Med. 2013;88:442-8.
11. **McLean M, Cilliers F, Van Wyk JM.** Faculty development: yesterday, today and tomorrow. Med Teach. 2008;30:555-84.
12. **Kern DE, Thomas PA, Howard DM, Bass EB.** Curriculum Development for Medical Education: A Six-Step Approach. Baltimore: Johns Hopkins University Press; 1998.
13. **Centra JA.** Types of faculty development programs. J Higher Educ. 1978;49:151-62.
14. **Sheets KJ, Schwenk TL.** Faculty development for family medicine educators: an agenda for future activities. Teach Learn Med. 1990;2:141-8.
15. **Kogan JR, Conforti LN, Bernabeo E, Iobst W, Holmboe E.** How faculty members experience workplace-based assessment rater training: a qualitative study (in press).
16. **Steinert Y.** Perspectives on faculty development: aiming for 6/6 by 2020. Perspect Med Educ. 2012;1:31-42.
17. **Swanwick T.** See one, do one, then what? Faculty development in postgraduate medical education. Postgrad Med J. 2008;84:339-43.

18. **Calkins S, Johnson N, Light G.** Changing conceptions of teaching in medical faculty. Med Teach. 2012;34:902-6.

19. **Steinert Y, Macdonald ME, Boillat M, Elizov M, Meterissian S, Razack S, et al.** Faculty development: if you build it, they will come. Med Educ. 2012;44:900-7.

20. **Steinert Y, Mann K, Centeno A, Dolmans D, Spencer J, Gelula M, et al.** A systematic review of faculty development initiatives designed to improve teaching effectiveness in medical education: BEME Guide No.8. Med Teach. 2006;28:497-526.

21. **Thomson O'Brien MA, et al.** Show allO'Sullivan PS, Irby DM. Reframing research on faculty development. Acad Med. 2011;86:421-8.

22. **Kogan JR, Hess BJ, Conforti LN, Holmboe ES.** What drives faculty ratings of residents' clinical skills? The impact of faculty's own clinical skills. Acad Med. 2010;86:S25-S8.

23. **Govaerts MJB, Schuwirth LWT, Van der Vleuten CPM, Muijtjens AMM.** Workplace-based assessment: effects of rater expertise. Adv in Health Sci Educ. 2011;16:151-65.

24. **Asch DA, Epstein A, Nicholson S.** Evaluating medical training programs by the quality of care delivered by their alumni. JAMA. 2007;298:1049-51.

25. **Asch DA, Nicholson S, Srinivas S, Herrin J, Epstein AJ.** Evaluating obstetrical residency programs using patient outcomes. JAMA. 2009;302:1277-83.

26. **Graber ML.** The incidence of diagnostic error in medicine. BMJ Qual Saf. 2013;Suppl 2:ii21-ii27.

27. **Singh H, Giardina TD, Meyer AND, Forjuoh SN, Reis MD, Thomas EJ.** Types and origins of diagnostic errors in primary care settings. JAMA Intern Med. 2013;173:418-25.

28. **Lieff SJ.** Evolving curricular design: a novel framework for continuous, timely, and relevant curriculum adaptation in faculty development. Acad Med. 2009;84:127-34.

29. **Bloom BS, Krathwohl DR.** Taxonomy of Educational Objectives: The Classification of Educational Goals, by a Committee of College and University Examiners. Handbook I: Cognitive Domain. New York: Longmans, Green; 1956.

30. **Anderson LW, Krathwohl DR, eds.** A Taxonomy for Learning, Teaching, and Assessing: A Revision of Bloom's Taxonomy of Educational Objectives. New York: Longman; 2001.

31. **Bixler B.** The ABCDs of writing instructional objectives. Available at: http://www.personal.psu.edu/bxb11/Objectives/ActionVerbsforObjectives.pdf. Accessed 29 June 2014

32. **Kassirer JP.** Teaching clinical reasoning: case-based and coached. Acad Med.2010;85: 1118-24.

33. **Eva KW.** What every teacher needs to know about clinical reasoning. Med Educ. 2005;39:98-106.

34. **Rencic J.** Twelve tips for teaching expertise in clinical reasoning. Med Teach. 2011;33:887-92.

35. **Kogan JR, Holmboe ES, Hauer KE.** Tools for direct observation and assessment of clinical skills of medical trainees: a systematic review. JAMA 2009;302:1316-26.

36. **Van der Vleuten CPM, Schuwirth LWT, Scheele F, Driessen EW, Hodges B.** The assessment of professional competence: building blocks for theory development. Best Pract Res Clin Obstet Gynaecol. 2010;24:703-19.

37. **Audétat MC, Beique C, Fon NC, Laurin S, Sanche G.** Clinical reasoning difficulties: a guide to educational diagnosis and remediation. Available at: http://healthsci.queen-su.ca/assets/ohse/Remediation_Guide.GRILLE_ang_final1er_sept11.pdf. Accessed 15 August 2014.

38. **Kogan JR, Conforti L, Bernabeo E, Iobst W, Holmboe E.** Opening the black box of clinical skills assessment via observation: a conceptual model. Med Educ. 2011;45:1048-60.

39. **Frank JR, Mungroo R, Ahmad Y, Wang M, De Rossi S, Horsley T.** Toward a definition of competency-based education in medicine: a systematic review of published definitions. Med Teach. 2010;32:631-7.

40. **Carraccio CL, Englander R.** From Flexner to the competencies: reflections on a decade and the journey ahead. Acad Med. 2013;88:1067-73.
41. **ten Cate O, Scheele F.** Competency-based postgraduate training: can we bridge the gap between theory and clinical practice. Acad Med. 2007;82:542-7.
42. **Holmboe ES, Hawkins RE, Huot SJ.** Effects of training in direct observation of medical residents' clinical competence: a randomized trial. Ann Intern Med. 2004;140:874-81.
43. **Jennett PA, Scott SM, Atkinson MA.** Patient charts and office management decisions: chart audit and chart stimulated recall. J Cont Educ Health Prof. 1995;15:31-9.
44. **Holmboe ES.** Medical record review and chart stimulated recall. In: Holmboe ES, Hawkins RE, eds. A Practical Approach to the Evaluation of Clinical Competence. Philadelphia: Elsevier; 2008.
45. **Wolpaw T, Papp KK, Bordage G.** Using SNAPPS to facilitate the expression of clinical reasoning and uncertainties: a randomized comparison group trial. Acad Med. 2009;84:517-24.
46. **Archer JC.** State of the science in health professional education: effective feedback. Med Educ. 2010;44:101-8.
47. **Thomson O'Brien MA, Freemantle N, Oxman AD, Wolf F, Davis DA, Herrin J.** Continuing education meetings and workshops: effects on professional practice and health care outcomes. Cochrane Database Syst Rev. 2001(2):CD003030. [PMID:11406063]
48. **Forsetlund L, Bjørndal A, Rashidian A, Jamtvedt G, O'Brien MA, Wolf FM, et al.** Continuing education meetings and workshops: effects on professional practice and health care outcomes. Cochrane Database Syst Rev. 2009;(2):CD003030. [PMID:19370580]
49. **Knowles MS.** Self-directed Learning: A Guide for Learners and Teachers. New York: Association Press; 1975.
50. **Schumacher DJ, Englander R, Carraccio C.** Developing the master learner: applying learning theory to the learner, the teacher, and the learning environment. Acad Med. 2013;88:1635-45.
51. **Knowles MS, Holton EF, Swanson RA.** The Adult Learner. 6th ed. Netherlands: Elsevier; 2005.
52. **Yardley S, Teunissen PW, Dornan T.** Experiential learning: AMEE guide No. 63. Med Teach. 2012;34:e102-e115.
53. **Ryan RM, Deci EL.** Self-determination theory and the facilitation of intrinsic motivation, social development and well being. Am Psychol. 2000;55:68-78.
54. **Brown JS, Collins A, Duguid P.** Situated cognition and the culture of learning. Educ Res. 1999;18:32-42.
55. **Kolb DA.** Experiential learning: experiences as a source of learning and development. New Jersey: Prentice Hall; 1984.
56. **Regehr G, Normal GR.** Issues in cognitive psychology: implications for professional education. Acad Med. 1996;71:988-1001.
57. **Sweller J, van Merrienboer JJ, Paas FGWC.** Cognitive architecture and instructional design. Educ Psych Rev. 1998;10:251-96.
58. **Steinert Y, Mann K.** Faculty development: principles and practice. J Vet Med Educ. 2006;33:317-24.
59. **Sargeant JM, Purdy A, Allen M, Nadkarni S, Watton L, O'Brien P.** Evaluation of a CME problem-based learning Internet discussion. Acad Med. 2000;75:S50-2.
60. **Mehta NB, Hull AL, Young JB, Stoller JK.** Just imagine: new paradigms for medical education. Acad Med. 2013;88:1418-23.

61. **Lucey C.** Clinical problem solving. Coursera. Available at: https://www.coursera.org/course/clinprobsolv. Accessed 3 June 2014.
62. **Medbiquitous.** Annual Conference 2014. Available at: http://www.medbiq.org/conference2014. Accessed 3 June 2014.
63. **Boillat M, Bethune C, Ohle E, Razack S, Steinert Y.** Twelve tips for using the objective structured teaching exercise for faculty development. Med Teach. 2012;34:269-73.
64. **Julian K, Appelle N, O'Sullivan P, Morrison EH, Wamsley M.** The impact of an objective structured teaching evaluation on faculty teaching skills. Teach Learn Med. 2012;24:3-7.
65. **Trowbridge RL, Snydman LK, Skolfield J, Hafler J, Bing-You RG.** A systematic review of the use and effectiveness of the Objective Structured Teaching Encounter. Med Teach. 2011;33:893-903.
66. **Flynn SP, Bedinghaus J, Snyder C, Hekelman F.** Peer coaching in clinical teaching: a case report. Fam Med. 1994;26:569-70.
67. **Ericsson KA, Krampe RT, Tesch-Römer C.** The role of deliberate practice in the acquisition of expert performance. Psychol Rev. 1993;100:363-406.
68. **Ericsson KA.** Deliberate practice and acquisition of expert performance: a general overview. Acad Emerg Med. 2008;15:988-94.
69. **Sullivan PB, Buckle A, Nicky G, Atkinson SH.** Peer observation of teaching as a faculty development tool. BMC Med Educ. 2012;12:26.
70. **Davis D, Thomson MA, O'Brien MAT, et al.** Impact of formal continuing medical education. Do conferences, workshops, rounds and other traditional continuing medical education activities change physician behaviour or health care outcomes? JAMA. 1999;282:867-74.
71. **Amin Z, Eng KH, Gwee M, Hoon TC, Rhoon KD.** Addressing the needs and priorities of medical teachers through a collaborative intensive faculty development program. Med Teach. 2006;28:85-8.
72. **Steinert Y.** Faculty development: from workshops to communities of practice. Med Teach. 2010;32:425-8.
73. **American Association of Medical Colleges.** MedEdPORTAL. Available at: https://www.mededportal.org. Accessed 2 February 2014.
74. **Society to Improve Diagnosis in Medicine.** Clinical Reasoning Toolkit. Available at: http://www.improvediagnosis.org/?ClinicalReasoning. Accessed March 2014.
75. **Wolpaw T, Côté L, Papp KK, Bordage G.** Student uncertainties drive teaching during case presentations: more so with SNAPPS. Acad Med. 2012;87:1210-7.
76. **Cahn PS, Benjamin EJ, Shanahan CW.** 'Uncrunching' time: medical schools' use of social media for faculty development. Med Educ Online. 2013;18:20995.
77. **Holmboe ES, Durning SJ.** Assessing clinical reasoning: moving from in vitro to in vivo. Diagnosis. 2014;1:111-7.
78. **Steinert Y, McLeod PJ, Boillat M, Meterissian S, Elizov M, Macdonald ME.** Faculty development: a 'field of dreams'? Med Educ. 2009;43:42-9.
79. **Barab SA, Barnett M, Squire K.** Developing an empirical account of a community of practice: characterizing the essential tensions. J Learn Sci. 2002;11:489-542.
80. **Jippes E, Steinert Y, Pols J, Achterkamp MC, van Engelen JML, Brand PLP.** How do social networks and faculty development courses affect clinical supervisors' adoption of a medical education innovation? An exploratory study. Acad Med. 2013;88:398-404.
81. **Baker L, Reeves S, Egan-Lee E, Leslie K, Silver I.** The ties that bind: A network approach to creating a programme in faculty development. Med Educ. 2010;44:132-9.

82. **Durning SJ, Hemmer P, Pangaro LN.** The structure of program evaluation: an approach for evaluating a course, clerkship, or components of a residency or fellowship training program. Teach Learn Med. 2007;19:308-18.

83. Kirkpatrick evaluation of training. In: Craig RL, Bittel LR, eds. Training and Development Handbook. New York: McGraw-Hill; 1967.

84. **Eva KW, Regehr G.** Self-assessment in the health professions: a reformulation and research agenda. Acad Med. 2005;80:S46-54.

85. **Davis DA, Mazmanian PE, Fordis M, Van Harrison R, Thorpe KE, Perrier L.** Accuracy of physician self-assessment compared with observed measures of competence: a systematic review. JAMA. 2006;296:1094-102.

86. **Myhre DL, Lockyer JM.** Using a commitment-to-change strategy to assess faculty development. Med Educ. 2010;44:516-7.

87. **Morrison EH, Rucker L, Boker JR, Hollingshead J, Hitchcock MA, Prislin MD, et al.** A pilot randomized, controlled trial of a longitudinal residents-as-teachers curriculum. Acad Med. 2003;78:722-9.

88. **Dunnington GL, DaRossa D.** A prospective randomized trial of a residents-as-teachers training program. Acad Med. 1998;73:696-700.

89. **Prislin MD, Fitzpatrick C, Giglio M, Lie D, Radecki S.** Initial experience with a multistation objective structured teaching skills evaluation. Acad Med. 1998;73:1116-8.

90. **Quirk M, Mazor K, Haley HL, Wellman S, Keller D, Hatem D, et al.** Reliability and validity of checklists and global ratings by standardized students, trained raters and faculty raters in an objective structured teaching environment. Teach Learn Med. 2005;17:202-9.

Lifelong Learning in Clinical Reasoning

Gurpreet Dhaliwal, MD

Physicians and educators agree that clinical reasoning is at the heart of clinical proficiency and is a core ability to be mastered during training and refined throughout a career. The importance of clinical reasoning has never been in doubt, but just about every other aspect of it—what it is, how to teach it, how to assess it—has been a subject of debate. This chapter adds and addresses another uncertainty in the field: How does an individual clinician develop excellence in clinical reasoning during training and extending throughout their career?

Reasoning is a critical procedure in medicine, but unlike central-line insertion or laparoscopic surgery, the medical literature contains no established approaches to improve it. This void leaves physicians who strive for excellence in their diagnostic decision-making with conventional wisdom (e.g., "see a lot of patients" or "read"), and leaves teachers and supervisors at a loss for strategies to develop their most promising clinicians (e.g., "keep doing what you are doing").

It is no secret that years of hard work (10 years or 10,000 hours in some professions [1]) are a prerequisite for superior performance, but it is unknown what that journey looks like for the individual clinician. Almost every physician accumulates experience, so what sets apart one clinician who reaches maximal potential from another who does not?

KEY POINTS

- There are no established approaches to optimizing clinical reasoning over a physician's career.
- Professionals reach their maximal potential when they continuously engage in activities that are specifically designed to improve performance.
- Methods that other professions use to optimize reasoning and judgment include point-of-care learning/progressive problem-solving, systematic feedback on decisions, simulation training, and deliberate practice.
- These methods can be integrated into medical training programs and daily clinical practice.

CHALLENGES

- Limited time to engage in mental training methods, such as feedback
- Limited opportunities to connect with colleagues and review cases or learning
- Information technology systems that do not facilitate learning opportunities (e.g., customized feedback on patient outcomes)
- Few extrinsic rewards for clinical/cognitive excellence

❖ Lessons From Other Professions

The acquisition of expert knowledge and judgment has been explored in other professions (e.g., firefighting, nursing, military, chess) (2, 3). Three key findings warrant emphasis.

First, experience alone does not produce expertise. For most complex tasks (e.g., writing, driving, medical procedures), adults tend to improve until they perform sufficiently, efficiently, and confidently, at which time they divert their mental energy elsewhere. As their learning curve flattens (Figure 8-1) they become an *experienced nonexpert* (4). Experts operate on a different trajectory and achieve their own maximal potential because they continuously engage in activities that are specifically designed to improve performance (5).

Second, experts in dynamic fields that require complex knowledge and judgment possess a large and rich repertoire of mental models (scripts) of the issues they face at work (2, 6). These scripts (e.g., for glaucoma, gout, or pneumonia) are templates in memory that allow the physician to recognize familiar situations and adapt previous solutions (pattern recognition) or to

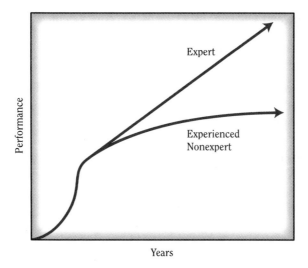

Figure 8-1 The different skill performance trajectories of experts and experienced nonexperts over a career.

identify novel scenarios that require analytical reasoning. Whether through the lens of cognitive psychology, education, naturalistic decision-making, or expertise science, a common theme emerges: Experts in professions are intentional learners who strategically strengthen their experience base (and thereby their scripts) by increasing the quantity or quality of their experiences related to real-world problems (7). This mindset and approach toward their work create a rich database from which patterns are readily recognized while fostering an adroit sense of when analysis is required (8).

Finally, decades of research have delivered this insight: It is hard, if not impossible, to teach professionals to *think* like experts, but they can be taught how to *learn* like the experts do. Once that learning takes hold, the expert thinking will follow (2).

This chapter outlines 4 mental training methods of expert professionals. Each involves a form of practice that can strengthen clinicians' experience base and improve clinical reasoning throughout a career (9). These methods make up a plan that can be adopted by practicing clinicians or trainees (and their teachers) who wish to invest their time wisely to achieve their maximum potential in clinical reasoning.

❖ Point-of-Care Learning

Physicians favor learning from the patient care problems they face at work (10). A purposeful approach to daily practice makes learning an explicit goal of the patient encounter rather than an incidental byproduct. With both routine and challenging cases, this requires deliberate mental steps to maximize script development.

Bereiter and Scardamalia characterize professional learning as a list of abilities to be acquired (4). Most professionals gradually check off the items on their to-do list (e.g., learn how to diagnose and treat cellulitis). As they develop efficiency and routinize tasks, these workers begin the path to becoming an experienced professional, and more specifically, an experienced nonexpert. Expert professionals also check off the items, but as their job becomes easier, they engage in progressive problem-solving by continually putting new challenges at the top of their list. They seek (or manufacture) problems that are slightly more nuanced or advanced versions of the ones they have recently mastered.

The typical cognitive action of an experienced physician who treats a patient with uncomplicated lower-extremity cellulitis is to activate previous knowledge, readily make the diagnosis, and prescribe familiar antibiotics. A physician with an intentional learning approach will diagnose and treat with the same expediency but will create a brief challenge where none existed: She will query a resource on mimics of cellulitis, consider how she might teach the subject better to her students, or discuss with a colleague her decision not to treat methicillin-resistant *Staphylococcus aureus*. This additional mental grappling with the case may increase the quality of the exposure and makes a stronger contribution to the physician's illness script for cellulitis. The clinician with this growth mindset habitually focuses on what is unknown rather than what is familiar in a given patient encounter (11).

An actionable goal for a clinician is to apply this form of mental engagement to a consistent fraction of cases each day. Because each day offers far more opportunities for learning than can be pursued (12, 13), the clinician must filter by some criteria (e.g., decision will affect patient outcome, a recurrent dilemma) to make the number of learning episodes realistic. The optimal time to pose a challenge or do a rapid information search is likely during or immediately after the patient encounter. Increasingly this form of real-time learning is done on handheld devices or computers, which bring efficiency but do not eliminate the barriers to information searching in real time posed by case complexity and time demands (14). Allowing days to pass, however, jeopardizes the ability to recall the critical cognitive challenge of the case and invites relegation by new, more immediate issues.

Looking up patient-driven questions in real time—the most familiar conceptualization of point-of-care learning—requires extra mental processing to make the new information stick. Efficient but intentional mental engagement (e.g., questioning, reflecting, discussing, recording) can help physicians who are so busy solving problems that they are unable to learn from the solutions (15). New learning is believed to be most effective in small increments; a small addendum of information allows the mind to review and, if necessary, undo part of its script, work with the new material, and be ready for future installments (16). A simple log of lessons learned (a minimalist version of a learning portfolio) facilitates reflection and permits re-exposure to the new knowledge in the future, either on scheduled review or at the time of future entries (17).

Almost all physicians seek to answer questions and learn in real time when patient care requires it. A physician with the intentional approach to learning develops a habit of reformulating her work into a brief cognitive challenge or problem, even when there is no immediate need to do so, in order to prepare her mind for future patient encounters. Sargeant and colleagues found evidence of this 2-track mindset in a cohort of outstanding physicians, where learning was an explicit goal rather than an incidental byproduct of work (18). This effortful and analytical approach that embeds micro-challenges and micro-learning into daily workflows makes incremental revisions and improvements to the illness scripts that drive clinical reasoning. This approach increases the likelihood that this knowledge can be accessed through nonanalytical channels in future patient care encounters.

❖ Seeking Systematic Feedback

Shanteau demonstrated that accurate feedback on decisions is essential for professionals to develop highly accurate intuition and judgment (19). Physicians make dozens of major decisions each day, but they have limited opportunities to link diagnostic and management judgments to patient outcomes. Obstacles include work patterns (e.g., rotating off service), time-limited interactions with patients (e.g., urgent care, hospital ward), and fragmentation in the health care system (e.g., readmission to another hospital) (20). When feedback is curtailed, multiple opportunities for learning and optimization are forfeited and the human tendency to equate the absence of feedback with positive feedback leads to a distorted and inflated self-assessment (21, 22).

When a physician discharges a patient with chest pain after excluding myocardial infarction but never learns the outpatient course or stress test results, he has not bolstered his knowledge or skill in assessing the likelihood of coronary artery disease. He may be fortunate to learn about outcomes by chance or through a critical event, but such random feedback is insufficient to optimize judgment. A deliberate learning approach for the same physician would be to manage patients with chest pain in the same manner, but also to check the electronic medical record monthly for his patients' recurrent admissions, cardiac events, or cardiac test results to calibrate judgments for future patients. In taking note of the outcomes he would focus analysis on the cognitive and affective factors that contributed to his decisions.

Operating under a "no news is good news" mindset conceals suboptimal outcomes and errors. All decision-makers—mediocre or great—inevitably commit errors. What distinguishes the latter group (in chess, sports, or the military) is that they methodically examine their own performance and capture as much wisdom as possible from their mistakes (23, 24).

Clinicians can develop their own systems to track decisions and outcomes (25) with a patient log, an electronic medical record alert, or planned review of discharge summaries. Physician groups can foster a culture where outcomes on others' decisions are shared routinely either electronically or at scheduled meetings. Whether this pursuit of feedback is individualized or shared among team members, dedicated time is required to search and review the electronic medical record. Handheld devices or electronic medical record systems can send reminders to clinicians at the appropriate time (e.g., 3 days or 3 months) to check the outcomes of a decision. Currently this task is left to the individual physician, but health systems should configure their health information technology systems to provide customized feedback and facilitate patient-level learning for their providers.

Importantly, outcomes must be systematically analyzed without overreaction or minimization (26–30). Physicians who make a wholesale change in their practice pattern on account of a single event are apt to fall prey to the availability heuristic, where a single salient event distorts probability assessments and errantly modifies judgment in the medium or long term. Focusing the reflection or analysis on the cognitive and affective factors that contributed to the decision (cognitive feedback) (31) rather than on the simple outcomes of good/bad or right/wrong (outcome feedback) is preferred for optimizing decision-making (32, 33). Consultation with a thoughtful colleague should be considered to increase the chance that the response and learning for future encounters are properly calibrated.

Physicians who seek to optimize their judgment should replace random feedback with a systematic method to track their decisions across a wide range of routine and complex cases. While the experienced physician becomes increasingly confident, the physician with an intentional learning approach becomes increasingly accurate.

❖ Simulation

Top chess masters spend more hours in simulation than in actual tournament play; they carefully analyze published chess games and recreate the steps of the match, playing move by move alongside the published expert (34). Top athletes regularly review films of previous games, including their own, scrutinizing minute-by-minute decisions. Pilots spend hours in high-fidelity flight simulators. Medicine has embraced simulation for psychomotor skills like laparoscopic surgery or cardiopulmonary resuscitation but has yet to do so for the cognitive challenges that define our most important procedure: diagnosis. Clinicians can test and potentially improve their knowledge and decision-making by adopting a simulation-based approach to reading published cases that arrive in their inbox and mailbox every day (35).

The cognitive demands of a simulation exercise should approximate those of the real-life task in order to contribute to the mental scripts that will be accessed in future work situations. Paper and computer cases are unlikely to replicate all of the contextual and messy features of real-world cases, including challenges of data collection, a low ratio of signal to noise in data, time pressures, and the simultaneous care of multiple patients.

In the real world, undifferentiated patients do not declare the key elements of their case or the organ system, consultant, or final test that will provide the diagnosis but still hold substantial value. These are the key challenges faced by the diagnosing physician (36). Therefore, the first step of expert learning from a case report is to recreate authenticity by deliberately avoiding the title, the specialty designation of the author, summary points prominently featured in text boxes, and early glimpses of images. Challenge and simulation follows from repeatedly stopping to solve the same diagnostic and management challenges that faced the treating physicians (like the chess master playing move by move). The reader must make a commitment at those key junctures—in his mind or in the margin of the paper—before going further, so that comparison can be made to the actual events or the authors' commentary on the case.

Likewise, when reading short vignettes or image quizzes, the clinician should adopt a simulation mindset to solve the problem without looking at the multiple-choice answers because few patients come through the door presenting a menu of options. Instead, the physician has to generate the potential diagnoses from scratch. Immediately scanning the answer options in a multiple-choice question bypasses this critical and challenging cognitive step. Much more can be learned from reviewing the answer options after generating an unassisted differential diagnosis. When the reader makes a selection in this way, he or she endures a struggle that replicates the one faced by the diagnosing clinicians. This approach, like that taken with a full-length case report, emphasizes that the journey is as important as the final destination when imprinting the clinical experience in memory (37).

This purposeful approach to reading cases is an effortful but accessible method that strengthens the clinician's experience base (38). A recent review of virtual patient experiences affirms that their greatest strength is the enhancement of clinical reasoning (39). Internet sites and medical journals publish online cases that force readers to solve them using this type of iterative and interactive manner (Table 8-1), with challenges and learning embedded throughout the case (40–42).

Table 8-1. Examples of Regularly Published Medium- and Full-Length Case Reports Available for Study

Journal	Journal Website	Section Title
The New England Journal of Medicine	www.nejm.org	Case Records of the Massachusetts General Hospital; Clinical Problem Solving; Interactive Medical Cases
JAMA	http://jama.jamanetwork.com/journal.aspx	Clinical Challenge
The Lancet	www.thelancet.com	Case Report; Morning Report at the Royal Free
BMJ	www.bmj.com	Endgames
BMJ Case Reports	http://casereports.bmj.com	Entire publication
Journal of General Internal Medicine	www.sgim.org/jgim-home	Exercises in Clinical Reasoning; Clinical Vignettes
Journal of Hospital Medicine	www.journalofhospitalmedicine.com	Clinical Care Conundrums
The American Journal of Medicine	www.amjmed.com	Images in Dermatology; Images in Radiology; Diagnostic Dilemma; ECG Image of the Month; Physical Findings
Mayo Clinic Proceedings	www.mayoclinicproceedings.org	Residents' Clinic
Cleveland Clinic Journal of Medicine	www.ccjm.org	IM Board Review
Consultant	www.consultant360.com	Multiple sections

❖ Deliberate Practice

In many professions, outstanding performers continually strive for a new level of achievement through deliberate practice. This form of training involves defining a high-value skill that lies beyond their level of competence, focusing concentration and practice explicitly on that specific task, and integrating feedback to close the gap between current and goal performance (3). Many areas of medical knowledge and skill that serve as the basis of judgment (e.g., social history, cardiac auscultation, chest radiograph interpretation) can be optimized in this way. While the original concept of deliberate practice focused on the development of specific skills, each of the aforementioned mental training methods embraces the core principle of deliberate practice, which is the consistent engagement in activities specifically designed to improve performance.

Classic descriptions of deliberate practice highlight the initial role of a coach. However, this is not practical for most physicians (43). Instead, the contemporary clinician who seeks to intentionally and rapidly improve a skill is likely to use technology in order to make deliberate practice feasible.

For instance, a clinician could record an impression of every cardiac murmur heard over a 6-month span and compare initial impressions to the echocardiogram, and then return to the bedside to auscultate the heart again. A primary care physician may have a strong desire to improve her skills in diagnosing rashes. Rather than hoping that she will get better with time, she makes improvement an explicit goal over the next 4 months. Her deliberate practice approach could include taking digital pictures of all unknown rashes in her clinic and referencing the original image when seeing the patient again in follow-up or when reviewing dermatology consultation notes. She could also sign up for a skin image to be emailed to her each week and commit to taking the quiz (in the manner described in the simulation section) until she has a 75% correct rate for 8 consecutive weeks.

We describe our daily work as being in the practice of medicine, but for enduring growth and improvement we should ask: What are we doing that is deliberate practice? Instead of waiting for incremental learning to happen from experience, a physician adopting the deliberate practice approach should seek or create high-value training experiences. An actionable goal is to always have a single skill that is being developed through deliberate practice, which can come in the form of focused self-study, arranged clinical experience, or online training. Because feedback is a defining element of deliberate practice, this strategy can be incorporated into case tracking described above (see under "Seeking Systematic Feedback").

❖ Conclusion

Many professions have established methods to improve high-stakes performance. Musicians rehearse, athletes scrimmage and practice, soldiers do drills, and pilots enter flight simulators (and in this regard, medical proceduralists have followed suit). Nothing in medicine is higher stakes than reasoning effectively, but we have yet to establish methods that refine and enhance this key ability.

Continuing medical education, licensing, and certification requirements are isolated measures that aim to maintain competence and raise the standard of the experienced professional through compulsory participation by all physicians. Conversely, committing to a program of continuous improvement in diagnostic decision-making is voluntary, with no extrinsic pressure to do so. It is also a solitary enterprise (although it can be enhanced immensely by a coach or collaboration with colleagues). In every field where it has been studied, expert performance results from sustained, individual practice rather than profession-wide actions.

An unanswered question for the clinician striving for clinical reasoning excellence has always been: Practically speaking, what should lifelong learning look like for me? Until the infrastructure of physician communities, information technology, and practice reorganization are in place to provide optimal learning environments, the strategies outlined here (Table 8-2) can provide a practical action plan for the clinician who aspires to transition from good to great knowledge and judgment.

Table 8-2. Comparison of Lifelong Learning Approaches of Experienced Nonexpert Clinical Reasoners and Expert Clinical Reasoners

Method	Experienced Nonexperts	Experts
On-the-job learning	Look up/consult when needed	Constantly examine margin of knowledge
Feedback	Random and focused on outcome only	Systematic and focused on cognition leading to outcome; regular self-audit with case log
Case studies	Occasional reading activity; casual approach to solving case	Prioritized reading activity; approach case as simulation exercise
Skill development	Expect that improvement will come with time	Self-study with deliberate practice until improvement confirmed

"Practical" refers to accessibility rather than ease. Continuous professional development demands time and effort beyond that required for daily patient care. There has never been a skill or profession where exceptional performance is achieved without extra time and effort, and there is no reason to believe that clinical reasoning is an exception to that rule (44). With practice, however, these methods can become streamlined and integrated into professional or personal routines and can replace time spent on equally time-consuming but lower-yield educational efforts (45). Training programs should consider how they might integrate these approaches into the regular curriculum (e.g., scheduled follow-up of patient outcomes, tracking of deliberate practice, faculty development to routinize point-of-care learning and challenges) so that students and residents develop these approaches as habits that take hold in the formative stages of their professional development. Training programs that foster these approaches among their faculty members and in their health care information technology system can leverage 2 powerful forces—role modeling and environment—to promote uptake of these methods by their trainees.

This learning program has limitations. Its scope is limited to the individual clinician's knowledge and judgment surrounding diagnostic decision-making. Readers and researchers are encouraged to consider how these same training methods could extend to communication and professionalism skills that are obligatory for true clinical excellence (46). The questions that are triggered by practice are often messy, convoluted, and "not in the book" and consequently require a broad range of sources of information ranging from the most reputable to the most practical (47, 48). Finally, few studies of superior performance among physicians verify these literature-based strategies (21, 49, 50). Systems-based interventions, such as cognitive training (51), diagnostic checklists (52), and computer-based diagnostic support (53), have been proposed to mitigate diagnostic error. These interventions are all derived from sound theoretical principles, but like the approaches described herein, remain to be tested and proven in medicine.

What motivates this voluntary effort to move beyond competence? Intrinsic motivators include personal quest for mastery, enjoyment from learning, job satisfaction, enhancement of teaching, and better patient outcomes. Some physicians view the charge to perform at their maximal potential as a moral and ethical duty to the patients they care for. Physicians who signal their commitment to continuous improvement of themselves and their thinking have a strong platform from which to lead, inform, influence, and motivate the professional development and activities of clinicians around them. Modern licensing and certification requirements endorse these individual learning efforts and demonstrate the standard of professional development that will be expected in the future (54–56).

Professionals can become experts—instead of just experienced practitioners—when they shift from reliable performance to relentlessly trying to improve. This distinction is not an added pressure, but it is an opportunity to shift the balance between self-assurance and self-improvement. A physician's commitment to continually monitor and improve his or her performance even when it is outwardly acceptable to others is likely a decision some make early in a career, but there is no statute of limitations on when it can be adopted and its large potential gains realized.

REFERENCES

1. **Ericsson KA, Krampe RT, Tesch-Römer C.** The role of deliberate practice in the acquisition of expert performance. Psychol Rev. 1993;100:363–406.
2. **Klein G.** Sources of Power: How People Make Decisions. Cambridge, MA: MIT Press; 1998.
3. **Ericsson KA, Charness N, Feltovich PJ, Hoffman RR, eds.** The Cambridge Handbook of Expertise and Expert Performance. New York: Cambridge University Press; 2006.
4. **Bereiter C, Scardamalia M.** Surpassing Ourselves. Peru, IL: Open Court; 1993.
5. **Ericsson KA.** Deliberate practice and the acquisition and maintenance of expert performance in medicine and related domains. Acad Med. 2004;79(10 Suppl):S70-81.
6. **Norman G.** Research in clinical reasoning: past history and current trends. Med Educ. 2005;39:418-27.
7. **Custers EJ, Regehr G, Norman GR.** Mental representations of medical diagnostic knowledge: a review. Acad Med. 1996;71(10 Suppl):S55-61.
8. **Moulton CA, Regehr G, Mylopoulos M, MacRae HM.** Slowing down when you should: a new model of expert judgment. Acad Med. 2007;82(10 Suppl):S109-16.
9. **Dhaliwal G.** Clinical excellence: make it a habit. Acad Med. 2012;87:1473.
10. **Campbell C, Parboosingh J, Gondocz T, Babitskaya G, Pham B.** Study of the factors influencing the stimulus to learning recorded by physicians keeping a learning portfolio. J Cont Educ Health Prof. 1999;19:16–24.
11. **Dweck CS.** Mindset. New York: Random House; 2006.
12. **Covell DG, Uman GC, Manning PR.** Information needs in office practice: are they being met? Ann Intern Med. 1985;103:596-9.
13. **Gorman PN, Helfand M.** Information seeking in primary care: how physicians choose which clinical questions to pursue and which to leave unanswered. Med Decis Making. 1995;15:113-9.
14. **Cook DA, Sorensen KJ, Wilkinson JM, Berger RA.** Barriers and decisions when answering clinical questions at the point of care: a grounded theory study. JAMA Intern Med. 2013;173:1962-9.
15. **Regehr G, Mylopoulos M.** Maintaining competence in the field: learning about practice, through practice, in practice. J Contin Educ Health Prof. 2008;28 Suppl 1:S19-23.
16. **Rushmer R, Kelly D, Lough M, Wilkinson JE, Davies HT.** Introducing the learning practice–II. Becoming a learning practice. J Eval Clin Pract. 2004;10:387-98.

17. **Parboosingh J.** Learning portfolios: potential to assist health professionals with self-directed learning. J Cont Educ Health Prof 1996;16:75-81.
18. **Sargeant J, Mann K, Sinclair D, Ferrier S, Muirhead P, van der Vleuten C, Metsemakers J.** Learning in practice: experiences and perceptions of high-scoring physicians. Acad Med. 2006;81:655-60.
19. **Shanteau J.** Competence in experts: the role of task characteristics. Organ Behav Human Decis Process. 2009;53:252-62.
20. **Schiff GD.** Minimizing diagnostic error: the importance of follow-up and feedback. Am J Med. 2008;121(5 Suppl):S38-42.
21. **Croskerry P.** The feedback sanction. Acad Emerg Med. 2000;7:1232-8
22. **Berner ES, Graber ML.** Overconfidence as a cause of diagnostic error in medicine. Am J Med. 2008;121(5 Suppl):S2-23.
23. **Eva KW.** Diagnostic error in medical education: where wrongs can make rights. Adv Health Sci Educ Theory Pract. 2009;14 Suppl 1:71-81.
24. **Lehrer J.** How We Decide. New York: Houghton Mifflin Harcourt; 2009.
25. **Kahneman D, Klein G.** Conditions for intuitive expertise: a failure to disagree. Am Psychol. 2009;64:515-26.
26. **Duffy FD, Holmboe ES.** Self-assessment in lifelong learning and improving performance in practice: physician know thyself. JAMA. 2006;296:1137-9.
27. **Sacchi S, Cherubini P.** The effect of outcome information on doctors' evaluations of their own diagnostic decisions. Med Educ. 2004;38:1028-34.
28. **Regehr G.** Self-reflection on the quality of decisions in health care. Med Educ. 2004;38:1025-7.
29. **Ernst E.** Science, clinical practice, and a synthesis of both. Am J Med. 2008;121:2.
30. **Crandall B, Wears RL.** Expanding perspectives on misdiagnosis. Am J Med. 2008;121(5 Suppl):S30-3.
31. **Croskerry P.** The importance of cognitive errors in diagnosis and strategies to minimize them. Acad Med. 2003;78:775-80.
32. **Balzer WK, Doherty ME, O'Connor RO.** The effects of cognitive feedback on performance. Psych Bull 1989;106:410-33.
33. **Wigton RS, Poses RM, Collins M, Cebul RD.** Teaching old dogs new tricks: using cognitive feedback to improve physicians' diagnostic judgments on simulated cases. Acad Med. 1990;65(9 Suppl):S5-6.
34. **Charness N, Krampe RT, Mayr U.** The role of practice and coaching in entrepreneurial skill domains: an international comparison of life-span chess skill acquisition. In: Ericsson KA, ed. The Road to Excellence: The Acquisition of Expert Performance in the Arts and Sciences, Sports, and Games. Mahwah, NJ: Erlbaum; 1996:51–80.
35. **Norman G.** The American College of Chest Physicians evidence-based educational guidelines for continuing medical education interventions: a critical review of evidence-based educational guidelines. Chest. 2009;135:834-7.
36. **Peile E.** Integrated learning. BMJ. 2006;332:278.
37. **Peile E.** More to be learnt from the discussion than the diagnosis. BMJ. 2003;326:1136.
38. **Peile E.** Commentary: Learning out of your depth. BMJ. 2009;339:b5180.
39. **Cook DA, Triola MM.** Virtual patients: a critical literature review and proposed next steps. Med Educ. 2009;43:303-11.
40. **Pappas G, Falagas ME.** Free internal medicine case-based education through the World Wide Web: how, where, and with what? Mayo Clin Proc. 2007;82:203-7.
41. **Peile E.** Interactive case report. Commentary: Learning from interactive case reports. BMJ. 2003;326:804-7.

42. **McMahon GT, Solomon CG, Ross JJ, Loscalzo J, Campion EW.** Interactive medical cases – a new journal feature. N Engl J Med. 2009;361:1113.

43. **Gawande A.** Personal best. Top athletes and singers have coaches. Should you? The New Yorker. 3 October 2011. Available at: http://www.newyorker.com/reporting/2011/10/03/111003fa_fact_gawande. Accessed 9 July 2014.

44. **Ericsson KA, Prietula MJ, Cokely ET.** The making of an expert. Harv Bus Rev. 2007;85:114-21, 193.

45. **Davis DA, Thomson MA, Oxman AD, Haynes RB.** Changing physician performance. A systematic review of the effect of continuing medical education strategies. JAMA. 1995;274:700-5

46. **Worrall P, French A, Ashton L.** Advanced Consulting in Family Medicine. Abingdon, Oxon, UK: Radcliffe Publishing; 2009.

47. **Cervero RM.** Place matters in physician practice and learning. J Contin Educ Health Prof. 2003;23 Suppl 1:S10-8.

48. **McDonald CJ.** Medical heuristics: the silent adjudicators of clinical practice. Ann Intern Med. 1996;124(1 Pt 1):56-62.

49. **Dhaliwal G.** Medical expertise: begin with the end in mind. Med Educ. 2009;43:105-7.

50. **Ericsson KA.** An expert-performance perspective of research on medical expertise: the study of clinical performance. Med Educ. 2007;41:1124-30.

51. **Croskerry P.** Cognitive forcing strategies in clinical decision making. Ann Emerg Med. 2003;41:110-20.

52. **Ely JW, Graber ML, Croskerry P.** Checklists to reduce diagnostic errors. Acad Med. 2011;86:307-13.

53. **Umscheid CA, Hanson CW.** A follow-up report card on computer-assisted diagnosis – the grade: C+. J Gen Intern Med. 2012;27:142-4.

54. **Institute of Medicine Committee on Planning a Continuing Health Professional Education Institute.** Redesigning Continuing Education in the Health Professions. Washington, DC: National Academies Press; 2010.

55. **Parboosingh JT, Gondocz ST.** The Maintenance of Competence Program of the Royal College of Physicians and Surgeons of Canada. JAMA. 1993;270:1093.

56. **Duffy FD, Lynn LA, Didura H, Hess B, Caverzagie K, Grosso L, et al.** Self-assessment of practice performance: development of the ABIM Practice Improvement Module (PIM). J Contin Educ Health Prof. 2008;28:38-46.

9

Remediation of Clinical Reasoning

D. Michael Elnicki, MD, FACP
Joan M. Von Feldt, MD, MSEd

❖ Introduction

The word *remediate* comes from Latin and means "to heal again." In modern usage, remediation is an attempt to "put right" or to reform through active correction of performance and/or behavior. As one educator put it, "if the goal is to help overcome their perceived deficiencies, and not simply eject them from the program, then remediation ... can be reviewed as the elevation of feedback and evaluation to a higher level" (1). Both the Liaison Committee on Medical Education and the Accreditation Council for Graduate Medical Education have directed educational programs to address the remediation of their learners (Table 9-1) (2, 3). This chapter emphasizes the identification and correction of clinical reasoning deficits, using conceptual frameworks described in Chapter 2, as a foundation on which to build a remediation strategy. First we describe the scope of remediation generally and then specifically for clinical reasoning. Next we discuss several standard frameworks for remediation. To clarify the frameworks, we use real cases to demonstrate the remediation processes for clinical reasoning. The cases highlight various tools that allow the struggling learners to improve their clinical performance (also see Chapter 4).

KEY POINTS

- Clinical reasoning deficits can often be simplified into categories to aid in the remediation process. These include illness script knowledge and organization, data collection, hypothesis generation, data integration, interpretation, and application.
- Correctly diagnosing the deficits is critical for successful remediation. Most learners will succeed with remediation.
- The steps of remediation include identifying the clinical reasoning deficit(s), diagnosing the details of the deficit, establishing a learning plan, coaching and remediation, and reassessment and monitoring.
- The learning plan during remediation is a multistep process that includes review, reflection, individual and group activities, deliberate practice, regular feedback, and reassessment.

❖ The Scope of the Problem

The remediation of learners is uncommon but is of critical importance. A remediation program for residents found that about 3% of all residents over a 10-year period required its services (4). At the medical student level, a national survey of internal medicine clerkship directors reported that 0% to 15% of students struggled during their core clerkship, and 0% to 11% struggled during their fourth year (5). Importantly, struggling learners

Table 9-1. Accreditation Agencies and Remediation

Liaison Committee for Medical Education, ed 31 (www.lcme.org/publications/functions.pdf)	Each student should be evaluated early enough during a unit of study to allow time for remediation. It is expected that courses and clerkships provide students with formal feedback during their experiences so that they may understand and remediate deficiencies.
Accreditation Council for Graduate Medical Education: Institutional Requirements 2007; 11.D. 4.d) (http://www.acgme. org/acgmeweb/Portals/0/ irc_IRCpr07012007.pdf)	The sponsoring institution must provide residents with fair, reasonable, and readily available written institutional policies and procedures for grievance and due process.

may require remediation in more than 1 competency or skill. One study found a mean of 2.1 and 1.6 deficits for medical students and residents, respectively (6). Medical educators are frequently dissatisfied with remediation processes (7). A structured review of remediation in medical education found a "paucity of evidence to guide best practices in medical education at all levels" and highlighted the need for further study (8).

In transitioning from general remediation to clinical reasoning remediation, several concepts deserve emphasis. Guerrasio and colleagues found clinical reasoning deficits to be a common reason for remediation, affecting about a third of learners undergoing remediation (6). Remediating clinical reasoning is felt to be more difficult than doing so for clinical skills (9), and the amount of time needed to remediate a clinical reasoning deficit in one study was 20 hours (3). A lack of faculty preparation and lack of structure in the process are felt to be important reasons for difficulty in remediating clinical reasoning deficits (10).

❖ Challenges

The remediation of clinical reasoning performance is problematic for many reasons. The clinical reasoning process is expansive, and difficulties in clinical reasoning may also appear as problems in other areas, such as basic clinical skills, communication, professionalism, or inadequate knowledge base. The clinical reasoning process is often inferred from diagnostic decisions made by learners. Often, these thought processes are not articulated, leaving those charged with assessing learners to intuit the clinical reasoning process. Yet through direct observation of patient care, review of written notes, and oral presentations, evaluators can make judgments on the adequacy of learners' clinical reasoning. Adequate sample sizes of learners' reasoning processes are needed, however, to avoid false conclusions (see Chapter 6).

A preceptor needs access to the learners' clinical thinking in order to facilitate the development of learners' clinical reasoning. This process may be difficult to accomplish in traditional clinical situations. Some studies of traditional case presentations to preceptors have shown that learners focus mainly on factual information and seldom express their clinical reasoning or diagnostic uncertainties (11, 12). Experienced clinicians may not recognize the clinical reasoning process they themselves used in a particular case because their expertise often involves rapid processes, primarily pattern recognition, rather than the slower hypothetico-deductive reasoning of beginning learners (13). The rapid pace of clinical rotations also does not lend itself to in-depth assessment of clinical reasoning. However, both students and preceptors consider the opportunity to reflect about the reasoning process as one of the most valued aspects of the educational encounter (14). Hopefully, the time and resource investment by medical schools in incorporating clinical reasoning exercises into clinical experiences for students may identify struggling learners earlier.

The very structure of medical education presents an additional challenge in remediating clinical reasoning. Despite improvements in recent years, current medical training in the preclerkship years still involves memorizing large amounts of information, with a limited emphasis on transferring that information to clinical contexts. When students arrive in the clerkship years, they may rely on housestaff and attending physicians to formulate differential diagnoses and plans because many feel inadequately prepared to do so. A study of clerkship directors inquired about competencies that students needed to acquire in their preclerkship education. Of the competencies listed, the clerkship directors felt areas of clinical reasoning (like probabilistic thinking) were most commonly deficient (15). Some medical schools have responded to this perceived problem with active early learning strategies, such as problem-based learning, which have demonstrated improvement in some aspects of clinical reasoning (e.g., more comprehensive increased use of hypothesis-driven reasoning and basic science in their diagnostic justifications) (16, 17) and courses that introduce clinical reasoning early in the curriculum.

Frameworks to Aid in Determining and Remediating Clinical Reasoning Deficits

The process of remediating learners with clinical reasoning deficits might be easier if medical educators agreed upon a single framework that summarized problems and outlined solutions. However, as one author recently lamented, "no established conceptual framework or structured approach regarding clinical reasoning difficulties and their identification and remediation has emerged" (18). The complexity of and lack of a gold standard for the clinical reasoning process, as well as the need to infer clinical reasoning from behaviors (see Chapter 4 and Chapter 6), have led to attempts to dissect and simplify reasoning into smaller components that provide achievable, concrete tasks for struggling learners to practice. For example, rather than saying, "You need to work on your reasoning skills," a remediation coach can say, "Let's work on your ability to represent a clinical problem. This is a critical component of clinical reasoning." Although this simplification is valuable in remediation, the actual process is nonlinear and iterative. We present here three types of frameworks—taxonomies of clinical reasoning, dual process theory, and knowledge organization—that may help structure the remediation of clinical reasoning.

Many authors (18–21) have created clinical reasoning taxonomies to facilitate this process, as outlined in Table 9-2. They each highlight specific aspects of a complex, multistep process. Diagnostic error can occur

Table 9-2. Taxonomies of Clinical Reasoning

Author	Step	Example
Audétat et al. (2013)	Data collection Hypothesis generation	Unable to generate adequate hypotheses Unfocused data gathering
	Hypothesis refinement and testing	Premature closure Lacking prioritization
	Diagnosis and developing management plan	Problems with synthesis and integration of data Inadequate management plan
Bowen (2006)	Data acquisition	History and physical examination
	Problem representation	Summarizing, articulating
	Hypothesis generation	Probabilistic thinking
	Selecting illness script	Matching characteristics
	Diagnosis	Synthesis and application
Bordage (1999)	Data gathering	History and physical examination
	Data integration	Over- or underestimating meaning of findings
	Situational	Fatigue vs. stress

in any (or multiple) of these components of clinical reasoning, including inadequate or faulty data collection, problem representation, hypothesis generation, data synthesis, and application. Learners can err while collecting data. The data can be misinterpreted, leading to faulty hypotheses. They may synthesize or integrate the information inaccurately. They may generate inadequate or incorrect hypotheses or differential diagnoses. Learners may lack adequate illness scripts to match the clinical data to the correct diagnosis. Learners must recognize the possibility of uncertainty in the diagnosis and embrace the concept of a "working diagnosis." Finally, the information must be put into action appropriately, or it can result in an inadequate management plan.

Like the structure provided by dividing clinical reasoning into components, dual process theory may provide a framework for educators to remediate struggling learners. Dual process theory describes clinical reasoning as the interplay between nonanalytic and analytic thinking (see Chapter 2). It may be helpful for remediators and struggling learners (i.e., those at risk for failing) to recognize that both nonanalytic and analytic reasoning skills need to be developed. Although experts and novices use the same reasoning processes, novices often lack the knowledge and knowledge organization to recognize more than typical presentations of common diseases non-analytically. As a result, they may rely on less efficient analytic approaches (e.g., hypothetico-deductive reasoning) to solve problems (22). Remediators can stress that students should build knowledge of illness scripts (i.e., knowledge of disease presentations) by encouraging them to see lots of patients and to mentally rehearse clinical reasoning with virtual cases to build their nonanalytic skills. At the same time, remediators should foster analytic skills given that combining the dual processes seems to improve diagnostic accuracy (23).

Given that knowledge is critical to clinical reasoning expertise, the third framework provides a method for assessing a learner's knowledge organization. Bordage and colleagues studied semantic discourses (i.e., the meaning of student clinical reasoning dialogues) of novices and experts as they discussed cases and assigned a specific level of discourse organization (reduced, dispersed, elaborated, compiled) to the learners and their discussions. They discovered that novices tended to have reduced or dispersed discourses regarding diseases, whereas intermediates and experts tended to have elaborated or compiled discourses, as described in Box 9-1 (24).

Box 9-1. Classifying Learners' Knowledge Structure

1. **Reduced.** Learners with little knowledge or understanding of the clinical problem cannot make connections between the features of the case and stored knowledge. Because knowledge is not triggered, it is impossible to distinguish absent knowledge from inaccessible knowledge. In response to the question, "What do you think about this problem?" the learner says very little of consequence, or essentially, "I don't know."

2. **Dispersed.** Learners with this type of discourse response to the question "What do you think?" talk about separate features of the case, which trigger associations with pathophysiology or diagnoses but fail to reflect consideration of other features and connect back to the case. Thus, the features present for a patient with pneumonia would be considered individually. Fever might trigger a list of diagnoses where fever is a prominent feature. Shortness of breath might trigger a whole new list of diagnoses in

continued

Box 9-1. Classifying Learners' Knowledge Structure (continued)

which dyspnea is characteristic. Knowledge is abundant but the coherence provided by the clinical context of the case is ignored, yielding extensive diagnostic considerations without prioritization or any effort to make a plausible diagnosis.

3. Elaborated. This is characterized by the transformation of specific case features into abstract, synthesized terms. "I started feeling poorly a few days ago" becomes "acute," for example. These abstract descriptors, called semantic qualifiers, have 2 characteristics. First, they can easily be paired with an opposite quality: *acute* versus *chronic*; *productive* versus *nonproductive cough*; or *ill-appearing* versus *well-appearing*. Second, the descriptors most often fall into categories typically used to characterize the problem during the medical interview: onset ("When did your symptoms start?"—*acute* vs. *subacute* vs. *chronic, sudden* vs. *gradual*), site ("What is bothering you?"—*unilateral* vs. *bilateral, localized* vs. *disseminated, monoarticular* vs. *polyarticular*), course ("Do your symptoms come and go?"—*episodic* vs. *continuous, recurrent* vs. *resolved*), severity ("How would you describe your discomfort?"—*severe* vs. *mild, sharp* vs. *dull*), and context (*young* vs. *older, male* vs. *female, smoker* vs. *nonsmoker*). In addition, learners with elaborated discourse organization are actively comparing and contrasting diagnostic considerations with the features of the case. These oral presentations tend to be easy to follow and are well organized and concise.

4. Compiled. Clinical case discourse in this category tends to be brief and highly synthesized, and often extends beyond the available features, showing evidence of searching for elements missing from a well-developed understanding of the problem. Fewer diagnostic considerations are entertained. At first it may be difficult to distinguish a lucky guess or premature closure from compiled discourse organization. Upon further questioning ("Did you consider anything else as an explanation for his symptoms?"), the

continued

> ## Box 9-1. Classifying Learners' Knowledge Structure (continued)
>
> learner with compiled discourse organization can compare and contrast highly relevant diagnoses with the features of the case. Reduced and dispersed discourse organizations are associated with difficulty making an accurate diagnosis, but elaborated and compiled organizations are associated with diagnostic accuracy.
>
> Used with permission from Bowen JL, Smith CS. The journey from novice to professional: how theories of learning can enhance teaching. In: Ende J, ed. Theory and Practice of Teaching Medicine. Philadelphia: American College of Physicians; 2010:10-1.

Briefly, reduced knowledge is characterized as inadequate or absent. Dispersed knowledge is associated with long lists without prioritization or connection to the patient being considered. The elaborated and compiled structures are associated with dynamic associations that allow immediate search for elements of a pattern. Armed with these categories, a remediator can select strategies that best fit the struggling learner (e.g., reduced learners focus on building their knowledge base, while dispersed learners focus on chunking knowledge and prioritizing patient data). Success in diagnostic reasoning is associated with diversified sets of semantic axes, which are methods of organizing clinical findings by using descriptive words (i.e., qualifiers) that help to more narrowly define a symptom (e.g., *acute* vs. *chronic, dull* vs. *stabbing*). Difficulties can be associated with lack of recognizing semantic characteristics of a case (25). When students develop expert-type knowledge structure, they show increased odds of diagnostic success (26).

Each of these frameworks has value and utility in structuring the remediation of struggling learners. None of them, however, is comprehensive or applies to all learners and all reasoning deficits. As such, we suggest being mindful of all three types of framework and attempting to tie remediation strategies to the frameworks, while also recognizing that none should be used as the sole basis of a remediation program.

❖ Remediation Strategies

Several steps exist in the process before remediation can begin. First, care must be taken to correctly diagnose the learner's deficit and to ensure that a clinical reasoning deficit actually exists. Educators need to be aware that multiple deficits may coexist in a learner. Physical or emotional stress, such as health, family, or financial problems, may impair anyone's reasoning and may be sufficient to have the appearance of a reasoning deficit. Similarly, substance abuse can negatively affect the learner's clinical reasoning capacity. Illness can affect performance, and frequently learners are reluctant to notify anyone that they are ill. The stress of a new environment or difficult social interactions can render a learner unable to manage routine clinical tasks; once these issues are resolved or stable, more intensive remediation may be unnecessary (20). A useful mnemonic for evaluating struggling learners is to first exclude *drugs*, *disease*, and *distractions* (DDD).

Other defects in the cognitive process may also appear to be reasoning deficits. Some learners may have passed through earlier courses without gaining an adequate base of knowledge or clinical skills. Without these tools, their reasoning will be faulty. Learners may possess knowledge at the reduced or dispersed levels and cannot readily apply their knowledge to clinical situations in the way that those with elaborated or compiled knowledge can (22, 27). Excessive cognitive load may overwhelm learners and retard their progress toward mastering material (28). Again, educators need to be aware that multiple deficits may coexist in a learner.

In designing the remediation program itself, a review of the remediation literature can provide valuable guidance, specifically that remediation programs should contain multiple components (8). The first step is assessment to identify deficiencies. This assessment may require the use of multiple assessment tools. Second, the deficit must be diagnosed and a learning plan agreed upon. Third, the learner, in collaboration with an advisor, develops a remediation plan. Fourth, the learner should receive individualized instruction with deliberate practice, feedback, and reflection. Finally, the learner needs reassessment and establishment of competency (9). These concepts will be developed further during the subsequent case descriptions.

The general goal of remediation efforts in clinical reasoning might be encapsulated in the phrase "to help students become more effective and efficient learners." The learner who requires remediation may have developed learning strategies that have led to success in previous educational settings but are less effective in the clinical setting. Student success in and acclimatization to a technology-driven, immediate-solution environment in high school or college may hamper learning in the clinical setting. Therefore, remediators should focus on students' learning strategies. Redirecting the learner to more focused reading, more reflective exercises, and increased comfort with uncertainty may assist the transition.

This may also help with deficits as seen through the lens of the previously described remediation frameworks.

The following paragraphs provide details on helping students become better learners and amplify the components of a successful remediation effort. As learners' deficits differ, so will the emphasis needed on these remediation components. Nevertheless, it is helpful to consider each when remediating a learner.

Becoming a "Better Learner"

Focused Readings

Although failing a clerkship exam is common, clerkship directors struggle with remediating this problem. A study of internal medicine clerkship directors found that nearly half (42%) had no specific remediation strategy for such students (29). Often, students are simply told to "read more," with no further direction. However, motivated students are already spending long hours reading. Guiding the student through specific reading assignments from quality sources and then reviewing the assigned readings reinforces what they read. Asking the students to apply what was learned by specific exercises, such as critically appraised topics (CATs). A CAT is a short summary of evidence on a topic of interest, usually focused on a clinical question by using the PICO (Problem, Intervention, Comparison, Outcome) format. The best available evidence is sought, and a brief conclusion is written (30). Concept mapping can help to increase information retention (31). Concept mapping arranges the most general concept at the top. Then links to the less inclusive concepts are drawn and circled. The lines linking the concepts have accompanying words that explain the relationship, if needed (e.g., cause-effect; direction). This exercise improves elaborated knowledge. Students can be encouraged to read about symptoms, rather than diseases, and to compare and contrast features of different conditions for both similarities and important differences (19).

Review the Basics

Frequently, a review of clinical decision-making is a critical component of the remediation process. Because clinical reasoning courses are frequently inserted into an already packed curriculum, understanding of basic reasoning principles has not been grasped. Reminding students of the dual process framework, including nonanalytic (e.g., pattern recognition, heuristics) and analytic (e.g., survey method using a mnemonic like VITAMIN BCD or RICHMOND) (Table 9-5) reasoning strategies may set the basic groundwork that is critical to successful remediation. These concepts are likely best reviewed in small chunks, with the educator tasked to supervise the learning, as part of the learning plan, rather than forcing learners to read their old medical school syllabus on the introductory course. Students should be encouraged to engage in deliberate practice in order to optimize improvement. In this approach, learners address specific, defined tasks under supervision and receive timely and specific feedback from a mentor or coach. This approach is used in numerous fields outside medicine, with demonstrated efficacy. A helpful exercise includes reviewing a recent admission (within the past week or 2) and the diagnostic strategies that the learner used when she or he admitted the patient. This exercise helps the coach recognize the (deficient) reasoning of the learner and also offers an opportunity for reflection. In our experience, struggling learners have not "followed up" to see what happened to the admitted patient and what diagnosis was eventually made. When follow-up is emphasized, illness scripts can be built on the experience of the admitting resident (night float) who frequently doesn't get follow-up of the patient during admission.

Increase Reflection
Learners may lack skill in reflection and self-assessment, and these skills should become part of the remediation process. A key aspect of the dual processing framework is to be aware of one's thinking processes and to consider means of improving. Although learners typically struggle with global self-assessment, studies have demonstrated better results with self-monitoring and more granular assessments (32). This approach emphasizes a more focused and real-time awareness of ability. Durning and colleagues have described microanalytic techniques that encourage self-regulatory behaviors, and the authors have included examples of remediation in their work (33). These techniques allow learners to analyze their performances more effectively and engage in better self-regulated learning. These structured approaches to improve clinical reasoning can move learners forward along the Dreyfus model, from rule-driven novices to competent practitioners and ultimately to reflective master clinicians (34). See Chapter 10 for further description of these techniques.

Narrative medicine, where learners develop reflective essays based on cases they encounter, is an important tool that can be used for many different educational activities. Mamede and colleagues have shown that forced diagnostic reflection improved diagnostic accuracy among internal medicine residents in complex cases (35, 36). The experience of writing facilitates reflection and may tap reservoirs of thought previously inaccessible to the writer (37). The process of reviewing what one has written with a coach/mentor or a small group may also facilitate discussion of (potential) personal struggles in a psychologically safe environment.

Considering Group Activities That Encourage the
Learner to Express Uncertainty

Uncertainty clouds all aspects of medical training, including the following: 1) uncertainties based on the concern that even in our information-intensive world, there are gaps in knowledge and skills, especially around evidence-based medicine, 2) uncertainties that stem from the illness and patient presentation, and 3) uncertainties connected with distinguishing between lack of knowledge or skill and the complexity of medicine. As difficult as it is for experienced physicians, uncertainty presents an added challenge for young physicians. These physicians are often unsure about their knowledge and skills or whether the relevant knowledge even exists, and they struggle with distinguishing between these two possibilities (38).

Practice inquiry is a method that may help all learners, especially struggling learners, to distinguish between these uncertainties, develop reflection abilities, and feel more comfortable with uncertainty. Practice inquiry allows for clinicians to engage case-based clinical uncertainty in small group settings (39) and is aimed at enhancing clinical judgment through collegial collaboration. During prescheduled, dedicated time, clinicians with patient panels meet in facilitated small groups to discuss individual patients for whom they are experiencing clinical uncertainty, along with diagnostic, therapeutic, prognostic, ethical, and/or clinician–patient relationship dilemmas (39). The single-case format includes eight phases that, given a moderately complex case, is completed in 50 to 60 minutes. In this scenario, each group phase begins with a request or question from the group facilitator who starts discussion and guides inquiry, followed by initial responses from the case presenter or colleague group members.

Converting Knowledge to Accessible Matrices
in the Clinical Setting

Bordage would describe this process as helping the learner convert knowledge organization from dispersed to elaborate (25). Increasing knowledge strengthens clinical reasoning *if* the knowledge is organized into a network of clinical findings. For a clinician, pattern recognition based on well-developed knowledge scripts is important, and repetitive exposure to common conditions helps the learner develop these illness scripts. Multiple caveats exist, however. First, not all common clinical presentations are typical, and illness scripts themselves need some structure beyond the basic scaffolding. Second, in more advanced training years, uncommon conditions and atypical presentations may be much more frequent and, very importantly, context may cloud the clinical pattern. The struggling learner may rely heavily on pattern recognition and does not recognize when to switch to analytic mode. The experience at the institution of one of the chapter's authors is that learners regularly experience diagnostic error during their training. When these errors occur, they frequently contain at least one cognitive bias and one contextual factor that may have influenced the outcome (40). As remediation progresses, exercises that include clinical presentations with contextual complications that reinforce "slowing down" may help the learner recognize the need to abandon pattern recognition and switch to a more analytic mode (41).

Assessing Improvement

After concluding efforts to remediate learners, medical educators need to assess the success of their efforts. Using a scale like RIME (Reporter, Interpreter, Manager, Educator) (42) at the start of the process may provide a means of assessing growth at the completion of the remediation. Several tools have been developed for assessing learners' clinical reasoning abilities. Traditionally, oral exams, standardized patient exams, and content-rich multiple-choice questions have been used in this regard (43). Some newer techniques include chart-stimulated recall, script concordance tests, key feature exams, simulated patients, and concept mapping (44). The most appropriate measures will need to fit the learner's identified deficits and be practical under local circumstances (See Chapter 6).

Monitoring

Remediated learners sometimes remain "fragile." As they resume their course of study, advisors or mentors should follow their progress closely and observe it for signs of "relapse" or the emergence of new problems. Early intervention may make the overall process easier.

The next section presents 4 cases that exemplify the structure of the remediation process. They were selected to demonstrate different defects in the clinical reasoning process and were adapted from actual learners encountered by the authors. Each case is presented in a standard format that demonstrates the remediation steps mentioned earlier (Table 9-3).

❖ Examples

Case 1

Assessment to Identify Deficiencies
This assessment may require the use of multiple assessment tools.

P.G. was the first intern to come to our residency program from her medical school. Her transcripts from her medical school showed no difficulties, and she had excellent U.S. Medical Licensing Examination (USMLE) scores. However, several evaluations from early rotations at our program were critical of her clinical skills and knowledge. Specifically,

Table 9-3. Remediation Steps

Steps	Methods
Identify the struggling learner	Failure on shelf exam (student) Poor performance in clerkship (student) Poor performance on the wards (resident)
Identify deficiencies (may require the use of multiple assessment tools)	See Chapter 6 Competency committee in conjunction with a remediation or coaching committee of the department or institution
Diagnose the deficit(s) Create a learning plan	Structured interview Direct observation of history and physical examination (5–10) Objective Structured Clinical Examination Interviews with supervising faculty and residents Review of performance on standardized testing
Coaching and remediation	Reviewing the basics Reading techniques
Individualized instruction	Deliberate practice Reflective exercises Regular feedback Group activity with practice inquiry Practice questions/assessment
Reassessment and monitoring	Formal assessments Performance on the wards

nurses and attending physicians noted that she "seemed unsure of herself." They noted that she had good "book knowledge" but was unable to apply it or to prioritize. Further notes indicated that she seemed reluctant to give plans or assessments on rounds. These sentiments were expressed in the intensive care unit, on the general internal medicine ward services, and in her continuity clinic. Several evaluators noted that they thought she was sincere and seemed to be trying hard. All her assignments were completed; she was always punctual and eager to stay beyond expected times. She was discussed during the resident competency meeting, where it was felt that she was performing at the "reporter" level on the RIME scale (42), less than expected for an intern. There were concerns regarding her progressing to a supervising resident level.

Diagnosis of Deficits and Development of Learning Plan
The resident in this case demonstrated several defects in clinical reasoning. Before considering the deficits, however, strengths need to be noted.

In general, the learning plan should include identifying the learner's strengths and communicating them to the learner. This reassures learners that evaluators recognize skill sets and makes the remediation process less intimidating. First, the evaluators feel she had a good knowledge base, a conclusion based on her USMLE scores and comments from her evaluations. Second, she had a good work ethic and has demonstrated an eagerness to learn. However, direct observation by her attendings in multiple settings revealed an inability to apply or prioritize knowledge to patient care issues and a reluctance to articulate diagnostic hypotheses and management plans. According to Bowen's taxonomy (Table 9-2), she struggled with the clinical reasoning components of problem representation, hypothesis generation, and illness script selection. The basis for these struggles was felt to be an inadequate knowledge of illness scripts, and her knowledge organization was felt to be dispersed (Bordage framework, Box 9-1). After meeting with the resident, her advisor and program director did not identify any issues outside medicine that were playing a role in her difficulties.

Individualized Instruction
Instruction should include deliberate practice, feedback, and reflection.

P.G. and her advisor developed a learner contract. With use of the clinical reasoning framework highlighted by Bowen, remediation activities were focused in the following areas:

1. For her perceived deficit in knowledge structure, P.G. solved four questions from the American College of Physicians' Medical Knowledge Self-Assessment Program and provided rationales for the answers to her advisor monthly, so that her thought processes would become transparent.
2. In terms of data collection, she needed to demonstrate the ability to process information obtained from a patient history and physical examination in oral presentations and written histories and physical examinations. Both of these were regularly reviewed by her advisor.
3. Regarding problem representation, she was instructed to develop and present problem assessments on all her patients, copies of which were regularly reviewed.
4. In reference to hypothesis generation, she was instructed to show the ability to generate a differential diagnosis for the patient's symptoms and justify reasoning in her oral and written case presentations on her rotations. Copies of her history and physical examinations were reviewed with her advisor.
5. In terms of "managing" her patients, she was expected to develop and present a problem assessment and plan to investigate her

leading diagnostic possibilities for her patients. She needed to demonstrate the ability to prioritize patient-related tasks, in both inpatient and outpatient settings, including providing rationales for tests performed.

To monitor, assess, and provide feedback about her performance, the following educational strategy was used. Once a week the attending physician on service with her would discuss her performance by using learning prescriptions (45). These are learning tasks that are summarized in the format of a drug prescription. Attending physicians can "prescribe" a topic or clinical question to be clarified by the learner. Doing so in the clinical context would both improve her illness scripts (as applicable to Bowen's taxonomy) and knowledge organization (as applicable to the Bordage framework). On both inpatient services and in outpatient clinic, an attending physician would specifically observe and evaluate her clinical reasoning process and provide feedback. Weekly reflective journaling was mandated to help practice self-regulated learning skills. P.G. was also required to write a weekly reflection about a patient case. She presented these reflections to her advisor, who provided feedback at the end of each month. The reflective writings were structured in the following manner:

1. Define a problem or issue of interest you.
2. Describe what resources you used to solve the problem.
3. Describe what you learned.
4. State what you will do differently next time.

Reassessment and Establishment of Competence
P.G. completed her remediation plan with the motivation and determination that went beyond expectations. She took it upon herself to provide articles at morning report about patient care–related issues. She read several books related to the clinical practice of medicine. She became involved in 2 specific research projects in her field of interest. Her clinical evaluations improved dramatically, and her advisor's report to the competency committee at the end of her internship was entirely favorable. She realized that she could fulfill her potential and developed greater confidence in herself. She completed the residency program on schedule with no further issues and matched into a fellowship program.

Case 2
S.R. was a clerkship student near completion of his clerkship year. During the first 2 weeks of his inpatient rotation, the resident had a busy service and had not been able to dedicate the time he usually did to the student's presentations. The resident described that the student's presentation in the morning was usually a verbatim presentation of the night-float sign-out.

Significant elements of history were omitted, and the differential diagnosis was usually the one working diagnosis from the night float. One morning on attending rounds, it was clear that the student had not reviewed the previous admissions, which are easy to retrieve from the electronic health record. Further inquiry into the student's performance during other rotations indicated that he was perceived to have adequate knowledge by his supervisors and had passed all the National Board of Medical Examiners (NBME) subject exams. He generally made a good effort on his clinical rotations, but he had not achieved honors in any rotations.

Assessment to Identify Deficiencies
This assessment may require the use of multiple assessment tools.

Discussing the student's performance on other rotations with the other clerkship directors helped to identify a pattern of learning difficulties that made it easier to identify the specific learning deficits and focus the learning plan. A national survey of clerkship directors found that 77% report the information to a school of medicine promotions committee, and 64% felt that clerkship directors need to share information on struggling students (5). This process helps to validate opinions through obtaining multiple observations. Interviews with other supervising faculty members and clerkship directors identified this student's poorly organized knowledge, as described in the Bordage model, and difficulty extracting information from the medical record. These assessments were based on both direct observations and from analyzing written notes. In terms of the Bowen taxonomy, this student seemed to have inadequate illness scripts for common clinical problems. The committee helped formulate the plan, especially after they reviewed feedback from other rotations.

An interview between the student and a faculty coach helped to identify deficits. Recent histories and physical examinations that S.R. had written were provided by S.R., reviewed by the coach, and discussed. The coach used the SNAPPS (Summarize history and findings; Narrow the differential; Analyze the differential; Probe preceptor about uncertainties; Plan management; Select case-related issues for self-study) technique for precepting in the outpatient setting. SNAPPS is a learner-centered case presentation technique that depends mostly on the student, and can reveal areas for improvement (46). This independent assessment of the student with a structured tool helped to ensure objectivity initially and in reassessment. Although not a validated assessment tool, SNAPPS is helpful and widely used.

Diagnosis of Deficits and Development of Learning Plan
Once deficits are identified, focused remediation can occur. According to the Bowen taxonomy, script theory, and the SNAPPS technique to distill

the performance of this student (Table 9-2), his difficulties were primarily in identifying cues, generating hypotheses, and collecting data using hypotheses (19). He generated hypotheses only with prompting, so that when he collected data on his own, he seemed to ask multiple, unrelated questions in a "shot gun" type approach. Through use of the Bordage model, we also identified some gaps in medical knowledge structure that needed attention, as a lack of knowledge and poor knowledge organization impede hypothesis generation capabilities. He seemed unable to transfer his "book" knowledge to the clinical setting, not an uncommon problem for students. This seemed consistent with S.R.'s performance on NBME subject exams. From the committee discussions, improving his matrix of knowledge and helping him to develop schema on approaches to common problems would help to broaden the differential diagnoses. It was hoped that expanding his illness scripts would improve his ability to access and apply knowledge and identify where effort was needed in the differential diagnosis process. This example also highlights how using more than one framework of clinical reasoning, in this case the Bowen and Bordage models, may help identify several related but different issues with a learner's reasoning abilities.

First and most important, S.R. was reassured that with conscientious practice he would improve. A learning plan was designed that included selected readings on patients seen on the wards with specific reflective exercises and feedback. Studies have demonstrated that structured reading exercises emphasizing how findings are connected can improve comprehension and deep learning over controls. This is particularly true for advanced learners, such as medical students (47).

Individualized Instruction
Instruction should include deliberate practice, feedback, and reflection.

Having S.R. read topics with an eye to mimickers of disease helped focus his medical knowledge base and promote progression in his knowledge level to more advanced discourses. As mentioned previously, telling the student to read more is always good advice, but recommending areas of focus helps the struggling learner organize his or her reading and, by extension, his or her knowledge. Reading better starts with reading about symptoms, rather than diseases, and using approaches that mimic the way learners will need to use their knowledge with undiagnosed patients. This can, in turn, aid in both knowledge organization and strengthening of illness scripts. Through this type of reading, learners should develop algorithms or schema with which to approach common symptoms. For example, acute kidney injury may be prerenal, intrarenal, or postrenal; anemia can be microcytic, normocytic, or macrocytic. Coaches can help

Table 9-4. Symptoms: Chest Pain and Shortness of Breath

Presentation	Typical	Atypical
Common	Pneumonia	Bleeding gastric ulcer
Uncommon	Antineutrophil cytoplasmic antibody–associated vasculitis	Metastatic ovarian cancer

learners to embrace these algorithms by highlighting their benefits. Better reading also includes reading about 2 diseases, rather than 1, to learn what clinical findings discriminate a disease from another. This reading should include exploration of likelihood ratios to understand the value of tests (see the Rational Clinical Examination series in *JAMA* [http://jama.jama-network.com/collection.aspx?categoryid=6257]). We also recommended that he create the 2 × 2 table of common and uncommon presentations for every patient that he worked up; this will allow him to think about "horses and zebras" (Table 9-4) and further strengthen illness scripts and his ability to appropriately match a presentation with a script.

He reviewed various mnemonics that could help him develop a broader differential diagnosis, including survey methods, as shown in Table 9-5. Differential diagnoses had to include a minimum of 3 diagnoses and 2 organ systems when he presented patients, with evidence to support and refute each diagnosis. The evidence that he used had to be unique to the diagnosis (i.e., fever couldn't justify both pneumonia and pulmonary embolus). The student identified his reading activities as they related to the specific patients being considered, and he wrote down a few things from his readings that would help him include or exclude other diagnoses. All

Table 9-5. Mnemonic Aids for Broadening Differential Diagnoses

VITAMIN BCD	RICHMOND
V = vascular	R = respiratory/rheumatology
I = infectious	I = infectious disease
T = toxic/traumatic	C = cardiology
A = autoimmune	H = hematology
M = metabolic	M = metabolic/mental health
I = idiopathic/iatrogenic	O = oncology
N = neoplastic/nutritional	N = neurology/nephrology
B = behavioral	D = digestive
C = congenital/genetic	
D = degenerative	

of these activities additionally served to build important scripts with key distinguishing features of each of the diseases.

Data processing seemed overwhelming to S.R., and he would benefit from developing techniques to review old records. Some of the difficulty was that S.R. was not generating a differential diagnosis ahead of time, and therefore a focused review of the records looking for data that could support or refute the potential diagnoses was not organized. Helping him prepare the differential diagnosis before a record review, in essence helping him to generate hypotheses (a key component of the reasoning taxonomies [Table 9-2]) helped him become more efficient.

The coach met with S.R. every other week and, using a narrative journaling exercise during some of these sessions, allowed the student to reflect on his progress of initial evaluation and subsequent management of a specific patient and of diagnostic errors that may have occurred during a patient's care.

Reassessment and Establishment of Competence
S.R. was discussed again at his clerkship competency committee. A structured interview of a patient encounter using the same SNAPPS method that was used for his initial assessment was repeated. His performance on his NBME internal medicine subject exam was better than his performance on all the subject exams he had taken previously.

Case 3

Assessment to Identify Deficiencies
This assessment may require the use of multiple assessment tools.

T.S. was a third-year medical student in his internal medicine core clerkship. He had passed all his basic science courses and his Step 1 USMLE, albeit with a low score. His evaluations and discussions with his attendings on the internal medicine clerkship revealed a dispersed level of knowledge (Box 9-1), and his differential diagnoses missed important conditions. His presentations were brief and disjointed. However, his residents thought he had made a good effort and that he was available and eager to see new patients. His written histories and physical examinations were considered accurate and thorough. At the end of the clerkship, T.S. failed the NBME subject exam, but he passed the Objective Structured Clinical Examination. (This uses standardized patients and assesses clinical skills, such as history-taking, physical examination, and patient counseling. It is structurally similar to the Step 1 USMLE Clinical Skills exam).

At the clerkship advisory committee meeting, T.S. was noted to have struggled with several standardized exams. His assessment at the learning laboratory showed no identified learning disorder. Specifically, he was assessed by a psychologist with expertise in this field and demonstrated normal reading and comprehension skills. There were no signs of dyslexia or attention-deficit/hyperactivity disorder.

Diagnosis of Deficits and Development of Learning Plan

T.S. demonstrated a common problem in clinical reasoning. He seemed to have dispersed knowledge (Box 9-1) (24). He had difficulty applying his knowledge to patient care, effectively having a knowledge transfer problem as he appeared to be unable to access his knowledge in an efficient and effective fashion.

Individualized Instruction

Instruction should include deliberate practice, feedback, and reflection.

T.S. was asked to repeat a month of internal medicine clerkship and was paired with a senior clinician coach, who was known to be an excellent teacher. The coach gave T.S. articles related to his patients at the end of the day, which consisted of both original research and reviews on common internal medicine topics. Before beginning clinical duties, they would review an article describing how it applied to his specific patient. As part of this activity, he would briefly present the patient to his coach. He also completed an assigned reading list of common internal medicine conditions from an internal medicine textbook designed for clerkship students. He completed 2 critically assessed topics (CATs) (30) and developed 4 concept maps (31) about patient issues he had encountered. For example, the student performed literature searches on the preferred diagnostic testing approaches for suspected renal artery stenosis and the cost-effectiveness of various approaches to antiplatelet therapy as secondary prevention of stroke. The CATs helped him to briefly summarize patients, articulate a critical clinical question, find an answer in the medical literature, and apply that answer to his patient's care. He created concept maps demonstrating his understanding of the pathophysiology of chronic liver failure and another of pulmonary hypertension with right-sided heart failure. The concept maps seemed to help him integrate knowledge and relate them to a greater whole, raising his level of knowledge and solidifying illness scripts, including identifying the key features of specific diseases. They also helped to make his thinking more transparent to his coach and the course directors.

Reassessment and Establishment of Competence

T.S. scored 20% higher on his NBME subject exam retake, which was a passing level. His clinical evaluations from the repeated rotation included comments about his well-organized presentations. His management plans were felt to have improved, but he still needed to develop them beyond the initial round of tests and therapies. He also needed to make his thought processes more transparent. He subsequently did well in other clerkships.

Case 4

Assessment to Identify Deficiencies
This assessment may require the use of multiple assessment tools.

W.A. was a first-year pulmonary fellow who came from a well-regarded internal medicine residency program. Her letters of recommendation were strong. However, she struggled in her first year of fellowship, and faculty members were anxious when she was on-call because of concerns that patients might not be effectively managed. Rounds were excessively long as she presented clinic patients and newly hospitalized patients in excruciating detail (e.g., all components of the pulmonary physical examination were presented), but she couldn't present a focused differential diagnosis or management plan. The more history the patient had, the longer the presentation, and the more diffuse the presentations were. When asked why she couldn't develop a management plan quickly in the outpatient setting, she said that when she was on the wards as a resident she had more time to do this.

Diagnosis of Deficits and Development of Learning Plan
At both a competency meeting and a structured faculty meeting, W.A.'s performance was discussed. The faculty said she was earnest in her efforts and very professional, and they were not worried about substance abuse or illness. The fellowship program director was concerned that she was lonely and far from her family and that isolation could be affecting her performance. The faculty agreed that she had difficulty in problem representation (Table 9-2), specifically synthesizing and prioritizing the clinical data. For example, when the patient had several symptoms, she failed to focus the interview on the most important aspects. She failed to make connections between the different pieces of information, and she really struggled to integrate and synthesize the "big picture." As a result she usually had inadequate management plans. It became clear that these deficits were related to a lack of illness scripts (i.e., knowledge content and organization issue) for common pulmonary problems. Her knowledge organization appeared to be dispersed.

Individualized Instruction
Instruction should include deliberate practice, feedback, and reflection.

The program director engaged the other fellows and worked as a social director to address the issue of social isolation. Select faculty members were assigned to help her strengthen her illness scripts. After her presentations, she was asked to organize and summarize the presentation with key features, incorporating aspects of the semantic axis. She was coached to always present a summary statement that was 3 sentences long (1 sentence of history, 1 sentence of physical examination, and 1 sentence of laboratory results/data/imaging findings) and a differential diagnosis that included a minimum of 3 diagnoses, 1 of which was nonpulmonary. This improved her abilities in problem representation and hypothesis generation. W.A. was also asked to identify the reading that she had done in thinking about the patient and was encouraged to include key reading findings in her assessment and plan. Feedback on her clinic notes was more frequent, and she met with the fellowship program director more regularly than the usual schedule. As the illness scripts of the common pulmonary diseases became more familiar to her, W.A.'s presentations became more focused.

W.A. lacked confidence in her diagnostic skills, and the uncertainty of diagnoses made her uncomfortable. A session on practice inquiry was substituted for the usual case management conference, and she volunteered as the presenter. The practice inquiry session allowed her to feel comfortable in the uncertainty of the difficult diagnostic dilemma, and her confidence improved accordingly.

Reassessment and Establishment of Competence
As the year progressed W.A. developed more confidence in her clinical care and identified her unique strengths. Both her supervising attending physicians and nursing staff noted this change. She took an introductory quality improvement course where she excelled, and she developed a quality improvement project within the division. Her attention to detail was critical to her success in the quality arena and is an example of where a weakness can be turned into a strength.

❖ Conclusions

Remediating clinical reasoning deficits is difficult and time consuming, but not impossible. The remediation process needs to be open and nonthreatening. Most clinical reasoning deficits reside in the domain of knowledge content, organization, and transfer. Educators need to carefully diagnose the component of the clinical reasoning process that learners struggle with the most in order to guide them on how to improve. A methodical approach is critical to ensuring that all deficits are recognized. Remediation efforts need to be tailored to the problem at hand, the more specific the better. Multiple tools and techniques described here (also see Chapter 4) are available to aid in the remediation process. These techniques can be helpful to nonstruggling learners as well. The success or failure of these efforts needs to be appropriately assessed. Successfully remediated learners should undergo continued monitoring as they progress through their educational programs to guard against relapses or new difficulties. As clinical problems become more complicated and their roles more complex with advancing training, these learners may be tempted to revert to prior behaviors. The deficits are not always correctable, and a pathway must exist, usually through the dean's office or program director, to deal with such cases. Fortunately, failures are relatively few, and, from the authors' experiences, the rewards in cases where learners are successfully remediated are great.

REFERENCES

1. **Kimatian SJ, Lloyd SH.** Remediation and due process for trainees. Int Anes Clinics. 2008; 46:113-25.
2. **Liaison Committee on Medical Education.** Functions and Structure of a Medical School. 2013. Available at: www.lcme.porg/publications/functions.pdf.
3. **Accreditation Council for Graduate Medical Education.** Institutional Requirements. 2007. Available at: http://www.acgme.org/acgmeweb/Portals/0/irc_IRCpr07012007.pdf
4. **Zbieranowski I, Takahashi SG, Verma S, Spadafora SM.** Remediation of residents in difficulty: a retrospective 10-year review of the experience of a postgraduate board of examiners. Acad Med. 2013;88:111-6.
5. **Frellsen SL, Baker EA, Papp KK, Durning SJ.** Medical school policies regarding struggling medical students during the internal medicine clerkships: results of a national survey. Acad Med. 2008;83:876-81.
6. **Guerrasio J, Garrity MJ, Aagaard EV.** Learner deficits and academic outcomes of medical students, residents, fellows, and attending physicians referred to a remediation program, 2006-2012. Acad Med. 2014;89:352-7.
7. **Hauer KE, Teherani A, Kerr KM, Irby DM, O'Sullivan PS.** Consequences within medical schools for students with poor performance on a medical school standardized patient comprehensive assessment. Acad Med. 2009;84:663-8.
8. **Hauer KE, Ciccone A, Henzel TR, et al.** Remediation of the deficiencies of physicians across the continuum from medical school to practice: a thematic review of the literature. Acad Med. 2009;84:1822-32.
9. **Hauer KE, Teherani A, Kerr KM, O'Sullivan PS, Irby DM.** Student performance problems in medical school clinical skills assessments. Acad Med. 2007;82:S69-76.
10. **Audétat MC, Dory V, Nendaz M, et al.** What is so difficult about managing clinical reasoning difficulties? Med Ed. 2012;46:2016-227.
11. **Wiese J, Varosy P, Tierney L.** Improving oral presentation skills with a clinical reasoning curriculum: prospective controlled study. Am J Med. 2002;112:212-8.
12. **Dhaliwal G, Hauer KE.** The oral patient presentation in the era of night float admissions. JAMA. 2013;310:2247-8.
13. **Wolpaw TW, Glover PB, Papp KK.** An exemplary model of learning in the rheumatology outpatient setting. Arthritis Rheum. 2001;44:S208.
14. **O'Malley PG, Kroenke K, Ritter J, Dy N, Pangaro L.** What learners and teachers value most in ambulatory educational encounters: a prospective, qualitative study. Acad Med. 1999;74:186-91.

15. **Windish DM, Paulman PM, Goroll AH, Bass EB.** Do clerkship directors think medical students are prepared for the clerkship years? Acad Med. 2004;79:56-61.

16. **Aaron S, Crocket J, Morrish D, et al.** Assessment of exam performance after change to problem-based learning: differential effects by question type. Teach Learn Med. 1998;10:86-91.

17. **Hmelo CE.** Cognitive consequences of problem-based learning for the early development of medical expertise. Teach Learn Med. 1998;10:92-100.

18. **Audétat MC, Laurin S, Sanche G, et al.** Clinical reasoning difficulties: a taxonomy for clinical teachers. Med Teach. 2013;35:e984-e989.

19. **Bowen JL.** Educational strategies to promote clinical diagnostic reasoning. N Engl J Med. 2006;355:2217-25.

20. **Bordage G.** Why did i miss the diagnosis? Some cognitive explanations and educational implications. Acad Med. 1999;74:S138-43.

21. **Goldszmidt M, Minda JP, Bordage G.** Developing a unified list of physicians' reasoning tasks during clinical encounters. Acad Med. 2013;88:390-7.

22. **Mandin H, Jones A, Woloschuk W, Harasym P.** Helping students learn to think like experts when solving clinical problems. Acad Med. 1997;72:173-9.

23. **Ark, TK, Brooks LR, Eva KW.** The benefits of flexibility: the pedagogical value of instructions to adopt multifaceted diagnostic reasoning strategies. Med Educ. 2007;41:281-7.

24. **Bordage G, Connell KJ, Chang RW, Gecht MR, Sinacore JM.** Assessing the semantic content of clinical case presentations: studies of reliability and concurrent validity. Acad Med. 1997;72:S37-9.

25. **Bordage G.** Elaborated knowledge: a key to successful diagnostic thinking. Acad Med. 1994;69:883-5.

26. **McLaughlin K, Coderre S, Mortis G, Mandin H.** Expert-type structure in medical students is associated with increased odds of diagnostic success. Teach Learn Med. 2007;19:35-41.

27. **Baker EA, Connell KJ, Bordage G, Sinacore J.** Can diagnostic semantic competence be assessed from the medical record? Acad Med. 1999;74:S13-5.

28. **Schumacher DJ, Englander R, Carraccio C.** Developing the master learner: applying learning theory to the learner, the teacher, and the learning environment. Acad Med. 2013;88:1635-45.

29. **Torre D, Papp KK, Elnicki M, Durning S.** Clerkship directors' practices with respect to preparing students for and using the National Board of Medical Examiners Subject Exam in Medicine: results of a United States and Canadian survey. Acad Med. 2009;84:867-71.

30. **Sackett DL, Straus SE, Richardson WS, Rosenberg W, Haynes RB.** Evidence-Based Medicine: How to Practice and Teach It. 2nd ed. Edinburgh: Churchill Livingstone; 2000.

31. **Daley BJ, Torre DM.** Concept maps in medical education: an analytical literature review. Med Ed. 2010;44:440-8.

32. **Eva KW, Regehr G.** Exploring the divergence between self-assessment and self-monitoring. Adv Health Sci Educ. 2010;16:311-29.

33. **Durning SJ, Cleary T, Sandars J, et al.** Viewing "strugglers" through a different lens: how a self-regulated learning perspective can help medical educators with assessment and remediation. Acad Med. 2011;86:488-95.

34. **Carraccio CL, Benson BJ, Nixon LJ, Derstine PL.** From the educational bench to the clinical bedside: translating the Dreyfus developmental model to the learning of clinical skills. Acad Med. 2008;83:761-7.

35. **Mamede S, van Gog T, van den Berge K, et al.** Effect of availability bias and reflective reasoning on diagnostic accuracy among internal medicine residents. JAMA. 2010;304:1198-203.

36. **Mamede S, Schmidt H, Penaforte J.** Effects of reflective practice on the accuracy of medical diagnoses. Med Educ. 2008;42:468-75.

37. **Charon R, Hermann N.** A sense of story, or why teach reflective writing? Acad Med. 2012;87:5-7.

38. **Atkinson P.** Training for Certainty. Soc Sci Med. 1984;19:949-56.

39. **Sommers LS.** Practice inquiry: uncertainty learning in primary care practice. Springer Science & Buisness Media. 2013;9:177-214.

40. **Ogdie AR, Reilly JB, Pang WG, et al.** Seen through their eyes: residents' reflections on the cognitive and contextual components of diagnostic errors in medicine. Acad Med. 2012;87:1361-7.

41. **Reilly JB, Ogdie AR, Von Feldt JM, Myers JS.** Teaching about how doctors think: a longitudinal curriculum in cognitive bias and diagnostic error for residents. BMJ Qual Saf 2013;22:1044-50.

42. **Pangaro L.** A new vocabulary and other innovations for improving descriptive in-training evaluations. Acad Med. 1999;74:1203-7.

43. **Ilgen JS, Humbert AJ, Kuhn G, et al.** Assessing diagnostic reasoning: a consensus statement summarizing theory, practice, and future needs. Acad Emerg Med. 2012; 19:1454-61.

44. **Huang GC, Newman LR, Schwartzstein RM.** Critical thinking in health professions education: summary and consensus statements of the Millennium Conference 2011. Teach Learn Med. 2014;26:95-102.

45. **Prystowsky JB, DaRosa DA.** A learning prescription permits feedback on feedback. Am J Surg. 2003;185:264-7.

46. **Wolpaw T, Cote L, Papp KK, Bordage G.** Student uncertainties drive teaching during case presentations: more so with SNAPPS. Acad Med. 2012;87:1210-7.

47. **McNamara DS.** Strategies to read and learn: overcoming learning by consumption. Med Educ. 2010;44:340-6.

10

Innovations and Future Directions

Jeffrey S. La Rochelle, MD, MPH, FACP
Anthony R. Artino Jr., PhD
Dario M. Torre, MD, PhD, MPH, FACP

❖ Introduction

This chapter presents examples of several new educationally grounded approaches to clinical reasoning that are important advances in the field and may expand our ability to teach and assess clinical reasoning. The development of clinical reasoning involves the ability to collect and integrate data, generate hypotheses, and appreciate "the relationship between each piece of data and each hypothesis" to rule out or confirm a diagnosis (1). Many exciting innovations are occurring throughout the spectrum of medical education, and we focus on those within 3 major areas: concept maps, self-regulated learning (SRL), and virtual patient panels. Although not entirely novel concepts, each innovation is grounded in educational theory and represents significant advances in teaching clinical reasoning. Concept maps and SRL both provide insight on the translation of clinical data into problem representation, a critical but often underemphasized step in the diagnostic reasoning process, and facilitate learning and assessment (2, 3). Virtual patient panels add complexity and authenticity to the delivery of clinical content and can be combined with concept maps or SRL to further enhance clinical reasoning. All the innovations emphasize the importance of process over obtaining a single correct answer, whether it is a diagnosis, treatment, or finding. We outline each of these

---

KEY POINTS

- New teaching innovations should be grounded in educational theory.
- Innovations should emphasize the clinical reasoning process rather than only the correct answer.
- Assessments should target specific clinical reasoning activities and be administered during those activities, as opposed to long afterwards.
- Understanding how a decision was made often promotes meaningful learning opportunities.
- Innovations in assessment and teaching may be augmented by combination with new methods in content delivery.

---

innovations in the context of educational theory and then examine some current applications along with future directions.

❖ Concept Maps

Concept maps are a visual representation of the learner's cognitive structures. They are characterized by ideas (concepts) connected by linking words that establish meaning within a network of interrelated and integrated knowledge structures (Figure 10-1).

Theoretical Framework

Cognitivism is a major theoretical framework that supports the application of concept mapping to the teaching and assessment of clinical reasoning. David Ausubel distinguishes meaningful learning from rote learning. Meaningful learning occurs when learning can be related to both previous knowledge and a preexisting cognitive structure, while rote learning is not linked to preexisting knowledge and remains isolated (4). In this context, meaningful learning is more likely to be retained. Ausubel defines concept learning, where related words combine to form propositions that actually constitute concepts; hence, "propositional learning largely involves learning the meaning of a composite idea generated by combining into sentences single words each of which represents a concept" (4). In other words, 2 concepts are related by a linking word, or proposition, that creates a meaningful relationship between concepts. Ultimately, concepts and linking words create a knowledge network in which concepts acquire meaning through the use of appropriate and accurate linking words (Figure 10-1).

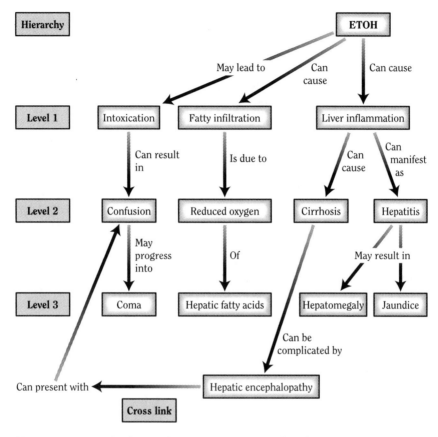

Figure 10-1 Example of a simple concept map using ethanol (ETOH) consumption as the main concept.

The development of relationships between concepts to acquire and develop new knowledge is an integral aspect of the theoretical foundation for concept maps.

Many of the cognitive principles described by Ausubel, specifically within the framework of meaningful learning, have been applied and further elaborated by Novak and Gowin with their work on concept mapping (4, 5). Through concept mapping, learners construct an organized visual schema or framework of meaningfully related concepts. Mapping can help a learner organize information, assess existing knowledge gains, develop insights into new and existing knowledge, and transfer knowledge to new experiences.

Concept mapping is also consistent with constructivism theory. From this perspective, learning occurs within the individual with respect to the process of constructing meaning from experience. According to Dewey, who first described the connections between experience and learning,

"Education is a development within, by, and for experience" (6). For Dewey, the experience must have 2 key principles: continuity and interaction. Continuity means that experience should be seen as a continuum in which "every experience both takes up something from those which have come before, and modifies in some way the quality of those which come after" (6).

Gagné, in his work on instructional design and conditions of learning theory, identifies 5 categories of human performance generated by learning outcomes: intellectual skills, verbal information, cognitive strategies, motor skills, and attitudes. Many elements of these categories include learning activities and performances that occur in concept mapping. Intellectual skills involve discrimination among concepts, verbal information concerns the acquisition of a body of knowledge (declarative knowledge), cognitive strategies entails the ability to think about what was learned and how to analyze and solve problems, and attitudes refer to an internal state that influences the learner's choices of action. Therefore, such learning outcomes outlined by Gagné are all performances that learners undertake in concept mapping learning activities (7).

Structure and Techniques Based on Learner's Tasks

Building on the theoretical framework previously outlined, concept maps are graphic representations of learner's knowledge structures. In this context, concepts represent events or objects that occur with regularity and are graphically presented in a hierarchical fashion from most inclusive to most specific. For example, in Figure 10-1, the overarching concept is ethanol, which includes all the concepts below (e.g., liver inflammation, intoxication). Concepts are related by propositions, or linking words, that give additional meaning to and establish relationships among concepts. For example, in Figure 10-1, the concepts "fatty infiltration" and "reduced oxidation" are given additional meaning by the proposition "is due to." This establishes a meaningful relationship between these concepts for the learner. Learners may use concept maps to build on what they already know; as a result learners and instructors have an opportunity to share, discuss, and revise their understanding of concepts, propositions, and the relationships between new and existing knowledge. Propositions may link concepts vertically or cross-link concepts horizontally. For example, Figure 10-1 shows a cross-link between the concepts of "hepatic encephalopathy" and "confusion" that further enhances the understanding of the topic for the learner. Crosslinks also represent the learner's ability to synthesize conceptual information from different sections of the map, integrate knowledge structures across different domains in the map, and begin to create their own unique meaning. The complexity and appropriateness of the hierarchical structure, along with the development of new crosslinks, are key features to creative thinking and the formation of new and meaningful knowledge in concept maps.

Two main types of mapping techniques have been used, with differences based on the degree of learner "directedness," or how much information or guidance the learner receives in constructing the map. For concept maps with greater directedness, the teacher provides some of the concepts, propositions, and crosslinks, and the learner must fill in the blanks (Figure 10-2) (8). Exercises involving maps with a high degree of directedness have the advantages of being less time-consuming to complete and easier to administer and score; however, the structure can affect the learners' cognitive processes, limiting the teachers' ability to assess the learners' inherent knowledge structures by providing a clinical reasoning scaffold (9).

Alternatively, concept maps with a low degree of directedness are created entirely by the learner, who determines the inclusion and relationships for the concepts, linking lines, propositions, and hierarchy

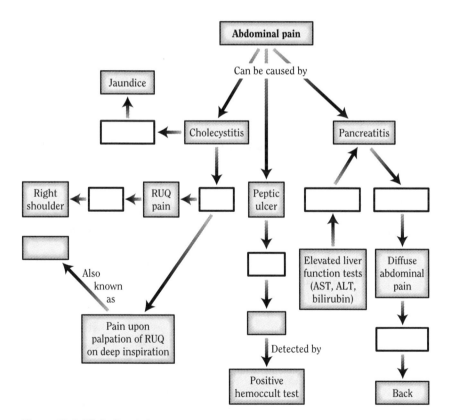

Figure 10-2 High-directedness map.

Some concepts and links are provided to the learners. ALT = alanine aminotransferase; AST = aspartate aminotransferase; RUQ = right upper quadrant.

to arrive at diagnostic possibilities (5). Teachers may adjust the directedness of the map to achieve their learning goals in the clinical reasoning process as matched to the learner or overall concept (Table 10-1). Maps with little directedness allow educators to discover a more in-depth view of the learner's process toward overall knowledge hierarchy (e.g., how links are created, what connections are made). A map with greater directedness focuses less on the hierarchical process and allows the teacher to inquire about a learner's knowledge and clinical reasoning skills about a specific area or set of concepts. For example, Figure 10-2 depicts several "blank" concepts (empty nodes that may be filled with concepts or linking words) around "pancreatitis," which allow for a focused assessment of knowledge and clinical reasoning regarding this specific domain of the overall concept map. Additionally, learners may be encouraged to use a highly directed concept map as scaffolding on which they can create additional concepts and links to further enhance their clinical reasoning.

Potential Use and Roles in Clinical Reasoning

Roberts describes 3 main concept mapping outcomes: to provide an additional resource for learning, to enable feedback, and to evaluate and assess conduct learning (5, 10). An advantage to concept mapping is the conduciveness of this process to individual as well as small group activities as an additional learning opportunity. In a study of such collaborative learning, Kinchin and Hay (11) found that students who produced

Table 10-1. Comparison of High- and Low-Directedness Concept Maps

Degree of Directedness	Time and Ease	Level of Learner	Knowledge	Reasoning
Low	More time-consuming for the student Increased difficulty for student	More advanced learner Familiar topic	Assess overall knowledge	Assess overall level of clinical reasoning
High	Quick to create and assess Easy for student to complete	Novice learner New topic	Assess specific domains within overall topic	Assess specific aspects (e.g., concepts, cross-links)

less sophisticated concept mapping structures benefited from students with more advanced structures, thus producing greater conceptual change. Although the study was not longitudinal, the findings may represent an example of meaningful learning whereby learners were able to associate prior knowledge with a new concept or linkage, in this case from a fellow learner, leading to the possibility of long-term retention. In relationship to feedback, concept mapping can assist the student in clarifying a topic, and teachers can use maps as a framework to provide feedback and identify student misunderstandings (10). This allows learners and teachers to assess their own reasoning processes by evaluating the quality of information obtained, monitoring for errors, analyzing inconsistencies, and providing remedial actions. Of note, the focus is on the process of clinical reasoning, and not on the ascertainment of a single correct answer.

The ability to integrate and synthesize critical clinical information and the correct use of pattern recognition are vital steps in making a correct diagnosis, and concept maps can be used as evaluation tools for identifying both valid and invalid learner thoughts and links. Concept maps can be used in formative assessments (where the teacher can assess the student's learning at a particular point) or summative assessments (to determine the student's understanding of a complete section or for a grade) (12). Concept mapping can provide educators with a meaningful learning strategy to foster the development of accurate reasoning processes. Overall, educators can use concept maps to assess the thinking process of students, identify gaps in knowledge or misconceptions, or delve into the learner's inaccurate information-processing and problem-solving skills. Concept maps also provide a different view of students' mind when students are challenged with problem-solving scenarios, providing opportunities for immediate and specific feedback.

Further research should explore concept mapping in groups, the learning impact of concept mapping longitudinally across the undergraduate and graduate curriculum, and even with the effect of mapping in interprofessional education. This would provide educators with the unique opportunity to identify a problem, target their efforts on specific areas of their students' weaknesses or strengths, give immediate and specific feedback, and ultimately assess the development and maturity of the students' clinical reasoning processes.

❖ SRL and SRL Microanalytic Approaches

Scholars and educators across specialties and disciplines have long tried to understand why individuals who seem to possess adequate knowledge often fail to display consistent learning and performance across activities (e.g., the classic "book smart" medical student who struggles in the clinical phases of training). In medical education, underperforming trainees represent a small but important subgroup of individuals who require disproportionate investments of time and resources on the part of faculty. Medical trainees may struggle for a variety of reasons, including personal issues (e.g., insufficient knowledge, personality disorders) and environmental constraints (e.g., subpar instruction, inadequate feedback) (see Chapter 9). Over the past 30 years, researchers from varied domains have explored the role that SRL, defined as a set of directed processes learners use to moderate their own learning and sustain their performance, plays in academic learning and performance (13, 14). More recently, medical education researchers have turned to theories of SRL—and, in particular, SRL microanalytic assessment techniques—to help understand and explain why and how some trainees succeed while others do not (15–17).

Framework for Assessing Clinical Reasoning
When trainees fail to demonstrate adequate performance across a range of clinical activities, such as clinical reasoning, medical educators typically look to test scores and direct observations to gather information about why trainees are struggling. Unfortunately, the data gleaned from tests and observations often provide limited diagnostic information about the strengths and weaknesses of individual trainees with respect to specific knowledge, skills, and attitudes (18). Furthermore, a recent meta-analysis suggests a paucity of evidence to guide best practices to identify and remediate underperformance in medical education settings (19).

One way to improve remediation activities is to create assessments that can reliably diagnose the underlying problems, or causal factors, that led to the performance deficits (19). Such assessments not only assist with remediation but can also form the foundation for the development of teaching strategies. In a general sense, the goal of such diagnostic assessments is to provide stakeholders with data that can be meaningfully interpreted and acted upon (18). Although many factors can negatively affect trainee performance, empirical studies from a variety of fields outside of medicine have revealed that individuals who perform poorly often exhibit deficits in SRL, such as maladaptive motivational beliefs and emotions (including low levels of confidence and high levels of negative affect [e.g., anxiety and boredom]), and regulatory deficits, such as poor planning, insufficient goal setting, ineffective self-monitoring, and infrequent use of effective learning strategies (14). Because SRL is considered a changeable state rather than a fixed trait, creating diagnostic assessments built around theories of self-regulation has potential value because data from such assessments provide detailed diagnostic information that can be used to devise remediation plans and teaching approaches. Furthermore, the successful use of SRL interventions in nonmedical education settings suggests that a self-regulation model of diagnostic assessment—which can lead to focused remediation and teaching—could be effective in medical education (20–22).

In the remainder of this portion of the chapter, we introduce a specific type of SRL assessment called SRL microanalysis, describe the characteristics of such assessments, and suggest ways to use assessment data to plan teaching and remediation strategies. We also include an example of how SRL microanalytic techniques can be used to assess clinical reasoning and explain its strengths and limitations. We begin by describing the theoretical foundation on which SRL microanalysis is built.

Social-Cognitive Approach

SRL has been defined as the degree to which individuals are active participants in their own learning processes (14). SRL is not a mental ability, like intelligence, nor an academic skill, like math proficiency. Instead, SRL is a set of self-directed processes that learners use to turn their mental abilities into academic skill and sustained performance. Models of SRL describe a recursive cycle of cognitive, motivational, and behavioral activities that are central to learning (23). Self-regulated learners are described as *active participants* in their learning who generate the thoughts, feelings, and actions necessary to attain their goals by deliberately planning, monitoring, and regulating their cognition, motivation, and behavior (24).

Over the past 30 years, theories of SRL have been developed to understand how students successfully adapt their cognition, motivation, and behavior to improve learning. Taken together, empirical investigations have consistently found that students who exhibit more adaptive self-regulatory beliefs and behaviors outperform their less adaptive classmates. That is, not only do highly self-regulated learners set goals, implement learning strategies, monitor goal progression, and establish productive environments for learning, but they also learn more and get better grades (25–29).

All of the many evidenced-based theories of SRL propose slightly different constructs and processes (13, 14, 30). Theories of SRL vary along many dimensions, including the role of motivation, the importance of the environment, and the use of cognitive strategies. For this chapter, we focus on a social-cognitive model of SRL because such models possess several key features that align well with many of the educational goals of medicine and several of the challenges associated with assessing and teaching clinical reasoning.

Social-cognitive theory is based on Bandura's model of reciprocal determinism, which states that student behaviors or skills, personal processes (beliefs and emotions), and environmental factors (classrooms and teachers) all interact and influence each other in reciprocal ways (31). Social-cognitive theory emphasizes the role of human cognition, with self-efficacy or confidence perceptions thought to be a key personal belief affecting individual behavior. For example, a medical trainee with low confidence in taking a medical history may exhibit low motivation and avoid such clinical activities, which in turn may produce negative feedback from his instructors. Conversely, if an instructor can identify the trainee's low self-efficacy and provide task-specific feedback on how to improve his history-taking skills, the student's perceptions of competence and confidence may increase while his anxiety about this activity diminishes. Ultimately, these enhanced personal beliefs and emotions may encourage greater behavioral engagement and motivation.

Another key assumption of social-cognitive theory is that "learning and behaviors are largely contextualized and thus what an individual thinks and does will often vary and change across contexts" (32). For example, a medical student may display acceptable skill when conducting a physical examination on an older patient, but that same trainee may show inadequate skill when examining a pediatric patient. From a teaching and assessment perspective, this context-specific assumption is critical because it implies that good self-regulation assessment tools should be tailored to specific contexts (17). That is, if we want to help struggling students improve their clinical reasoning skills, we must first assess their performance at a fine-grained, context-specific level.

Working from these social-cognitive assumptions, Zimmerman (33) developed a model of SRL that emphasizes the relationships between SRL processes and subprocesses. From this perspective, SRL is conceptualized as a 3-phase, cyclical loop (Figure 10-3) that surrounds any well-defined or discrete learning activity or event. In short, processes preceding action (forethought phase; before the activity) affect learning efforts (performance phase; during the activity), which, in turn, influence how learners react to and judge their performance success (self-reflection phase; after the activity).

Forethought processes, such as goal-setting and strategic planning, as well as motivational beliefs, such as self-efficacy perceptions, help to marshal an individual's efforts to learn. Once an individual engages in a task, such as studying for a licensing exam, interviewing a patient, or conducting a physical examination, the person typically solicits the use of performance phase processes such as using specific tactics to facilitate task performance (self-control) and tracking the effectiveness of these methods (self-observation). The information that an individual gathers from task

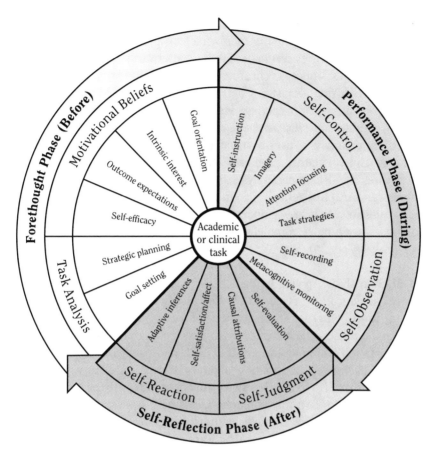

Figure 10-3 Zimmerman's 3-phase, cyclical loop conceptualizing the relationship between self-regulated learning process and subprocesses.

performance is used to judge whether he succeeded or failed (self-evaluation), to judge why this performance occurred (causal attributions), and do determine what he needs to do to improve future performance (adaptive inferences). Information garnered during the self-reflection phase is then fed back into the cyclical loop to influence later forethought phase processes.

Using Microanalytic Techniques

As opposed to traditional self-report measures that ask individuals to rate their beliefs and behaviors *after the fact* and in a decontextualized manner, microanalytic measures are customized and administered during particular activities, and they involve the use of context-specific questions targeting the various processes and subprocesses of the cyclical loop (Figure 10-3).

Thus, the purpose of SRL microanalysis is to evaluate how individuals approach (forethought), monitor (performance), and reflect (self-reflection) *during* specific activities, as opposed to long afterwards. A benefit of applying Zimmerman's 3-phase cyclical loop to assess SRL is that it allows one to assess SRL during almost any activity (e.g., a traditional exam, a study session, or a diagnostic reasoning activity). The only requirement is that the activity under investigation has a clear beginning, middle, and end (34).

SRL microanalysis uses focused questions to evaluate the beliefs, emotions, and regulatory processes employed by trainees. Some of the key features of SRL microanalysis include the use of 1) individualized administration; 2) theoretically grounded, highly contextualized questions; and 3) questions that are temporally linked to the phases of the cyclical SRL model (for a more complete description of the characteristics of SRL microanalysis, see 34).

SRL Microanalysis Applied to Medical Education

In medical education, evidence of the validity of SRL microanalysis is just starting to emerge. For example, in a recent qualitative pilot study, Cleary and Sandars (35) collected preliminary data that demonstrated the implementation and potential utility of SRL microanalysis for generating important diagnostic information about students' regulatory processes as they performed a clinical activity (venipuncture). In particular, the researchers developed a microanalytic assessment to evaluate the regulatory profiles of 2 groups of medical students: those who were successful in a venipuncture task and those who were unsuccessful in this task. The authors' SRL microanalytic questions showed good inter-rater reliability and revealed that students who successfully completed the venipuncture task had high levels of strategic thinking before, during, and after the task; that is, they focused on the strategies and technique needed to draw blood. On the other hand, students who struggled with the task tended to focus less on strategy and more on the broad outcome of "drawing blood." Cleary and Sandars noted that "SRL microanalysis provides medical educators a potential assessment instrument to evaluate the extent to which medical students regulate their behaviors during medical activities" (35).

More recently, Artino and colleagues (36) have applied SRL microanalysis to a clinical reasoning activity. Table 10-2 provides examples of several of the microanalytic questions used. Altogether, 71 students completed the study, and the results revealed that most students in the early stages of learning diagnostic reasoning were aware of and thought about at least 1 key diagnostic reasoning process or strategy while solving a clinical case, but a much smaller fraction of these students set goals or developed plans that incorporate such strategies. Additionally,

Table 10-2. Sample Microanalytic Questions for the Clinical Reasoning Task

Phases of SRL Feedback Loop	SRL Processes	Assessment Questions
Forethought (before)	Self-efficacy	How confident are you that you can determine the most likely diagnosis for this patient on your first attempt? [Likert-type item]
	Goal setting	Do you have a goal (or goals) in mind as you prepare to do this activity? If so, please explain. [Open-ended item]
	Strategic planning	What do you think you need to do to perform well on this activity? [Open-ended item]
Performance (during)	Metacognitive monitoring	As you have been going through this process, what has been the primary thing you have been thinking about or focusing on? [Open-ended item]
Reflection (after)	Causal attributions	Why do you think you were unable to arrive at the correct diagnosis? [Open-ended item]
	Adaptive inferences	You now have a chance to reanalyze the case. What do you think you need to do to arrive at the correct diagnosis? [Open-ended item]
	Anxiety	How anxious are you about not being able to come up with the correct diagnosis? [Likert-type item]

results from several regression analyses suggested that, after adjustment for prior achievement and verbal reasoning ability, students' strategic planning explained significant additional variance in several short- and longer-term performance outcomes, including course grade, second-year grade point average, and U.S. Medical Licensing Examination Step 1 and National Board of Medical Examiners internal medicine subject exam (R^2 change of 0.15, 0.14, 0.08, and 0.10, respectively). On the basis of these results, Artino and colleagues concluded that medical students who focus on task-specific processes as they approach a diagnostic reasoning task (i.e., during strategic planning) tend to achieve better performance outcomes than their counterparts who do not. Using such data, medical educators have insight into the reasons why some trainees succeed in clinical activities—such as diagnostic reasoning—while others do not.

Improve Remediation and Teaching

Research on SRL microanalysis and its practical applications are still very much in their infancy, particular within the field of medical education. As discussed above, a primary purpose of microanalytic protocols is "to generate reliable information about students' regulatory processes that can be used by educators and practitioners to inform the development of academic interventions or to guide instruction" (37). Indeed, in educational contexts outside of medicine, greater emphasis has been placed on linking formative assessments to intervention development. Moreover, recent work suggests that teachers value microanalytic forms of assessment data because such information can be used to plan instructional interventions and remediation activities (38).

Recently, Cleary and Platten developed an SRL intervention, called the Self-Regulation Empowerment Program, and collected preliminary evidence of how teachers can use SRL microanalytic protocols to guide tutoring sessions with high school students who are struggling in science courses (39). Results from this work suggested that changes in SRL processes were closely linked to shifts in academic achievement. Although promising, this case study has important methodologic limitations. Thus, more work is clearly needed to systematically investigate the links between interventions that use SRL microanalytic assessments and improvements in student learning and performance.

In medical education, researchers and practitioners are just now beginning to appreciate the potential uses of SRL microanalysis to inform efforts to improve learning and performance in medical trainees (17, 40). Sandars has argued that "Using microanalysis of SRL processes as an 'assessment for learning' is based on obtaining a picture of which key SRL processes are being employed, or not being employed.... A coaching approach can then be used to help the learner specifically develop the SRL processes that are not being fully utilized" (40). In fact, Sandars and his colleagues have recently put forth an integrative model for teaching medical students how to make an appropriate clinical diagnosis. The proposed model includes microanalytic assessment methods to help teachers identify the main processes involved in generating an accurate clinical diagnosis. This information is then used to provide focused feedback to help students improve their clinical decision-making skills. Systematic research is now needed to support (or refute) the effectiveness of such an approach.

❖ Virtual Patient Panels

According to the Association of American Medical Colleges Group on Information Resources, most medical schools across the United States and Canada are using some form of virtual patient software. In fact, use of virtual patients in some format has been available to medical schools for over 40 years (41). Although early implementation was hampered by technologic limitations, there has been a global trend in the increased use of virtual patients, with recognition that many cross-cultural issues affect the development of cases appropriate for an increasingly diverse learner population (42). Recently, the European Commission has partially funded an online repository of virtual patient cases, called eViP, with the goal of creating 320 cases accessible under a common creative license to share across institutions (43). Early uses of virtual patients were limited to assessments of history and communication skills, but modern software platforms allow for the collection of more robust data on how a learner approached a problem and reached a diagnosis (41). In fact, one of the most effective uses for virtual patients may be to facilitate and understand the development of clinical reasoning (44). Learner encounters with virtual patients are equivalent to encounters with standardized patients in terms of learning potential and comfort, and in many ways, virtual patients may be better suited for deliberate practice over a variety of content areas and environmental contexts (44, 45). Instead of having a single virtual patient addressing individual topics, the use of a panel of virtual patients fully embedded into an integrated curriculum may not only improve clinical reasoning grounded in educational theory but also enhance professional identity formation (46, 47).

The use of virtual patient panels is breathing new life into the experiential learning model that Kolb developed over 30 years ago. Experiential learning emphasizes the experience as the source of learning, which can be enhanced through active participation of learners who have a meaningful role (48). Learners first conceptualize the experience in an abstract sense and may even verbalize an approach to a particular problem before the actual experience. This is followed by a transformation of the experience into learning through reflection and active experimentation, where the learner can attempt different approaches to a similar problem or apply a similar approach to a slightly different problem. Experiential learning has clear ties with the theory of situated cognition, which also endorses the belief that individuals learn through experience. More specifically, learning is inextricably bound to thinking and doing, wherein the environment plays a crucial role in the learning process (47). The context of the learning experience, to include the activity, the people involved, their culture, their body language, and other factors not only contribute to the learning process but are an integral part of learning. Therefore, educational experiences more closely aligned with the actual clinical practice may improve learning from both an experiential and situated cognition theoretical view point (47).

Many examples of programs using a variety of virtual patient innovations are grounded in educational theory, and studies are assessing the optimal use and standard design for these cases to be shared internationally. In one of the earlier applications, Orr and colleagues implemented a panel of virtual patients for students in a Doctor of Pharmacy program and found this approach improved overall knowledge and communication skills in their learners (49). The innovation allowed learners to interact via weekly emails with a panel of virtual patients, who were portrayed by faculty and community pharmacists, during a single semester. The goals of the innovation were to develop clinical assessment skills, enhance communication skills, expand topic-specific knowledge, and facilitate small group interactions. Learners were evaluated on their responses to patients in terms of their clinical reasoning, timeliness, and communication skills. In addition, learners received feedback from their virtual patients and from their peers within each small group. This innovation represents a fairly simple application of experiential learning and situated cognition as described above. Learners were engaged in a realistic, but controlled, experience interacting with patients in real time, similar to their actual practice as pharmacists. The additions of small group interactions to discuss patient issues and peer-to-peer assessments regarding their responses helped foster a sense of community and professional identity. A limitation of this early innovation is that interaction with virtual patients was limited to email, which may reduce some of the authenticity of this experience. In addition, there is a high burden on faculty members to portray each of the virtual patients, monitor learner responses, and provide responses and feedback. A challenge for these types of innovations is in the creation of appropriate assessment tools that will accurately measure the quality of patient interactions and clinical reasoning.

A more recent innovation with virtual patient panels significantly advanced the application of educational theory into practical learning. Salminen and colleagues developed a pilot curriculum for senior medical students using virtual patient panels under the premise that situational examples are critical in the development of clinical reasoning (50). The goals of their innovation were to embed the teaching of clinical reasoning and communication skills into a virtual patient model as formative learning with the addition of learner self-reflection. The innovation was designed around the theory of experiential learning, and began with learners developing a pre-experience strategy consistent with abstract conceptualization as the first step to understanding the experience. This was followed by the concrete experience of the actual virtual patient encounter, which involved the gathering of historical information, obtaining physical examination information, and the development of a preliminary diagnosis with an assessment on plan for treatment. Learners were then asked to reflect on the outcomes of their virtual patient encounters and on their pre-experience strategies in approaching the encounter consistent with the first step in transforming the experience into learning, or reflective observation. Finally, learners were able to apply this learning to the next encounter and, in a sense, actively experiment within a controlled environment to fully transform the experience into long-term learning. The pilot was deemed a success as the overall approach supported self-directed learning and reflective thinking, and the learners felt engaged with the authenticity of the virtual patients (50).

Perhaps the most robust innovation using virtual patient panels is the Evolve clinic, developed by Hughes and colleagues at the Michigan State University College of Osteopathic Medicine (51). The goals of the Evolve curriculum are to create a longitudinal learning process, promote professional development, integrate practical applications into the learning environment, and develop critical thinking skills. The Evolve clinic is designed as a longitudinal curriculum spanning 4 years in which learners interact with the same panel of virtual patients, developing a continuity of care experience that models a team approach to patient care. In this curriculum, the virtual patients are computer-generated avatars, and faculty serve as guides overseeing individual learners and their group practices. The Evolve clinic begins with students learning what to ask patients based on a series of signs and symptoms, and the complexity and severity of the patient issues can be modified over time. In this way, learning can be enhanced by controlling the virtual environment, and by incorporating consequences associated with learner choices, enhancing the overall development process consistent with tenets of situated cognition (47, 52). Importantly, the cases often have more than 1 correct answer, which allows for the development of clinical reasoning in a more realistic context. The evaluation can focus on the development of clinical reasoning through the identification of patterns and approaches to problems instead of simply identifying a correct diagnosis. This is an important step forward in the evaluation and development of clinical reasoning, consistent with the development of a decision-making process and identification of areas of weakness in a learners approach to a clinical problem (41, 44). An important part of the Evolve clinic is that students are placed in small "group practices" that meet regularly in a clinical setting. Students are required to wear professional attire and their white coats as if they were actually seeing patients in clinic. Additionally, students both work independently and as medical home teams, furthering the authenticity of the encounter while providing opportunities for both autonomy and competence in a controlled and safe setting conducive for exploration and learning.

❖ Summary

This chapter has presented just a few of the many innovations in the teaching of clinical reasoning that are ongoing in medical schools in the United States and the world. We introduced the use of concept maps that allow visualization of knowledge hierarchy, which not only strengthen established connections but facilitate the creation of new associations for learners. This innovation is grounded in theory and moves away from the emphasis on a single correct answer while focusing more on the process of clinical reasoning. Variations in the "directedness" of the concept map allow for probing of current understanding and probing of a learner's clinical reasoning process. Concept map exercises with mixed small groups of medical, pharmacy, and nursing students may represent an opportunity for enhancing interprofessional education. Concept maps can be used to assess the reasoning ability of a learner in a variety of settings to include virtual clinic encounters associated with a panel of virtual patients.

SRL further delves into understanding the process of learning and clinical reasoning. There are clear implications for how we teach material and how we remediate struggling learners, with an emphasis on strategic planning and task-specific processes as an essential first step when approaching a complex clinical encounter. Again, as demonstrated in concept maps, finding a single correct answer is not the goal, and there is more emphasis on the process of clinical reasoning. As with concept maps, SRL has many applications and can be formally integrated into the pre-experience strategy and self-reflection aspects of the virtual patient encounters.

Finally, virtual patient panels represent a controlled immersion in the clinical experience, providing a safe environment for early learners to develop their professional identity and join the community of physicians. Realistic branching of cases allows for multiple "correct" paths that may lead to slightly different outcomes. The inclusion of learners from other disciplines into a medical home model can provide a unique and powerful addition to interprofessional education.

A common theme among these innovations is that the integration of sound educational theory and practice should promote meaningful learning opportunities. New teaching methods should be grounded in theory and rigorously evaluated for their impact beyond just learner approval.

An important challenge is to develop equally innovative evaluation tools and rubrics to match these new teaching methods. As seen with each of the innovations described, these rubrics should focus less on obtaining a single correct diagnosis and more on the strategic approach to clinical problems, patterns of questioning, the clinical decision-making process, learner self-reflection, and professional identity formation (41, 44). We should be moving well beyond filling out a checklist or multiple-choice test designed at obtaining a single correct answer with regard to clinical reasoning. Rather, our educational interventions should be grounded in theory and focus on understanding and teaching the process of clinical reasoning to better equip our learners for the future practice of medicine.

REFERENCES

1. **Eva KW.** What every teacher needs to know about clinical reasoning. Med Educ. 2004;39:98-106.
2. **Groves M, O'Rourke P, Alexander H.** The clinical reasoning characteristics of diagnostic experts. Med Teach. 2003;25:308-13.
3. **Higgs J, Jones MA, Loftus S, Christensen N.** Clinical Reasoning in the Health Professions. 3rd ed. Oxford: Butterworth-Heinemann-Elsevier; 2008.
4. **Ausubel DP.** Educational Psychology: A Cognitive View. New York: Holt, Rinehart and Winston; 1968.
5. **Novak JD, Gowin DB.** Learning How to Learn. New York: Cambridge University Press; 1984.
6. **Dewey J.** Experience and Education. New York: Collier Books; 1938.
7. **Gagné RM, Briggs LJ, Golas KC.** Principles of Instructional Design. 5th ed. Belmont, CA: Thomson-Wadsworth; 2005.
8. **Schau C, Mattern N.** Use of mapping techniques in teaching applied statistics courses. Am Stat. 1997;51:171-5.
9. **Ruiz-Primo MA.** Examining concept maps as an assessment tool. In: Canas AJ, Novak JD, Gonzalex FM, eds. Concept Maps: Theory, Methodology, Technology. Proceedings of the First International Conference on Concept Mapping, Pamplona, Spain, 2004:555-62.
10. **Roberts L.** Using concept maps to measure statistical understanding. Int J Math Educ Sci Technol. 1999;30:707-17.
11. **Kinchin IM, Hay DB.** How a qualitative approach to concept map analysis can be used to aid learning by illustrating patterns of conceptual development. Educ Res. 2000;42:43-57.
12. **Coffey JW, Carnot MJ, Feltovich PJ, Hoffman RR, Canas AJ, et al.** A summary of literature pertaining to the use of concept mapping techniques and technologies for education and performance support. Technical Report submitted to the US Navy Chief of Naval Education and Training. Pensacola, FL: Institute for Human and Machine Cognition; 2003.
13. **Boekaerts M, Pintrich PR, Zeidner M.** Handbook of Self-Regulation. San Diego, CA: Academic Press; 2000.
14. **Zimmerman BJ, Schunk DH, eds.** Handbook of Self-Regulation of Learning and Performance. New York: Routledge; 2011.

15. **Brydges R, Butler D.** A reflective analysis of medical education research on self-regulation in learning and practice. Med Educ. 2012;46:71-9.

16. **Cleary TJ, Durning SJ, Hemmer PA, Gruppen LD, Artino AR.** Self-regulated learning in medical education. In: Walsh K, ed. Oxford Textbook of Medical Education. Oxford, United Kingdom: Oxford University Press; 2013:465-77.

17. **Durning SJ, Cleary TJ, Sandars JE, Hemmer PA, Kokotailo P K, Artino AR.** Viewing "strugglers" through a different lens: how a self-regulated learning perspective can help medical educators with assessment and remediation. Acad Med. 2011;86:488-95.

18. **Rupp AA, Templin J, Henson RA.** Diagnostic Measurement: Theory, Methods, and Applications. New York: Guilford Press; 2010.

19. **Hauer KE, Ciccone A, Henzel TR, Katsufrakis P, Miller SH, Norcross WA, et al.** Remediation of the deficiencies of physicians across the continuum from medical school to practice: a thematic review of the literature. Acad Med. 2009;84:1822-32.

20. **Cleary TJ, Zimmerman BJ.** Self-regulation differences during athletic performance by experts, non-experts and novices. J Appl Sport Psychol. 2001;13:61-82.

21. **DiBendetto MK, Zimmerman BJ.** Constructand prective validity of microanalytic measures of students' self-regulation of science learning. Learn Individ Differences. 2013;26:30-41.

22. **Kitsantas A, Zimmerman BJ.** Comparing self-regulatory processes among novice, non-expert, and expert volleyball players: a microanalytic study. J Appl Sport Psychol. 2002;14:91-105.

23. **Azevedo R.** Using hypermedia as a metacognitive tool for enhancing student learning? The role of self-regulated learning. Educ Psychol. 2005;40:199-209.

24. **Lajoie SP, Azevedo R.** Teaching and learning in technology-rich environments. In: Alexander PA, Winne PH, eds. Handbook of Educational Psychology. 2nd ed. Mahwah, NJ: Lawrence Erlbaum Associates; 2006:803-21.

25. **Pintrich PR, De Groot EV.** Motivational and self-regulated learning component of classroom academic performance. J Educ Psychol. 1990;82:33-40.

26. **Pintrich PR, Garcia T.** Student goal orientation and self-regulation in the college classroom. In: Maehr ML, Pintrich PR, eds. Advances in Motivation and Achievement: Goals and Self-Regulatory Processes. Greenwich, CT: JAI; 1991:371-402.

27. **Zimmerman BJ, Bandura A.** Impact of self-regulatory influence on writing course attainment. Am Educ Res J. 1994;31:845-62.

28. **Zimmerman BJ, Martinez-Pons M.** Development of a structured interview for assessing student use of self-regulated learning strategies. Am Educ Res J. 1986;23:614-28.

29. **Zimmerman BJ, Schunk DH, eds.**Self-Regulated Learning and Academic Achievement: Theoretical Perspectives. 2nd ed. Mahwah, NJ: Lawrence Erlbaum Associates; 2001.

30. **Puustinen M, Pulkkinen L.** Models of self-regulated learning: a review. Scand J Educ Res. 2001;45:269-86.

31. **Bandura A.** Self-Efficacy: The Exercise of Control. New York: W.H. Freeman; 1997.

32. **Cleary TJ, Dong T, Artino AR.** Assessing contextualized, dynamic processes: the benefits and limitations of self-regulated learning microanalysis. Program of the Annual Meeting of the American Educational Research Association, Philadelphia, PA; 2014.

33. **Zimmerman BJ.** Attaining self-regulation: a social-cognitive perspective. In: Boekaerts M, Pintrich P, Zeidner M, eds. Handbook of Self-Regulation. Orlando, FL: Academic Press; 2000:13-39.

34. **Cleary TJ.** Emergence of self-regulated learning microanalysis: historical overview, essential features, and implications for research and practice. In: Zimmerman B, Schunk D, eds. Handbook of Self-Regulation of Learning and Performance. New York: Routledge; 2011: 329–345.

35. **Cleary TJ, Sandars J.** Self–regulatory skills and clinical performance: a pilot study. Med Teach. 2011;33:e368-e374.

36. **Artino AR, Cleary TJ, Dong T, Hemmer PA, Durning SJ.** Exploring clinical reasoning in novices: a self-regulated learning microanalytic assessment approach. Med Educ. 2014;48:280-91.

37. **Cleary TJ, Zimmerman BJ.** A cyclical self-regulatory account of student engagement: theoretical foundations and applications. In: Handbook of Research on Student Engagement. New York: Springer; 2012:237-57.

38. **Cleary TJ, Zimmerman BJ, Keating T.** Training physical education students to self-regulate during basketball free throw practice. Res Q Exercise Sport. 2006;77.2:251-62.

39. **Cleary TJ, Platten P.** Examining the correspondence between self-regulated learning and academic achievement: a case study analysis. Educ Res Int 2013;2013: article ID 272560.

40. **Sandars J.** Technology and the delivery of the curriculum of the future: opportunities and challenges. Med Teach. 2012;34.7:534-8.

41. **Cendan J, Lok B.** The use of virtual patients in medical school curricula. Adv Physiol Educ. 2012;36:48–53.

42. **Fors UG, Muntean V, Botezatu M, Zary N.** Cross-cultural use and development of virtual patients. Med Teach. 2009;31:732–8.

43. Electronic Virtual Patients. Available at: http://www.virtualpatients.eu/. Accessed 5 July 2014.

44. **Cook DA, Triola MM.** Virtual patients: a critical literature review and proposed next steps. Med Educ. 2009;43:303–11.

45. **Triola M, Feldman H, Kalet AL, Zabar S, Kachur EK, Gillespie C, et al.** A randomized trial of teaching clinical skills using virtual and live standardized patients. J Gen Intern Med. 2006;21:424-9.

46. **Edelbring S1, Broström O, Henriksson P, Vassiliou D, Spaak J, Dahlgren LO, et al.** Integrating virtual patients into courses: follow-up seminars and perceived benefit. Med Educ. 2012;46:417-25.

47. **Schumacher DJ, Englander R, Carraccio C.** Developing the master learner: applying learning theory to the learner, the teacher, and the learning environment. Acad Med. 2013;88:1635-45.

48. **Kolb D.** Experiential Learning: Experience as the Source of Learning and Development. Englewood Cliffs, NJ: Prentice-Hall; 1984:231–41.

49. **Orr KK.** Integrating virtual patients into a self-care course. Am J Pharm Educ. 2007;71:30.

50. **Salminen H, Zary N, Björklund K, Toth-Pal E, Leanderson C.** Virtual patients in primary care: developing a reusable model that fosters reflective practice and clinical reasoning. J Med Internet Res. 2014;16:e3.

51. **Michigan State University College of Osteopathic Medicine.** Experiential clinic idea EVOLVES to help students integrate basic and clinical sciences. Available at: http://com.msu.edu/Events%20and%20News/Archived%20News/2013/09September/ Experiential%20clinic%20idea%20EVOLVES%20to%20help%20students%20 integrate%20basic%20and%20clinical%20sciences%20.htm. Accessed on 5 April 2014.

52. **Round J, Conradi E, Poulton T.** Improving assessment with VPs. Med Teac. 2009;31:75963.

11

Afterword: Teaching Clinical Reasoning—Where Do We Go From Here?

Steven J. Durning, MD, PhD, FACP

Joseph J. Rencic, MD, FACP

Robert L. Trowbridge Jr., MD, FACP

Lambert Schuwirth, MD, PhD

While clinical reasoning is at the heart of a clinician's work, knowing how to teach it effectively may be the Holy Grail of medical education. Although everyone acknowledges the importance of knowledge in clinical reasoning expertise, the scope of what constitutes clinical reasoning is remarkable and leads to debate about how to best teach it, learn it, and assess it. Indeed, the very term *clinical reasoning* is so broad it may be used to refer to practically any form of thought that clinicians use to ultimately arrive at a diagnosis (diagnostic reasoning) or patient-specific plans (therapeutic reasoning).

In this book, we focus specifically on diagnostic reasoning and we thus use the terms *diagnostic reasoning* and *clinical reasoning* interchangeably throughout. The spectrum of such reasoning includes the process of deliberate hypothetico-deductive reasoning: the stringing together and analyzing of the building blocks of the clinical problem, like the meticulous process of solving the multiplication of two 3-digit numbers by hand. Clinical reasoning also includes the nonanalytical process of recognizing a problem as a whole, like when we do not have to think twice when we recognize a door to be a door and we immediately know how to operate it despite the wide variety of shapes and forms that a door can take. Additionally, clinical reasoning includes patient and environmental factors, as well as one's motivation and emotional state. All of these can shape and modify the clinician's thinking in conscious and unconscious ways, resulting in variable clinician performance across seemingly similar clinical situations.

One could now think that with such a broad concept and so many different views on how to approach clinical reasoning, it would be impossible to teach it, but we do not believe that this is the case. Take, for example, the complexity of learning a language with the vast vocabulary and byzantine grammatical rules that govern it—yet sure enough, there are millions of 2-year-olds who slowly but surely develop mastery. Similarly, there are various aspects to teaching and learning clinical reasoning that work, and much is known and shared in the pages that are before you.

Our understanding of clinical reasoning has been strengthened by recent scholarship based on theoretical and conceptual insights from multiple fields. The study of clinical reasoning shares features with the study of diagnostic errors, decision-making, and judgment, which have also benefited from these recent developments. One of the important highlights of this book is that our understanding and definition of clinical reasoning has evolved in conjunction with epistemologic theories. Historically, clinical reasoning focused on the clinician's brain ("the world inside the clinician's head") but has now expanded to include patient and environmental factors ("the clinician's head inside the world") (1). We believe that the definition of clinical reasoning will continue to evolve because it is a complex construct that can be further informed and transformed by new theoretical lenses. For this book, we have used the following working definition: the cognitive and noncognitive process by which a health care professional consciously and unconsciously interacts with the patient and environment to collect and interpret patient data, weigh the benefits and risks of actions, and understand patient preferences to determine the diagnosis and plan of care for a patient.

Given that clinical reasoning is a multifaceted, evolving construct, the editors have been careful not to label clinical reasoning as a "skill," avoiding the false suggestion that reasoning is a single technical ability, divisible from knowledge and noncognitive attributes, such as attitude or motivation. The literature has demonstrated repeatedly that expert performance in clinical reasoning is not generic and cannot be disentangled from well-organized knowledge. Indeed, the book cites literature showing that an expert can see 2 patients with the same chief complaint as well as history and physical examination facts (or nearly identical) and yet come to 2 different diagnostic decisions. This is known as the phenomenon of context specificity. Recent work in clinical reasoning also highlights that excellence in clinical reasoning is a "state" rather than a "trait"—clinical reasoning abilities are situation specific, resting with a particular patient in a specific setting with specific resources and interactions with both the patient and the environment.

This book has synthesized insights about teaching clinical reasoning, pulling from the medical education literature as well as from the fields of psychology, education, expertise, and systems analysis. We have included topics that are germane to teaching and included theory, assessment, curricula, remediation, and faculty development. The goal has been to provide a "landscape" of where the field began and where it stands now, recognizing that there remains much that we do not know about the best approach to teaching clinical reasoning. With these ideas in mind, we review the highlights of the book and discuss future directions in teaching clinical reasoning.

As noted above, the study of clinical reasoning has also been informed by work from diverse fields and theoretical perspectives. We began with a review of these concepts. This work continues to emerge, and we believe that social cognitive theories are particularly likely to lead to important advances because they provide a means of exploring variation in work-based performance, including the above-mentioned phenomena of context specificity.

We subsequently outlined why a longitudinal, integrated curriculum in clinical reasoning is needed. The "siloization" of medical school curricula has made clinical reasoning an "orphan" topic in many medical schools rather than a focal point of the entire curriculum. Our experience suggests that many pathophysiologic courses still have a disease-based rather than symptom-based focus, making the translation of learning to clinical settings where patients present with symptoms and findings, not known diseases, more challenging. Fortunately, there has been a recent trend toward building clinical reasoning courses within medical schools, but these may only produce yet another silo if not integrated into the larger curriculum. Theoretical and experimental insights have provided valuable content to be taught within clinical reasoning curricula. We believe that the core of any clinical reasoning curricula should include knowledge of diseases, starting with typical presentations of common diseases, then moving to atypical presentations of common diseases and uncommon diseases.

We then discussed how curricular design can also be informed by the diagnostic error literature, which continues to make important contributions to the understanding of clinical reasoning. Through highlighting the importance of the system and cognitive dispositions to respond as well as providing support for both nonanalytical and analytical reasoning, this area of study provides a meaningful lens through which to view advancements in the field. It is important to recognize that cognitive errors are common among both experienced clinicians and novices; an improved understanding of how the clinical reasoning process works, and how it may be derailed, is likely to help both teachers and learners alike.

In considering how clinical reasoning is taught and learned, it becomes clear that few subjects in medicine provide a more telling example of the complex interactions between the concepts of teaching and learning than clinical reasoning. Clinical reasoning is learned (thankfully) despite shortcomings in our teaching. Explicit instruction (e.g., teaching) in this field is difficult and at times not available to the teachers' introspection. We thus outlined several practices and educational techniques from a variety of fields to assist the teacher, but clearly more research is needed to further refine our practice.

The assessment of clinical reasoning is similarly difficult. As described previously, clinical reasoning is a complex construct that encompasses many abilities. Therefore, there is no magic bullet or Holy Grail instrument that will determine competence in clinical reasoning. The chapters on assessment and remediation highlighted the need for multiple instruments and large sampling to aid in reliably assessing clinical reasoning. Given the complexity of the construct of clinical reasoning, learners need to be followed, instructed on which areas of performance need to be addressed, and given the opportunity to make improvements. This becomes particularly important with learners moving from the classroom to the clinical arena as they progress though undergraduate and graduate medical education and beyond. These chapters also direct attention to the evolving and at times nonlinear nature of clinical reasoning and provide examples of methods that can be used to improve assessment and remediation practices. These ideas include assessing intermediate steps, including traditionally noncognitive aspects (e.g., motivation), and using frameworks that include the interactions that occur in practice.

The chapter on faculty development pointed out that few existing faculty development programs specifically focus on clinical reasoning and that there is great need for our community to study, publish, and disseminate faculty development efforts. The reader is encouraged to review the digital supplemental material to provide some assistance with this, but more is needed.

We also provided suggestions for how the teacher/clinician might embark on a lifelong "program" of reasoning improvement. Using the principles of deliberate practice theory with practice activities that may be meaningful for medicine, specific recommendations were made for how the busy clinician may emphasize improving his or her abilities in clinical reasoning as part of his or her daily work.

The final chapter provided some thoughts on future directions in the teaching, assessment, and remediation of clinical reasoning. Several techniques were described in detail, with acknowledgment that these are only a few of the exciting and innovative developments that may improve our teaching and learning of clinical reasoning in future years. It also acknowledged that virtual and simulated learning will likely play a vital role in the future of clinical reasoning teaching.

In conclusion, we provide several recommendations for advancing the scholarship in the field of clinical reasoning. In doing so, we use Boyer's framework for scholarship to categorize this agenda (2).

❖ Discovery Agenda

Recommendation: Continue to seek explanations for the variance underlying case and context specificity. Social cognitive theories provide one potential lens for exploring the latter phenomena that should be investigated further.

Recommendation: Place a greater emphasis on the study of developing clinician's abilities in clinical reasoning. Indeed, the statements "few existing [insert the topic in teaching] programs specifically focus on clinical reasoning" and "there is a need to study and disseminate" resound through all of the chapters, as clear steps are needed to move forward. Where possible, this should be accompanied by the study of the effect of such programs on patient outcomes.

❖ Integration Agenda

Recommendation: Recognize the lenses that we bring to the construct of clinical reasoning (e.g., information processing, situativity) and continue to seek new methods and theories that may increase the power of the explanatory model of clinical reasoning and inform the development of new techniques in teaching and assessment.

Recommendation: Seek to further integrate the fields of diagnostic reasoning (e.g., cognitive psychology focus) and therapeutic reasoning (e.g., medical decision-making focus) and capitalize on concepts common to both fields

❖ Application Agenda

Recommendation: Elevate the teaching and learning of clinical reasoning to the level of a "foundational science" in undergraduate medical education. It should be infused throughout the curriculum and included from the outset of medical education.

Recommendation: Recognize the critical need for a national (or international) curricula of virtual cases that provide opportunities for deliberate practice of typical presentations of common diseases, atypical presentations of common diseases, typical presentations of uncommon diseases, and atypical presentations of uncommon diseases. There should be multiple examples of a given disease that highlight the diversity of presentations to learners. With the electronic resources at our disposal, the only apparent limitation to building such a database is developing the collaborative network, which we acknowledge may be challenging.

Recommendation: Seek optimal ways of combining current assessment instruments to construct means of assessing the clinical reasoning abilities of learners of varying levels of experience. What can be particularly vexing in terms of clinical reasoning assessment is nonanalytic reasoning and recent developments of biologic measures to assess clinical reasoning show promise in this area.

Recommendation: Provide clinicians with regular and broad-based feedback on their diagnostic performance by building electronic health records with active feedback mechanisms regarding patient outcomes.

Recommendation: Faculty development programs specific to teaching clinical reasoning need to be constructed and disseminated. Participation in such programs is likely to have a salutary effect on the clinical reasoning abilities of the faculty themselves. Indeed, teaching has recently been acknowledged as a deliberate practice activity for clinical reasoning.

REFERENCES

1. **Durning SJ, Artino AR.** Situativity theory: a perspective on how participants and the environment can interact: AMEE Guide no. 52. Med Teach. 2011;33:188-99.
2. **Boyer E.** Scholarship Reconsidered: Priorities of the Professoriate. San Francisco: Jossey-Bass; 1990.

Glossary

Affective bias (also called visceral bias): irrational preference driven by physicians' emotions about their patients that can induce cognitive errors. Positive and negative emotions can lead to this bias.

Analytic reasoning (system 2 thinking, slow thinking): slow, conscious, effortful thinking; examples include causal reasoning and hypothetico-deductive reasoning.

Anchoring: narrow focus on aspects of a patient's presentation to support a diagnostic hypothesis, even if other concurrent features or subsequent information refutes the hypothesis; has also been described as focusing on a specific diagnosis despite the presence of contradictory information.

Availability bias: tendency to think that diagnoses that come to mind immediately are more likely or more common; may be the result of recent or powerful experiences.

Bayesian reasoning: analytic form of clinical reasoning that stresses Bayes theorem, which states that the post-test odds of an event are equal to the pretest odds of an event multiplied by the likelihood ratio (LR) of a test result. For example, if the pretest odds of a pulmonary embolism based on the Wells score are 1:3 (probability of 25%) and the D-dimer result is negative with a LR of 0.1, then the post-test odds are 1:30. Therefore, the post-test probability is 3% (the probability equivalent of odds of 1:30).

Blind obedience: inappropriate deference to the recommendations of authority, from direct superiors or "expert" consultants, even in the absence of a sound rationale or in the face of contradictory data.

Causal reasoning: reasoning approach in which the clinician uses basic science concepts (pathophysiology, anatomy, biochemistry) to develop or confirm diagnostic hypotheses.

Cognitive bias: cognitive dispositions or preferences that can affect judgments and decisions in a subconscious manner; examples include availability bias and confirmation bias.

Chunking (see also encapsulation, a form of chunking):   cognitive process of grouping and relating bits of information. Chunking is an information processing tactic that prevents cognitive overload. Chunks vary dramatically in size and organization and are affected by ongoing knowledge gains and experience.

Clinical reasoning: cognitive processes by which a health care professional consciously and unconsciously interacts with the patient and environment to collect and interpret patient data, weighs the benefits and risks of actions, and understands patient preferences to determine a working diagnostic and therapeutic management plan whose purpose is to improve a patient's well-being.

Cognitive load theory: theory that describes the limitations of human working memory, stated to be 7 ± 2 (or 4 ± 2) bits or pieces of information.

Confirmation bias: tendency to seek out findings that are likely to support a suspected diagnosis and avoid those that may contradict it.

Content specificity: experimental observation that specific case content dramatically affects diagnostic accuracy.

Context specificity: observation that an individual's performance on a particular patient presentation (e.g., gout in a 70-year-old man in the clinic) only weakly correlates with performance on the same presentation in a different context (e.g., a 70-year-old man who presents to the clinic the next day or who comes to the emergency department with gout); that is, performance depends on the specific context.

Control value theory: theory providing an integrative framework for viewing the relations among motivation, emotion, and performance in academic settings.

Deductive reasoning: see hypothetico-deductive reasoning.

Deliberate practice: sustained engagement in component parts of an activity, typically under the direction of a coach (at least initially) who provides substantive feedback on the learner's performance with the purpose of achieving expert performance.

Diagnostic error:
  1. missed opportunity in the diagnostic process that occurs when the correct diagnosis could have been made earlier on the basis of information available at the time or, at the very least, further evaluation should have been undertaken given the available information, or
  2. situation when the clinician had at his or her disposal all of the information necessary to make the diagnosis but made the diagnosis later (delayed diagnosis), made a different diagnosis (wrong diagnosis), or missed the diagnosis altogether (missed diagnosis).

Diagnostic momentum: tendency of a diagnostic label to become propagated by multiple intermediaries (patients, physicians, nurses, other team members) over time; what might have begun as a possible "working diagnosis" becomes an "established diagnosis."

Diagnostic reasoning: aspect of clinical reasoning that includes the cognitive processes and practices used in the collection and analysis of a patient's symptoms, signs, and laboratory and radiologic findings, with the goal of determining their cause.

Diagnostic reliability: consistency in making the correct diagnosis, assuming adequate data are available at the time that the clinician selects it.

Distributed cognition: theory for viewing thinking in groups—thinking does not "sit" in the head of any one individual in the group (e.g., how a crew navigates a ship).

Dual process theory: theory that describes cognitive processes as the interplay of 2 reasoning approaches: nonanalytic (fast, subconscious, system 1) and analytic (slow, conscious, system 2).

Encapsulation: merging of multiple facts about a concept (e.g., a syndrome) under 1 term or phrase that working memory can use as only 1 bit of information (e.g., congestive heart failure is an encapsulation of a syndrome characterized by cardiac dysfunction, orthopnea, paroxysmal nocturnal dyspnea, elevated jugular venous pressure, crackles in the lungs, lower extremity edema). Encapsulation has the potential to reduce cognitive load.

Framing effect: susceptibility of diagnosticians to be disproportionately influenced by how a problem is described, by whom it is described, or even the environment where an encounter takes place.

Heuristics: mental short-cuts or rules of thumb that are used subconsciously in approaching a situation or problem.

Hindsight bias: tendency to ascribe predictability when events are viewed in retrospect and when the outcome is already known; examiners may be more likely to be critical of clinical care, for example, if a poor patient outcome was known to result from this care.

Hypothetico-deductive reasoning: method of analytic thinking; process of positing an answer (hypothesis) and then assessing whether that individual answer adequately explains the observed symptoms, findings, and any obtained test results; if so, the hypothesis is confirmed. For example, a clinician considers pulmonary embolism as a cause of dyspnea and pleuritic chest pain. The physician deduces that the patient should have a positive finding on computed tomographic pulmonary angiography and orders the test, which shows a pulmonary embolism.

Illness script: schema (mental model) that categorizes a disease by its clinical findings, risk factors, pathophysiology, and natural history; each individual clinician develops idiosyncratic illness scripts based on his or her knowledge and experiences of a disease.

Inductive reasoning: thinking approach that starts with symptoms or observations and then generalizes these to a larger framework, which explains them. For example, in diagnostic reasoning, a clinician uses clinical findings, risk factors, natural history, and basic science knowledge to develop a hypothesis that adequately explains them.

Information processing theory: group of theories that describes how humans acquire and organize knowledge by using the analogy of computer processing (see key theories within information processing theory [i.e., dual process theory, cognitive load theory]).

Metacognition: process of examining one's thought processes and feelings, including factors that may influence conclusions and behavior; "thinking about one's thinking."

Nonanalytic reasoning (system 1 thinking): cognitive process that is typically fast, low effort, and subconscious (e.g., pattern recognition).

Pathophysiologic reasoning: see causal reasoning.

Odds to probability conversion equation: odds/odds + 1.

Premature closure: settling on a final diagnosis before it is fully verified or before the data necessary to make a diagnosis have been reviewed. Many types of cognitive bias can lead to premature closure.

Problem representation: synthesis of the key aspects of a clinical presentation as determined by the clinician that includes the important discriminatory factors of the history, physical examination, and laboratory/imaging studies; it is often expressed as a summary statement.

Remediation: process of improving or remedying the performance of a learner in a domain where deficiencies exist.

Schema: cognitive framework that helps organize and interpret information.

Script theory: theory that pertains to how one develops an illness script (see illness script).

Self-regulated learning theory: construct of learning that describes 3 key phases: preparation for the task and assignment of value, performance with concurrent self-monitoring, and post hoc self-reflection and critique of performance.

Semantic competence: ability to use semantic qualifiers correctly and appropriately for a broad array of symptoms or findings in multiple different contexts.

Semantic qualifier: word or phrase that specifies the meaning of a symptom or finding with the purpose of defining the patient's problem as clearly and specifically as possible (e.g., acute, unilateral).

Situated cognition: theory that argues that thinking is located in the specifics of a given situation and therefore is shaped by and emerges from interactions with the environment and participants.

Situated learning: theory that argues that learning occurs through meaningful participation within a community of individuals (community of practice).

Situativity theory: group of social cognitive theories that incorporate the participants, the environment, and their interactions.

Summary statement: brief synthesis of the clinical data (history, physical, laboratory, imaging) that includes only key information and excludes nonpertinent distractors; an approximation of the problem representation aspect of script theory.

System 1 thinking: see nonanalytic reasoning.

System 2 thinking: see analytic reasoning.

Visceral bias: see affective bias.

Zone of proximal development: knowledge or skills that a learner cannot master on his or her own but can with aid of a teacher's guidance (e.g., educational scaffolding for learning exercises).

Index

Note: Page number followed by *f*, *t*, or *b* indicates figures, tables, or boxes, respectively.